Legal & Disclaimer s

The information and contents herein are not designed to replace or take the place of any form of medical or professional advice and are not meant to replace the need for independent medical, financial, legal or other professional advice or services, as may be required. The content and information in this book have been provided for educational and entertainment purposes only.

The content and information in this book have been compiled from reliable sources and are accurate to the author's best knowledge, information, and belief. The author cannot guarantee this book's accuracy and validity and cannot be held liable for any errors and/or omissions. Further, changes will be periodically made to this book when needed. It is recommended that you consult with a health professional who is familiar with your personal medical history before using any of the suggested remedies, techniques, or information in this book.

Table of contents

Introduction.................................1

Chapter 1: The History and Science of the Keto Diet2

A Prescription for Seizures 2

Ketones Are the Key...2

The Macro on Keto Diet 3

What's the MCT Diet?.........................3

The Advantages of the Keto Diet 3

Foods You Can Eat.............................5

Foods Need to Avoid........................7

The Most Common Mistakes on The Keto Diet 8

Chapter 2 Ketogenic Breakfast Recipes 11

Almond Bread 11

Almond Coconut Cereal.....................11

Almond Porridge.............................11

Asparagus Frittata Recipe 12

Avocados Stuffed with Salmon 12

Bacon and Brussels Sprout Breakfast 13

Bacon and Lemon spiced Muffins.............13

Bacon and Seasoned Mushroom Skewers......14

Breakfast Burrito.............................14

Breakfast Cauliflower Mix......................15

Breakfast Chia Pudding.........................15

Breakfast Chicken Muffins 16

Breakfast Sandwich...........................16

Brussels Sprout Gratin with Pork Crust...........17

Cauliflower Breakfast Bread 18

Cauliflower Cakes.............................18

Cheesy Asparagus Delight....................19

Cheesy Sausage Quiche 19

Chia Cereal Nibs................................20

Chicken Chowder served with Cheddar Cheese20

Chorizo and Cauliflower Breakfast mix..........21

Coated Asian Salad 21

Coated Green Bean Salad 22

Coated Simple Buffalo Wings.....................22

Coconut Biscuits.............................23

Coconut Milk Soup...........................23

Cold Apple Salad 24

Creamy Eggs and Asparagus with Cayenne

Pepper....................................24

Delicious Chicken Muffins 25

Easy Scrambled Eggs 25

Fried Asparagus with Sauce 26

Hash Casserole 26

Hemp Porridge 27

Her bed Frittata with Bacon 27

Hot Broccoli Soup............................27

Hot Green Bean Casserole 28

Keto Breakfast Burger 29

Keto Veggie Frittata 29

Mexican Casserole with Cilantro Topping 30

Minted Meatball Pilaf...........................31

Mixed Nuts Breakfast Bowl 31

Mixed Veggie Breakfast Bread....................32

Mushroom Breakfast Bowl......................32

Nutritious Breakfast Salad......................33

Oven baked Sausages and Eggs..................33

Oven-Baked Eggs and Sausage Mix 34

Serrano Poached Eggs 34

Shrimp Pasta with Chopped Basil.................35

Simple Sausage Muffins 35

Simple Spinach Frittata 36

Simple Tomato Soup with Topping................36

Smoked Salmon with Green sauce................37

Spaghetti Casserole Italian style....................37

Spiced Avocado Muffins 38

Spiced Lunch Curry...........................39

Spinach Rolls with Mayonnaise...................39

Steak Bowl served with Chipotle Adobo Sauce40

Tasty Breakfast Muffins 41

Tasty Granola Breakfast...........................41

Zucchini Noodle Soup with Lime Wedges 42

Chapter 3 Ketogenic Vegetable Recipes 43

Arugula and Chorizo Salad Recipe.................43

Avocado n Egg Salad 43

Broccoli Stew with lemon flavor 44

Brussels Sprouts Soup with chicken stock......44

Buttered Asparagus...........................44

Butternut Squash Salad 45

Cabbage and Brussels Sprouts Salad 45

Cabbage with Coconut aminos Salad.............46

Capers Eggplant Medley 46

Casserole Of Cauliflower.............................47

Celery and Walnuts Salad Recipe.................47

Chard Chicken Soup....................................47

Cheesy Asparagus Fries...............................48

Cheesy Asparagus Frittata...........................48

Cheesy Eggplant Soup.................................49

Cheesy Poached Eggs with collard greens 49

Cheesy Zucchini Cups.................................50

Coconut Asparagus Soup 50

Coconut Spring Greens Soup 51

Collard Greens with Cherry Tomatoes 51

Creamed Asparagus and cheese....................52

Creamed Spinach Soup................................52

Creamy Broccoli Soup.................................53

Creamy Cauliflower Soup.............................53

Creamy Eggplant Soup................................54

Creamy Roasted Bell Peppers Soup 54

Delicious Cauliflower Soup 55

Fast Salad For Lunch 55

Garlic-Squash and Mushrooms Mix...............56

Green Beans n Stock Saucy Casserole 56

Grilled Eggplant Onion Salad 57

Hot Arugula Keto Soup 57

Hot Catalan Greens....................................58

Kale with Pumpkin seed Salad 58

Lemony celery with parsley stew...................59

Lettuce and Tomato Salad Recipe.................59

Mushroom Chops Stew................................60

Oven-Baked Radishes 60

Pan-fried Collard Greens and Ham 60

Parmesan Fennel Soup 61

Pork With Cinnamon...................................61

Pumpkin Soup (Keto) 62

Pureed creamy celery soup 62

Pureed Pumpkin Soup 63

Roasted Bell Peppers Soup Recipe with Parmesan 63

Roasted Lemon Asparagus 64

Roasted Tomato Cream................................64

Seasoned Keto Cabbage Soup.......................64

Sesame Alfalfa Sprouts Salad 65

Sesame Mustard Greens 65

Sliced Swiss Chard Pie.................................66

Slow cooked Mixed Vegetable Soup..............66

Sour cream and celery soup..........................67

Spiced Collard Greens and Butternut Soup....68

Spicy Cabbage Soup 68

Spinach and Mustard Greens Soup 69

Spinach Stew Recipe 69

Spinach, Broccoli and Cauliflower Soup.........70

Stewed Eggplant..70

Stir-Fried Mustard Greens...........................71

Stress-free Cheesy Tacos.............................71

Sweet Coconut Cauliflower Mix 72

Sweet Mushroom Cream 72

Swiss Vegetable Soup.................................73

Tangy Poblano Soup 73

Tasty Onion and Tomato Soup.....................74

Tomato Soup (Keto)...................................74

Vegetable Lunch Pate.................................75

Watermelon Radish Salad 75

Wraps Filled With Tomato, Avocado & Turkey76

Zucchini And Hot Avocado Soup 76

Chapter 4 Ketogenic Snacks and Appetizers Recipes 77

Almond Broccoli Biscuits 77

Almond Flaxseed Muffins.............................77

Artichoke, Tomato and Mozzarella Appetizer 78

Asian Mint Chutney: Side Dish 78

Baked Chia Seeds 79

Balsamic Zucchini Chips 79

Beef Spicy Shots 80

Blueberry, Jalapeno and Pepper Salad...........80

Braised Eggplant Dish: Side Dish 81

Broccoli and Cheddar Biscuits 81

Brussels sprouts with Bacon and Cream Cheese82

Cauliflower with Side Salad..........................83

Cheesy and Olives Bombs 83

Cheesy Bread sticks....................................83

Cheesy Snack Italian Style........................84

Cider and Cashew Hummus..........................84

Coconut Almond Bars 85

Coconut Avocado Dip..................................85

Creamy Smoked Salmon and Dill Spread........86

Creamy Spinach and Onion Dip 86

Creamy Spinach Dip with Garlic....................86

Delicious Caramelized Bell Peppers: Side Dish87

Dessert With Bacon 87

Easy Cheese Sauce: Side Dish 88

Easy Tuna Cakes 89

Eggplant, Olives and Basil Salad....................89

Fresh Tomato, Onion and Jalapeno Pepper Salsa 90

Fresh Veggie Bars......................................90

Green Beans And Avocado with Chopped Cilantro 91

Italian Pizza Dip..91

Jalapeno Cheesy Balls 92

Keto Veggie Noodles: Side Dish 92

Minty Zucchini Rolls....................................93

Mushrooms Stuffed with shrimp mixture.......93

Oven-baked Crackers 94

Pan-Fried Cheesy Sticks 94

Pan-fried Italian Meatballs..........................95

Parmesan Basil Dip 95

Parmesan Chicken Wings............................95

Parmesan Spinach Balls 96

Pecan with Maple syrup Bars........................97

Plum and Jalapeno Salad with Basil...............97

Seasoned Easy Fried Cabbage......................98

Sesame Zucchini Spread 98

Shrimp Salad with Tomato and Radish 99

Shrimp wrapped with prosciutto 99

Simple Tomato Tarts 99

Special Tomato And Bocconcini: Side Dish ...100

Stir-Fried Queso..100

Tasty Avocado Spread 101

Chapter 5 Seafood & Fish Recipes 102

Arugula Cod 102

Baked Calamari Mix with Sauce 102

Baked Eggplant, Sardines and Artichokes Salad103

Baked Fish with Mushrooms 103

Balsamic Calamari Salad............................. 104

Butter Glazed Mussels................................ 104

Cake up Tuna 105

Caper Sauce Salmon.................................. 105

Catfish with Okra Mix................................. 106

Citrus Rich Octopus Salad 106

Cod La Pan–roasted................................... 107

Coriander Shrimp with Salad 107

Crab Cakes with Sauce 108

Cream Cheese Salmon Sushi 108

Creamy Clam Chowder Luncheon 109

Creamy Salmon With Tinge 109

Crispy Calamari Rings 110

Crusted Coconut Salmon Nuggets................ 110

Delicious Cod Salad 111

Delicious Monk fish with Sauce 112

Fish Ginger Soup 112

Flounder with Shrimp Etouffee 113

Fresh Catfish Mix with Pineapple Salsa 114

Freshly Made Calamari Salad 114

Greek Sardine Mix Salad 115

Grilled Lemon Catfish................................. 115

Halibut With Simple Baking......................... 116

Her bed Catfish with Salad 116

Hot Balsamic Salmon Mix............................ 117

Hot Cod Pie 117

Hot Sardine Soup....................................... 117

Hot Shrimp with Pepper Mix........................ 118

Italian Style Clams Delight........................... 118

Juicy Salmon Skewers................................ 119

Kale and Salmon Salad 119

Lobster with Avocado Mix............................ 120

Luscious Herbed Clams 120

Mackerel with Sauce 120

Maple Glazed Salmon Fillet.......................... 121

Mediterranean Cod Salad 121

Mix of Kimchi 122

Mixed Fish with Cauliflower Pie.................. 122

Monk fish and Tomato-Garlic Sauce 123

Oysters With Plain Grilling 124

Parmesan Shrimp Skewers............................124

Red Shrimp Stew..124

Roll in Salmon 125

Sage Shrimp Kebabs and Tomato Salad 125

Salad Of Shrimp and Asparagus 126

Salmon Crust Fillet..127

Salmon Fillets..127

Salmon Mix Salad..128

Salmon with Mushroom Shrimp Filling.........128

Sardine Cucumber Salad 129

Sardines Tapenade Mix.................................129

Sea Bass with Capers 130

Shrimp and Asparagus with Lime Flavor.......130

Shrimp and Eggs Salad Mix 131

Shrimp Mayo Side Salad 131

Shrimp Mushroom Medley.............................132

Shrimp, Calamari with Avocado Sauce 132

Simple Baked Catfish with Salad...................133

Simple Sardines and Cucumber Mix 134

Smoked Salmon with Eggs Salad..................134

Spicy Salmon Fillets with Salad 134

Tangy Pepper Filled Oysters 135

Tomatoes Stuffed With Tuna & Cheese 135

Tuna Salad Mix..135

Tuna with Arugula Sauce 136

Chapter 6 Ketogenic Poultry Recipes .. 137

A pot filled Roasted Chicken 137

Almond Butter Chicken Stew 137

Artichokes and Chicken Breast Mix..............138

Arugula Chicken Bowls..................................138

Bacon, Chicken and Broccoli mix 139

Baked Turkey Delight 139

Balsamic-Plum Chicken Mix..........................140

Cauliflower Turkey Soup 140

Cheese Rich Turkey Bowls.............................140

Cheesy Chicken and Kale Casserole 141

Chicken Chilies Soup 141

Chicken Fajitas With Paprika.........................142

Chicken Gumbo Recipe 143

Chicken in Creamy Sauce Recipe.................. 143

Chicken Italian Style Servings....................... 144

Chicken Masala Curry.................................... 144

Chicken Mushroom Sautee 145

Chicken Soup, Chinese Style......................... 146

Chicken Soup, Indian Style 146

Chicken Stroganoff 147

Chicken Thighs with Mushrooms and Cheese147

Chicken with Green Onion Sauce Recipe 148

Chicken with Mustard Sauce 148

Chicken with Olive Tapenade and Garlic...... 149

Chicken with Sour Cream Sauce 149

Chipotle Spiced Chicken 150

Chunky Chicken Cheese Soup 150

Cranberry Turkey Salad 151

Creamy Italian Chicken Soup........................ 151

Creamy Turkey Spinach Medley 152

Duck Breast Salad.. 152

Duck Breast with Vegetables........................ 153

Easy Chicken Stir–fry 153

Flavorsome Turkey Chili................................ 154

Fried Chicken... 154

Garlic Chicken Meatloaf 155

Grilled Wings with Green Sauce.................... 155

Hot Wings (Buffalo Sauce Style)................... 156

Leek and Chicken Mix................................... 157

Lemon Chicken and Fennel Salad................. 157

Lettuce Wrapped Turkey 158

Luscious Chicken thigh Stew 158

Mango Habanero Chicken............................. 159

Mayonnaise Chicken Salad........................... 159

Mexican Cheesy Casserole 160

Minced Chicken Burgers................................ 160

Olive Braised Chicken.................................... 161

Oregano Chicken Breasts 161

Pan-Fried Sour Chicken Thighs..................... 162

Pan-seared Duck Breast Recipe.................... 162

Parmesan Chicken Cal zone.......................... 163

Passata Chicken Soup.................................... 163

Pecan–Crusted Chicken................................ 164

Pepperoni Chicken Bake................................ 164

Salsa Chicken with Veggies spray..................165
Savory Chicken Recipe 165
Seared Cheesy Meatballs...............................166
Simple Chicken Salad 166
Skillet Chicken and Mushrooms Recipe.......167
Spiced Turkey Mix...167
Spinach Artichoke Chicken............................168
Stuffed Chicken Breast Recipe 168
Turkey and Cranberry Salad Recipe 169
Turkey Chili Recipe...169
Turkey Pie...170
Turkey Soup 171
Turkey Squash Curry 171
Turkey Stuffed Chive Rolls............................172
Turkey Tarragon Bake....................................172
Turkey Zucchini Lasagna 173

Chapter 7 Ketogenic Meat Recipes 174
Almond Glazed Beef Meatloaf......................174
Avocado-Beef Zucchini Cups 174
Awesome Pilaf 175
Bacon Burger..176
Baked beef with mushroom bowls 177
Baked beef with mushrooms and celery 177
Baked lamb chops with cranberry tomato sauce...178
Baked lamb with fennel and figs..................178
Baked Parmesan veal with tomatoes sauce..179
Baked pork sausage and mushrooms 179
Baked veal and green beans 181
Beef Cabbage Casserole................................181
Beef Keto Stew...182
Beef Patties with coconut flour 182
Braised veal and capers 183
Brisket and Beef Burgers...............................183
Cheesy ham and cauliflower soup bowls......184
Cheesy sausage with tomatoes....................184
Cheesy veal and beans..................................185
Cheesy veal dish..185
Coconut Smoked Beef Mix............................186
Creamy lamb sauce.......................................186
Creamy veal with mushrooms and squash ...187

Crusty Pork Cheese Pie...............................188
Dijon Beef Fillets and Coconut Sauce...........188
Garlic and Lemon Pork 189
Garlic Beef Chili...189
Garlic Beef Meatball Casserole 190
Garlicy sausage and tomatoes stew............191
Greek Beef Mix..191
Grilled Cajun Beef and Apricots Sauce.........192
Grilled Ginger Lamb Chops..........................192
Grilled lamb chops 192
Ground Beef Casserole with keto mayonnaise193
Ground Beef Goulash...................................194
Healthy Beef Pot Roast Recipes..................194
Healthy Beef with Tzatziki Recipe...............194
Healthy Italian Pork Chops Recipes 195
Healthy Lemon Pork Chops 196
Healthy Thai Beef Recipes...........................196
Herb Beef and zucchini soup bowls 197
Hot and spicy beef stew with olives............197
Italian Style Beef Casserole 198
Juicy Pork Chops with Stock Chicken...........198
Lamb and vegetables 199
Lamb Leg Curry 199
Lamb pot pie 200
Lemon Cranberry Pork Roast 200
Mediterranean Pork Recipes.......................201
Mexican Cilantro Beef Dish 201
Mint lamb...202
Mushroom Sauce with Meatballs 202
Nutmeg Meatballs Curry..............................203
Pan seared sausage and kale.......................204
Pan-Fried Chorizo Mix 204
Pork Rolls...205
Roasted Beef and pepperoncini...................205
Rosemary lamb bowls 206
Sauerkraut Soup and Beef...........................206
Seared beef soup bowls 207
Seared beef with peanut sauce...................208
Seared veal and capers................................208
Shredded lamb topped with lemon dressing209
Slow cook lamb chili.....................................209

Smokey Baked Pork...................................209
Spicy Beef and Scallops Mix...................210
Spicy Cinnamon Pork Chops 210
Spicy Mexican Luncheon..........................211
Stewed Beef...211
Sweet Jamaican Pork 212
Tasty Zucchini Noodles and Beef 212
Tomato–stuffed Squash and Beef 213
Turmeric Jamaican Beef Pies 213
Vegetable Beef Stew 214

Chapter 8 Ketogenic Side Dish Recipes 215

Almond Cheddar Soufflés 215
Asian Salad with Cucumber 215
Asian Style Braised Eggplant.....................216
Asparagus Deal 216
Avocado Fries with Almond Mix 217
Baked Brussels sprouts with ranch dressing.217
Baked Eggplant Salad with Oregano 217
Baked green bean fries 218
Baked Parmesan Egg plant and Tomatoes 218
Balsamic Steak Salad................................219
Bisque of Lobster 220
Broccoli with Parmesan Cheese.................220
Butternut Squash and Zucchini Indian Salad 221
Buttery Grilled Onions 221
Cajun Spaghetti Squash Pasta.....................222
Cauliflower and Hazelnuts Polenta.............222
Cauliflower rice with hot dogs.....................223
Cauliflower, Avocado and Spinach Dip with Sour Cream 224
Cheesy asparagus.....................................224
Cheesy creamy garlic mushrooms 225
Cheesy Twice-Baked Stuffed Zucchini..........225
Cheesy zucchini with parsley 226
Coco Keto Soup...226
Coco Meal Soup..227
Coconut Cauliflower Rice.............................227
Creamy Broccoli with Lemon and Almonds ..228
Creamy Cheese Sauce...............................228
Creamy Coconut Cauliflower Mash 229
Creamy Endive and Watercress Salad with

Chives 229
Creamy Sausage Gravy 230
Crispy Turnip Sticks 230
Curried Zucchini Noodles Soup 231
Fried Bacon and Swiss Chard 231
Fried Mushroom and Spinach 232
Garlic chili with cabbage and radish............232
Garlicky Brussels Sprouts with Mustard.......233
Green Beans And Vinaigrette Mix 233
Green Beans with Mashed Avocado 234
Hot Green Beans: Side Dish 234
Hot Special Side Dish.................................235
Irish Side Dish with Steak 236
Italian Flavored Zucchini and Tomatoes.......236
Keto Chowder Recipe 237
Keto Eggplant Salad with Toppings 237
Keto Mushrooms: Side Dish 238
Keto Rice Dish - Side Dish...........................238
Keto Stuffed Peppers...................................239
Mushroom and Arugula Salad with Prosciutto 239
Mushroom Salad with Parmesan 240
Mushroom, Almonds and Hemp Pilaf...........241
Okra and Tomatoes with Crispy Bacon.........241
Oven baked Baby Mushrooms 242
Oven baked zucchini and cream 242
Pan-fried bacon with lemony chard 242
Parmesan sprinkled garlic beans..................243
Roast green beans with cranberries..............243
Roasted cheesy mushrooms........................243
Roasted Mixed Olives.................................244
Rolls of Sausage Pizzas 244
Salad Bowl of Caprese With Tomato 245
Sauté Cabbage with Butter 245
Saute Edamame with Mint..........................246
Sauteed Broccoli with Parmesan.................246
Sautéed Kohlrabi with Parsley.....................246
Sautéed Mixed Vegetable with Pumpkin Seeds 247
Side Cauliflower Salad................................247
Spicy Green Beans and Vinaigrette 248
Stuffed Sausage with Bacon Wrappings.......248
Tasty Lunch Pizza......................................249

Turkey and Collard Greens Soup...................249
Warm Delicious Roasted Olives 250
Yummy Creamy Spaghetti Pasta: Side Dish...251
Yummy Muffins...................251
Zucchini and Squash Noodles with Peppers .252

Chapter 9 Ketogenic Dessert Recipes .. 253

Almond Lime Cheesecake...................253
Almond Mug Cake...................253
Almond Peanut Butter and Chocolate Brownies254
Almond Peanut Butter Fudge 254
Baked stuffed apples...................255
Cheesy Berry Mousse 255
Cheesy Caramel Custard 255
Chocolate Flavored Biscotti 256
Cocoa banana buns...................256
Cocoa Brownies 257
Cocoa Walnut Spread 257
Coconut Almond Bars 257
Coconut avocado blend with coconut butter258
Coconut Avocado Pudding...................258
Chocolate pudding...................259
Coconut Chocolate Cups...................259
Coconut Cookie Balls 259
Creamy Blueberry Scones...................260

Creamy Peach Cake 260
Creamy Ricotta Mousse 261
Lemon Flavored Mousse 261
Lemon rhubarb sauce 262
Lemony cherry jelly...................262
Lemony fairy cakes...................262
Lemony plum and dates blend...................263
Nutmeg Spiced Coconut Granola...................263
Quick bake cookies...................264
Slow cook blueberry lemon curd 264
Strawberries and cashew blend...................264
Strawberry Coconut Dessert 265
Strawberry Tart 265
Sweet and sour stew 265
Tasty Chocolate Pudding 266
Tasty cookie...................266
Vanilla Cheesecake...................266
Vanilla Chocolate Cookies 267
Vanilla Flavored Ice Cream 267
Vanilla pumpkin cookie 268
Vanilla Spiced Macaroons 268

Introduction

Greetings!! Thanks for getting this book, "The Keto Diet Cookbook for Beginners."
If you are considering the ketogenic diet or have started it and need a little help, this is the book for you. Maybe you aren't sure what's going on in your body or you're curious about what brands are keto-friendly. This book will clear all those questions up.

I love cooking, food, and I'm a keto dieter. I'm not a professional chef, doctor, or a nutritionist, but I've spent many hours researching the keto diet and cooking recipes. I'm no expert, but I would say I understand the diet more than most people. In this book, I've collected 500+ easy to make, delicious and common on the table recipes, moreover, the most essential information is written in a simple, easy-to-understand way. The keto diet can get confusing, especially once you get into the science side, but I hope I've had distilled everything in a way that's easy to grasp.

On the keto diet, you can eat food like delicious grass-fed steaks, full-fat butter, and baked goods sweetened with stevia. Sound like a diet you could get behind? Keep reading and let's learn more!

Chapter 1: The History and Science of the Keto Diet

Before we get into the specific foods you can and can't eat on the ketogenic diet and how to succeed, it's good to know where the diet came from and how it works on a scientific level. The keto diet has origins stretching back to ancient times, but it took a thousand years before scientists knew exactly what was going on.

A Prescription for Seizures

People have suffered from seizures and epilepsy for thousands of years. Back in ancient Greece and India, the most common treatment was to stop eating or drinking. For some reason, fasting seemed to be prevent whatever was causing the seizures. For centuries, that was what patients had to go through - fasting or seizures. In 1911, French doctors developed a diet that could relieve seizures. It was vegetarian and low in calories. A few decades later, another doctor began experimenting, and learned that a diet low in carbs and high in fat also prevented seizures. Why?

Ketones Are the Key

When you fast, your body begins producing compounds known as "ketones." These are distributed through the body as fuel, because the body needs something to continue functioning normally. These compounds also show up when you restrict your carb intake, because the body normally depends on carbs for energy. When you replace most of your carbs with fat, the body begins to turn fatty acids into ketones, and depends on those for fuel instead. Unlike carbs, however, excess ketones are not stored as body fat.

That doesn't mean you should stop eating carbs completely. That's actually very unhealthy, if not impossible. You can eat significantly less, however, and choose the quality of carbs. Refined carbs like sugar and white bread don't offer much nutrition, so they mostly end up as body fat. Complex carbs like vegetables and fruit are much higher in good minerals and vitamins, so the carbs you do eat on the ketogenic diet are always complex. Less carbs trigger ketosis, which is the name of the ketone-producing process. That is what prevents seizures and results in other benefits, which we'll discuss a bit later on.

The Macro on Keto Diet

Ketosis begins when your daily diet consists of a certain percentage of carbs, fat, and protein. That percentage is a mere 5-10% carbs, 15-20% protein, and 60-75% fat. For most people, that means eating just 20 grams of net carbs per day. For the record, a single slice of white bread has 13 grams. If you want to stay in ketosis, most meals should have just 7 net carbs per serving. What's the difference between net carbs and total carbs? Total carbs count fiber, while net carbs doesn't. That's why complex carbs like vegetables are a much better choice, because they may have a fairly large amount of carbs, they also have a lot more fiber than white bread or candy.

What's the MCT Diet?

In your exploration of the ketogenic diet, you might have seen the abbreviation "MCT" pop up. That stands for medium-chain triglycerides, which is the hot fat for the ketogenic diet. It's found mostly in coconut products - especially coconut oil - and in smaller amounts in cheese and butter. This fat has been shown to promote a lot of ketone production, so lots of people eager to get into ketosis will focus on getting as much of it as possible. The MCT diet adjusts the percentage a little, so you're getting 30-50% of your total daily calories from MCT oils. Because MCT is more effective at producing ketones, you can have more carbs and protein while staying in ketosis. This makes the diet easier for a lot of people. The MCT diet was created in the 1970's, but it's more popular in the United Kingdom than the US.

The Advantages of the Keto Diet

The keto diet has stayed popular for years, and it's because of the many benefits dieters report. Here are the top reasons to consider a low-carb diet:

The Diet Might Make It Easier to Lose Weight

When you cut out the highest-carb food from your diet, which includes sugar, you might experience weight loss. Combined with exercise, lots of people find they are finally able to reach their weight goals when on the ketogenic diet. This is because it isn't eating fat that makes people overweight; it's sugar and foods low in nutrients, but high in carbs.

By eating less carbs and more nutrients, losing weight can become much easier.

The Diet Can Provide A Boost Of Energy

When you eat high-carb foods, your blood sugar rises quickly, and then crashes. Throughout the day, this rollercoaster of highs and lows is exhausting, and makes it hard to be productive. When you switch to high-fat foods and snacks, your energy levels become more staple. You'll have more consistent energy through all your activities. Your mental clarity can also improve, since the brain is mostly fat, and loves the fat found in keto staples like salmon, avocados, nuts, and coconut oil.

You Won't Feel Hungry On The Keto Diet

A lot of diets are characterized by hunger. You are supposed to eat less and you end up feeling hungry all the time. That isn't a problem on the keto diet. The body uses fat and quality proteins a lot more efficiently than refined carbs, which rush through the system and leave you feeling empty quickly after eating. You won't need to snack during the day as much after filling keto meals, and that can result in weight loss, too.

The Diet Can Result In Healthier Skin And Hair

The keto diet is so effective at treating dry hair and skin, there's even a term for it: the "keto glow." Lots of people find that after switching to a keto diet, their hair becomes sleeker, shinier, and healthier. Dry or acne-scarred skin is also hydrated by all the good fats, while even finger and toenails can become stronger and healthier-looking. In addition to encouraging more foods that help hair and skin, cutting out sugar and processed foods on the keto diet most likely plays a role in the glow, as well.

The Diet May Help Protect Against Serious Diseases

While more studies are needed to support this reason, there is research out there that suggests the ketogenic diet may protect people from certain diseases. Healthy fats lower bad cholesterol, a major cause of heart disease, while losing weight is also healthy for the heart. As for the brain, at least one study showed that being in ketosis improves a person's memory. When given MCT oil, Alzheimer's patients' brains produced more ketones.

Foods You Can Eat

For being a restrictive diet, the list of foods you can eat is relatively extensive. All kinds of meat and seafood (ideally grass-fed, wild-caught, and organic) are allowed, while all full-fat dairy is also encouraged. You can eat lots of low-carb vegetables, as well, though you're more limited on fruit. A banana every now and then shouldn't throw you out of ketosis, however, but you should always be careful about what else you eat that day. Here's a fairly complete list of everything you're allowed to eat on the keto diet:

Meat/seafood:

Beef (ideally grass-fed)
Eggs (ideally cage-free and organic)
Fish/shellfish (ideally wild-caught)
Goat
Lamb
Organ meats
Pork (ideally free-range and organic)
Poultry (organic)

Vegetables/fruit:

Alfalfa sprouts
Avocado
Berries   (blackberries,   raspberries,
cranberries, etc)
Bell peppers
Bok choy
Broccoli
Button mushrooms
Cabbage
Cauliflower
Celery
Citrus (lemons, oranges, limes)
Cucumber
Eggplant
Garlic
Kale
Lettuce
Onions
Parsley
Radishes
Sea vegetables
Spinach
Swiss chard
Tomatoes
Watercress
Zucchini

Nuts/seeds (in moderation):

Almonds
Brazil nuts
Chia seeds
Flax seeds

Macadamia nuts
Pecans
Pumpkin seeds

Shredded coconut (unsweetened)
Sunflower seeds
Walnuts

Full-fat dairy:

Cheese (cheddar, parmesan, mozzarella, brie, ricotta, etc)
Cottage cheese
Cream cheese
Dairy-free milk alternatives (unsweetened almond milk, coconut milk, macadamia nut milk)
Greek yogurt (plain and unsweetened)
Heavy cream

Fats/oils:

Almond oil
Avocado oil
Cocoa butter
Coconut oil/coconut cream

Duck fat
Ghee (clarified butter)
Nut butters (in moderation)
Olive oil (cold-pressed extra-virgin)

Beverages:

Sparkling water + seltzers (w/out added sweeteners)
Unsweetened coconut water
Unsweetened coffee (or sweetened with natural o-calorie sweetener)
Unsweetened herbal tea (or sweetened with natural o-calorie sweetener)
Water

Baking/cooking supplies:

Almond flour
Baking   powder/baking
(aluminum-free)
Coconut aminos (soy sauce substitute)
Coconut flour
Erythritol/stevia blends
Fish sauce
Mayonnaise (w/out added sugar)

Monk fruit extract or powder
sodaPsyllium husk (a thickener)
Spices + herbs
Sugar-free ketchup
Sugar-free yellow mustard
Vinegar (white, wine, and apple cider)
Xanthan gum (in very small amounts)

Foods Need to Avoid

Knowing what to avoid on the ketogenic diet is determined by asking yourself two questions: Is it low-carb? Does it have artificial ingredients? Foods too high in carbs will throw you out of ketosis when you eat too much, while anything with artificial or processed ingredients also tends be too high in carbs, while also being just unhealthy. Here's what to avoid:

Processed meats:

Deli meat
Grain-fed meats

Hot dogs
Sausages

Grain:

Barley
Buckwheat
Corn
Oatmeal

Quinoa
Rice
Wheat
Wheat gluten

High-carb veggies and fruit:

Artichokes
Bananas
Carrots
Clementines
Dried fruit
Fruit syrups
Grapes
Jam/jelly
Kiwi

Mangos
Pears
Pineapple
Potatoes
Squash
Sweet potatoes
Watermelon
Yams

Low-fat or fat-free dairy:

Fake butter alternatives
Low-fat/fat-free cream cheese
Low-fat/fat-free sour cream
Low-fat/fat-free yogurt
Skim milk

Beans/legumes:

Black   Lentils
Chickpeas   Peas
Fava   White
Kidney

Certain oils:

Canola   Sesame
Corn   Soybean
Grapeseed   Sunflower
Peanut

Refined + artificial sweeteners:

Agave   Equal   Splenda
Aspartame   Honey   Sucralose
Cane sugar   Maple syrup   White sugar
Coconut sugar   Raw sugar
Corn syrup   Saccharin

Other:

Alcohol   Diet foods
Baked goods + treats   Fast food

The Most Common Mistakes on The Keto Diet

The ketogenic diet isn't the easiest to follow. You have to be careful to eliminate certain foods and ingredients like wheat and sugar, which like to hide in sometimes surprising foods, and you have to stick to your percentages of fat, protein, and carbs. People don't even think about certain things when they start out, which can make the diet harder or not as beneficial. Here are the most common mistakes to avoid (and what to do instead):

Mistake #1: Not planning ahead

You decide to go on the ketogenic diet and dive right in. Unfortunately, you still have a kitchen full of foods not allowed on the keto diet and no idea what to make for meals.

You also don't know what restaurants have keto-friendly options, or what brands you should look for at the store. This makes your new diet very difficult, and you always feel at a loss and tempted to break the diet. As soon as you make the decision to go keto, get rid of everything in your house that isn't keto-approved. Look up recipes and start meal-planning, so you know exactly what to get at the store. You'll feel much more prepared and less overwhelmed.

Mistake #2: Not anticipating the keto flu

The keto flu is what happens when your body transitions from burning carbs to burning fat. Symptoms include headaches, fatigue, and nausea. While most people get through it without too much trouble in a week or two, it can be uncomfortable, especially if you aren't prepared for it. If you go about your normal routine and don't know what to do when symptoms hit, you may start regretting your choice to go keto and back out. You'll feel discouraged and disappointed in yourself. If you accept that the keto flu is coming, however, you can do things to make it easier. Staying hydrated is very important, since you lose more water during this phase of the diet. You should also eat as much protein and fats as you need, without worrying about the percentages, and be sure to replenish your electrolytes (especially sodium) by drinking chicken broth with salt. If your symptoms are especially bad, it's okay to eat some clean carbs (like a sweet potato or high-carb fruit) to make the adjustment easier.

Mistake #3: Not adjusting your exercise routine

Some people worry that they can't build muscle on the keto diet, but you definitely can. You just have to adjust your routines and possibly the diet slightly to make the most of your workouts. Anaerobic exercise, which is intense and interval-based, isn't improved by the keto diet because it relies on carbs. You can still do this type of exercise, but you should eat 15-30 fast-acting carbs before and after a workout. Aerobic and cardio exercise, however, can improve with the keto diet and doesn't require any adjustments to your carb intake.

Mistake #4: Ignoring your electrolytes

Electrolytes are necessary to good health. On the keto diet, you lose them more than on other diets, especially during the first weeks of ketosis. Many people neglect these minerals, which can lead to potentially serious health problems. Be sure to get sodium, magnesium, potassium, and calcium through food or supplements, if necessary. Talk to your doctor about testing your levels, and be aware of how much you need per day for your best health.

Mistake #5: Not getting good sleep

Sleep is just as important to the body and mind as good food. Without good sleep, your health will suffer. A lot of people have terrible sleep habits, like getting distracted by their phone and computers in bed, never getting up at the same time, and so on. There's a lot you can do to improve your sleep quality. Make sure the room is completely dark and free from electronic blue lights, which have been shown to disrupt good sleep patterns. Start winding down an half or half-hour before bed, and turn off the TV and keep away from your phone and computer. Give your mind the chance to settle and prepare the body for sleep.

Mistake #6: Not finding support

When you change your diet dramatically, it will be hard. Lots of people believe they can do it alone, but they're soon overwhelmed and discouraged. It's very difficult to do anything by yourself; humans are built for community. To ensure long-term success, find a good support network, whether it's people who are going keto themselves, or are just really good listeners and cheerleaders. Consider looking online for a group on a website like MeetUp. You should also be clear with your family (if they aren't going keto with you) about what you need from them in terms of support. That might mean asking that they keep treats out of the house or that they agree to eating only keto meals if you're cooking. With good support, you'll find the motivation you need to stick to your diet.

Chapter 2 Ketogenic Breakfast Recipes

Almond Bread

Prep Time + Cook Time: 13 minutes Serves: 4

Ingredients:

- Salt
- Whisked egg, 1
- Almond flour, 1/3 cup
- Coconut oil, 2 ½ tbsps.
- Baking powder, ½ tsp.

Directions:

1. Rub a large microwave-safe mug with oil
2. Set a mixing bowl in position to combine baking powder, egg, oil, and salt with flour.
3. Set the mixture in a greased mug and microwave on high for 3 minutes
4. Allow the bread to cool before slicing
5. Enjoy

Nutrition:

Calories: 343, Fat: 38.5, Fiber: 0.4, Carbs: 0.8, Protein: 2.1

Almond Coconut Cereal

Prep Time + Cook Time: 5 minutes Serves: 2

Ingredients:

- Water, 1/3 cup
- Coconut milk, 1/3 cup
- Roasted sunflower seeds, 2 tbsps.
- Chia seeds, 1 tbsp.
- Blueberries, ½ cup
- Chopped almonds, 2 tbsps.

Directions:

1. Set a medium bowl in position to add coconut milk and chia seeds then reserve for five minutes
2. Plug in and set the blender in position to blend almond with sunflower seeds
3. Stir the combination to chia seeds mixture then add water to mix evenly.
4. Serve topped with the remaining sunflower seeds and blueberries

Nutrition:

Calories: 181, Fat: 15.2, Fiber: 4, Carbs: 10.8, Protein: 3.7

Almond Porridge

Prep Time + Cook Time: 15 minutes Serves: 1

Ingredients:

- Ground cloves, ¼ tsp.
- Nutmeg, ¼ tsp.
- Stevia, 1 tsp.
- Coconut cream, ¾ cup

- Ground almonds, ½ cup
- Ground cardamom, ¼ tsp.
- Ground cinnamon, 1 tsp.

Directions:

1. Set your pan over medium heat to cook the coconut cream for a few minutes
2. Stir in almonds and stevia to cook for 5 minutes
3. Mix in nutmeg, cardamom, and cinnamon
4. Enjoy while still hot

Nutrition:
Calories: 695, Fat: 66.7, Fiber: 11.1, Carbs: 22, Protein: 14.3

Asparagus Frittata Recipe

Prep Time + Cook Time: 40 minutes Servings: 4

Ingredients:

- Bacon slices, chopped: 4
- Salt and black pepper
- Eggs (whisked): 8
- Asparagus (trimmed and chopped): 1 bunch

Directions:

1. Heat a pan over medium heat, add bacon, stir and cook for 5 minutes.
2. Add asparagus, salt, and pepper, stir and cook for another 5 minutes.
3. Add the chilled eggs, spread them in the pan, let them stand in the oven and bake for 20 minutes at 350° F.
4. Share and divide between plates and serve for breakfast.

Nutrition: calories 251, carbs 16, fat 6, fiber 8, protein 7

Avocados Stuffed with Salmon

Prep Time + Cook Time: 10 minutes Servings: 2

Ingredients:

- Avocado (pitted and halved): 1
- Olive oil: 2 tbsps.
- Lemon juice: 1
- Smoked salmon (flaked): 2 ounces
- Goat cheese (crumbled): 1 ounce
- Salt and black pepper

Directions:

1. Combine the salmon with lemon juice, oil, cheese, salt, and pepper in your food processor and pulsate well.
2. Divide this mixture into avocado halves and serve.
3. Dish and Enjoy!

Nutrition:
calories 300m, fat 15, fiber 5, carbs 8, protein 16

Bacon and Brussels Sprout Breakfast

Prep Time + Cook Time: 22 minutes Serves: 3

Ingredients:

- Apple cider vinegar, 1½ tbsps.
- Salt
- Minced shallots, 2
- Minced garlic cloves, 2
- Medium eggs, 3
- Sliced Brussels sprouts, 12 oz.
- Black pepper
- Chopped bacon, 2 oz.
- Melted butter, 1 tbsp.

Directions:

1. Over medium heat, quick fry the bacon until crispy then reserve on a plate
2. Set the pan on fire again to fry garlic and shallots for 30 seconds
3. Stir in apple cider vinegar, Brussels sprouts, and seasoning to cook for five minutes
4. Add the bacon to cook for five minutes then stir in the butter and set a hole at the center
5. Crash the eggs to the pan and let cook fully
6. Enjoy

Nutrition:
Calories: 275, Fat: 16.5, Fiber: 4.3, Carbs: 17.2, Protein: 17.4

Bacon and Lemon spiced Muffins

Prep Time + Cook Time: 30 minutes Serves: 12

Ingredients:

- Lemon thyme, 2 tsps.
- Salt
- Almond flour, 3 cup
- Melted butter, ½ cup
- Baking soda, 1 tsp.
- Black pepper
- Medium eggs, 4
- Diced bacon, 1 cup

Directions:

1. Set a mixing bowl in place and stir in the eggs and baking soda to incorporate well.
2. Whisk in the seasonings, butter, bacon, and lemon thyme
3. Set the mixture in a well-lined muffin pan.
4. Set the oven for 20 minutes at 350°F, allow to bake
5. Allow the muffins to cool before serving

Nutrition:
Calories: 186, Fat: 17.1, Fiber: 0.8, Carbs: 1.8, Protein: 7.4

Bacon and Seasoned Mushroom Skewers

Prep Time + Cook Time: 30 minutes Servings: 6

Ingredients:

- mushroom caps - 1 pound
- bacon strips - 6
- Salt and ground black pepper, to taste
- sweet paprika - ½ tsp.
- Sweet Mesquite; for seasoning

Directions:

1. Use mushroom caps with salt, pepper, and paprika as seasoning.
2. Spear a bacon strip on a skewer. Spear a mushroom cap, and fold the bacon over it.
3. Continue this process until you get a mushroom and bacon braid.
4. Do this for the rest of the mushrooms and bacon strips.
5. Season with sweet mesquite, place all skewers on a grill that has been preheated over medium heat.
6. Cook for about 10 minutes, then flip. Cook for another 10 minutes.
7. Divide on different plates and serve.

Nutrition:

Calories: 47, Fat: 2.9, Fiber: 0.8, Carbs: 2.6, Protein: 3.6

Breakfast Burrito

Prep Time + Cook Time: 26 minutes Serves: 1

Ingredients:

- Medium eggs, 3
- Onion powder, 1 tsp.
- Garlic powder, 1 tsp.
- Cumin, 1 tsp.
- Ground beef, ¼ lb.
- Chopped cilantro, 1 tsp.
- Sweet paprika, 1 tsp.
- Julienned onion, 1
- Salt
- Coconut oil, 1 Tsp.
- Black pepper

Directions:

1. Set the pan over medium heat to brown the beef evenly.
2. Stir in the garlic, paprika, seasoning, onion powder, and cumin to cook for around 4 minutes
3. Set another bowl in position to whisk together the eggs, some pepper, and some salt.
4. Pour the eggs in a pan over medium heat to cook for 6 minutes
5. Set the egg burrito on a plate with beef mixture, add the onion and cilantro then roll

Nutrition:

Calories: 482, Fat: 24.8, Fiber: 2.4, Carbs: 11.3, Protein: 52.2

Breakfast Cauliflower Mix

Prep Time + Cook Time: 35 minutes Servings: 4

Ingredients:

- Ghee: 2 tbsps.
- Small yellow onion (chopped): 1
- Garlic (minced): 2 cloves
- Coconut aminos: 1 tbsp.
- Beef meat (lean and ground): 1 pound
- Sunflower seed butter ¼ cup
- Salt and black pepper
- Cauliflower head (grated): 1
- Water ½ cup
- Homemade mayonnaise: ½ cup
- Cumin (ground): 1 tsp.
- Jalapeno peppers (chopped): 3
- Eggs: 4
- Avocado (peeled, cored and chopped): ½
- Parsley (chopped): 1 tbsp.

Directions:

1. Heat a pan with the ghee over medium heat, add jalapeno, onions, and garlic, stir and cook for 3 minutes.
2. Add meat, salt, and pepper, stir and brown for another 5 minutes.
3. Add cauliflower, stir and cook for 2 minutes.
4. Add sunflower seed butter, water, mayo, amino, and cumin, stir and cook for another 5 minutes.
5. Pour 4 holes in this mixture, add crack an egg to each hole, sprinkle with salt and pepper, place in preheated broiler and cook for 10 minutes.
6. Spread this mixture over the plate, sprinkle with parsley and garnish with avocado and serve.

Nutrition: calories 288, fat 12, fiber 6, carbs 15, protein 38

Breakfast Chia Pudding

Prep Time + Cook Time: 40 minutes Serves: 2

Ingredients:

- Coconut cream, 1/3 cup
- Chia seeds, 1/3 cup
- Swerve, 1 tbsp.
- Water, 2 cup
- Vanilla extract, 1 tbsp.
- Cocoa nibs, 2 tbsps.
- Coffee, 2 tbsps.

Directions:

1. Set a small pot on fire with water to boil over medium heat.
2. Add in coffee then simmer for 15 minutes, remove from heat and strain in a bowl.
3. Stir in the coconut cream, cocoa nibs, vanilla extract, chia seeds, and swerve
4. Set into bowls then refrigerate for 30 minutes

Nutrition:

Calories: 149, Fat: 12.5, Fiber: 2.9, Carbs: 10.8, Protein: 2

Breakfast Chicken Muffins

Prep Time + Cook Time: 1 hour 10 minutes Serves: 3

Ingredients:

- Chopped green onions, 2 tbsps.
- Black pepper
- Boneless chicken breast, ¾ lbs.
- Salt
- Cayenne pepper powder, 1 tbsp. mixed with 3 tbsps. melted coconut oil
- Medium eggs, 6
- Garlic powder, ½ tsp.

Directions:

1. Rub the chicken breast with garlic powder, pepper, and salt then set on a well-lined baking tray.
2. Set the oven for 25 minutes at 425°F, allow to bake
3. Once fully baked, take the chicken meat to a bowl for shredding using a fork.
4. Combine the shredded chicken with half of cayenne pepper, coconut oil, and pepper powder. Coat evenly then reserve
5. Set a bowl in position to whisk together green onions, seasonings, eggs and the remaining pepper with oil
6. Divide the mixture to a muffin tray topped with shredded chicken.
7. Set the oven for 30 minutes at 350°F
8. Enjoy the muffins while still hot

Nutrition:

Calories: 338, Fat: 20.6, Fiber: 0.2, Carbs: 1.3, Protein: 35.3

Breakfast Sandwich

Prep Time + Cook Time: 20 minutes Serves: 1

Ingredients:

- Guacamole, 1 tbsp.
- Salt
- Butter, 2 tbsps.
- Medium eggs, 2
- Minced pork sausage, ¼ lb.
- Black pepper
- Water, ¼ cup

Directions:

1. Set a mixing bowl in position to combine the sausage mixture with some seasonings.
2. Mold the mixture into a patty and set on a clean working surface.
3. Set the pan over medium heat with someone tbsp. butter to cook the sausage patty until cooked evenly, reserve on a plate
4. Whisk an egg into two bowls with some seasonings.
5. Set a pan with the remaining butter over medium-high heat then put 2 greased biscuit cutters in the pan then add an egg in each

6. Set the water on a pan to cook the eggs for three minutes with the pan covered under reduced heat
7. Drain excess grease from the egg using paper towel
8. Set the sausage patty on one egg bun then spread the guacamole on top the finish with other egg bun

Nutrition:
Calories: 735, Fat: 66, Fiber: 0.5, Carbs: 1.7, Protein: 33.6

Brussels Sprout Gratin with Pork Crust

Prep Time + Cook Time: 45 minutes Servings: 4
Ingredients:
- Onions - 2 ounces, diced
- Garlic - 1 tsp., minced
- Brussels sprouts - 6 ounces, chopped
- butter - 2 tbsps.
- 1 tbsp. coconut aminos
- Salt and ground black pepper, to taste
- liquid smoke - ½ tsp.

For the sauce:
- cheddar cheese - 2. 5 ounces, grated
- A pinch of black pepper
- butter - 1 tbsp.
- heavy cream - ½ cup
- turmeric - ¼ tsp.
- paprika - ¼ tsp.
- A pinch of xanthan gum

For the pork crust:
- Parmesan cheese - 3 tbsps.
- pork rinds - ½ ounces
- sweet paprika - ½ tsp.

Directions:
1. Add some heat to the frying pan with 2 tbsps. butter over high heat followed by addition of the Brussels sprouts, salt, pepper, and stir gently. Cook the mixture for about 3 minutes.
2. Mix garlic and onion together, stir, and cook for 3 minutes.
3. Gently stir a mixture of liquid smoke and coconut aminos, then remove the heat, and keep it away for a while.
4. Heat another pan with 1 tbsp. butter; this time making use of medium heat, followed by the addition of heavy cream, and stir.
5. Pour some cheese, black pepper, turmeric, paprika, and xanthan gum in a pot, stir, and cook until it becomes thick again.
6. Add Brussels sprouts mixture, toss to coat, and divide into ramekins.
7. Add the Parmesan cheese with pork rinds, ½ tsp. paprika in a food processor. Ensure it is well pulsed.
8. Cut the crumbs into different parts on top of Brussels sprouts mixture, put some ramekins in the oven at 375°F
9. Bake the mixture for about 20 minutes.
10. Then serve.

Nutrition:
Calories: 258, Fat: 22.3, Fiber: 2, Carbs: 6.6, Protein: 9.9

Cauliflower Breakfast Bread

Prep Time + Cook Time: 35 minutes Servings: 6

Ingredients:

- Chopped spinach- 1 cup
- Chopped walnuts - ½ cup
- Chopped Oregano - 1 tbsp.
- A Ground black pepper and a pinch Salt to taste
- Melted coconut oil- 1 tsp.
- 1 cauliflower, head, riced
- 3 (Whisked) eggs
- Minced clove- 1 garlic
- Chopped yellow onion- 1

Directions:

1. With moderate or medium temperature, Heat a pan with the oil, add onion, mix properly and cook for 10 minutes.
2. While the oven is set to a temperature of 350° F, Put cauliflower, spinach, walnuts, eggs, garlic, oregano, salt, and pepper into the pan and mix carefully, compress into a small loaf pan, and bake for 15 minutes.
3. Slice, divide between plates and serve for breakfast.
4. Enjoy!

Nutrition: calories 200, fat 3, fiber 4, carbs 9, protein 7

Cauliflower Cakes

Prep Time + Cook Time: 30 minutes Servings: 4

Ingredients:

- Cauliflower head (florets separated): 1
- Nutritional yeast: 1 tsp.
- Eggs: 2
- Almond flour: 2/3 cup
- Turmeric powder: ½ tsp.
- Ghee: 2 tbsps.
- Salt and black pepper

Directions:

1. Place the cauliflower florets in a saucepan, add water to cover, simmer over medium heat, boil for 8 minutes, drain well, place the cauliflower in the food processor and pulse.
2. In a bowl, mix the cauliflower with flour, eggs, yeast, salt, pepper, and turmeric powder, stir well and make medium sized pies from this mixture.
3. Heat a pan with the ghee over medium heat, add the patties, cook on each side for 3 minutes, divide between the plates and serve for breakfast.
4. Dish and enjoy!

Nutrition: calories 200, fat 3, fiber 8, carbs 16, protein 7

Cheesy Asparagus Delight

Prep Time + Cook Time: 35 minutes Serves: 2

Ingredients:

- Feta cheese, ½ cup
- Olive oil, 1 tbsp.
- Chopped green onions, 2
- Asparagus spears, 12
- Minced garlic clove, 1
- Black pepper
- Medium eggs, 6
- Salt

Directions:

1. Set the pan over medium heat with some water to cook the asparagus for 8 minutes.
2. Drain the liquid then chop the asparagus then reserve
3. Set the pan over medium heat with some oil again to fry the onion; chopped asparagus then cook for 5 minutes as you stir gently.
4. Stir in the seasonings and eggs to cook for 5 minutes while covered
5. Set the asparagus spears on top of the frittata with sprinkled cheese on top.
6. Set the oven for 9 minutes at 350°F then allow to bake.
7. Enjoy.

Nutrition:

Calories: 384, Fat: 28.3, Fiber: 3.4, Carbs: 9.7, Protein: 25.5

Cheesy Sausage Quiche

Prep Time + Cook Time: 50 minutes Serves: 6

Ingredients:

- Eggplant slices, 5
- Salt
- Medium eggs, 6
- Black pepper
- Whipping cream, 2 tsps.
- Halved cherry tomatoes, 10
- Chopped parsley, 2 tbsps.
- Chopped pork sausage, 12 oz.
- Grated Parmesan cheese, 2 tbsps.

Directions:

1. Set the baking tray then align the sausages on it, then eggplant slices and then cherry tomatoes
2. Set a mixing bowl in position to whisk together the parmesan cheese, eggs, cream, and the seasonings.
3. Set the oven for 40 minutes at 375°F, then pour on the baking tray, allow to bake
4. Enjoy

Nutrition:

Calories: 275, Fat: 21.5, Fiber: 0.4, Carbs: 1.9, Protein: 17.7

Chia Cereal Nibs

Prep Time + Cook Time: 55 minutes Serves: 4

Ingredients:

- Cocoa nibs, 2 tbsps.
- Chia seeds, ½ cup
- Coconut oil, 2 tbsps.
- Water, 1 cup
- Vanilla extract, 1 tbsp.
- Hemp hearts, 4 tbsps.
- Psyllium powder, 1 tbsp.
- Swerve, 1 tbsp.

Directions:

1. Set a mixing bowl in a clean working surface to stir in water and chia seeds then reserve for 5 minutes
2. Stir in the psyllium powder, hemp hearts, swerve, vanilla extract, and oil
3. Mix in the cocoa nibs to make a dough.
4. Split the dough into two then mold to a cylindrical shape.
5. Set the molded dough in a lined baking sheet to flatten well the cover with a parchment paper.
6. Set the oven for 20 minutes at 285°F. Allow to bake.
7. Remove parchment paper and bake for 25 minutes.
8. Allow the cylinders to cool before serving.

Nutrition:

Calories: 324, Fat: 25.4, Fiber: 8.1, Carbs: 14.3, Protein: 12.8

Chicken Chowder served with Cheddar Cheese

Prep Time + Cook Time:4h and 10minutesServings: 4

Ingredients:

- chicken thighs - 1 pound, skinless and boneless
- canned diced tomatoes - 10 ounces
- chicken stock - 1 cup
- cream cheese - 8 ounces
- Juice from lime -
- Salt and ground black pepper, to taste
- jalapeño pepper - 1, chopped
- onion - 1, peeled and chopped
- fresh cilantro - 2 tbsps., chopped
- garlic clove - 1, peeled and minced
- Cheddar cheese, shredded, for serving
- Lime wedges, for serving

Directions:

1. Mix chicken with the tomatoes, stock, cream cheese, salt, pepper, lime juice, jalapeño, onion, garlic, cilantro in a slow cooker.
2. Stir gently, then cover, and cook on high heat for about 4 hours.
3. Remove the cover of the slow cooker and shred the meat.
4. Divide into different bowls.
5. Serve with cheddar cheese on top and some lime wedges on the side.

Nutrition:

Calories: 447, Fat: 28.5, Fiber: 2.1, Carbs: 9.3, Protein: 38.5

Chorizo and Cauliflower Breakfast mix

Prep Time + Cook Time: 55 minutes Serves: 4

Ingredients:

- Chopped green onions, 2 tbsps.
- Chopped canned green chilies, 12 oz.
- Whisked eggs, 4
- Chopped onion, 1
- Chopped chorizo, 1 lb.
- Garlic powder, ½ tsp.
- Salt
- Cauliflower head, 1
- Black pepper

Directions:

1. Set the pan to fry the chorizo and onion until browned for a few minutes over medium heat.
2. Stir in the green chilies to cook for some minutes then remove from heat
3. Set the blender on to process the cauliflower and the seasoning
4. Pour the mixture on a bowl then mix in chorizo mixture, eggs, garlic powder, and the seasoning.
5. Prepare the baking tray with some greasing and pour the mixture on it
6. Set the oven for 40 minutes at 375ºF, allow to bake
7. Allow the casserole to cool then top with green onion
8. Slice and enjoy

Nutrition:
Calories: 883, Fat: 52.8, Fiber: 26.7, Carbs: 68.2, Protein: 43.5

Coated Asian Salad

Prep Time + Cook Time: 25 minutes Servings: 4

Ingredients:

- ground beef - 1 pound
- coconut aminos - 2 tbsps.
- garlic cloves - 2, peeled and minced
- sesame seed oil - 2 tbsp.
- apple cider vinegar - 1 tsp.
- sesame seeds - 1 tsp.
- green onion - 1, chopped

Directions:

1. Heat a pan containing oil over medium heat, add the garlic, and brown for 1 minute.
2. Put beef into the mixture, then stir, and cook for about 10 minutes.
3. Make coleslaw mixture, add pour into a pan.
4. Toss to ensure it is well coated, and cook for 1minute.
5. Then add vinegar, sriracha, coconut aminos, salt, pepper, stir, and cook for about 4 minutes.
6. Add green onions and sesame seeds, then toss to coat.
7. Separate into different bowls and serve.

Nutrition:
Calories: 281, Fat: 14.3, Fiber: 0.2, Carbs: 1.5, Protein: 34.7

Coated Green Bean Salad

Prep Time + Cook Time: 15 minutes Servings: 8

Ingredients:

- white wine vinegar - 2 tbsps.
- mustard - 1½ tbsps.
- Salt and ground black pepper, to taste
- green beans - 2 pounds
- extra virgin olive oil - ⅓ cup
- Fennel - 1½ cups, sliced thin
- goats cheese - 4 ounces, crumbled
- Walnuts - ¾ cup, toasted and chopped

Directions:

1. Pour water into a saucepan, and sprinkle some salt. Boil the mixture over medium-high heat.
2. Add green beans to the mixture, cook for about 5 minutes, and move to a bowl containing ice water.
3. Drain the green beans properly and place in a salad bowl. Mix with some walnuts, fennel, and goat cheese and toss gently.
4. Mix vinegar with mustard, salt, pepper, oil, and whisk in a bowl.
5. Pour the resulting mixture over the salad, and to ensure it is adequately coated.
6. Then serve.

Nutrition:
Calories: 244, Fat: 19.1, Fiber: 6.5, Carbs: 14.1, Protein: 8.6

Coated Simple Buffalo Wings

Prep Time + Cook Time: 30 minutes Servings: 2

Ingredients:

- butter - 2 tbsps.
- 6 chicken wings, cut in half
- Salt and ground black pepper, to taste
- A pinch of garlic powder
- cayenne pepper powder - 3 tbsp
- olive oil - 4 tbsp
- A pinch of cayenne pepper
- sweet paprika - ½ tsp.

Directions:

1. Mix chicken pieces with half of the hot sauce, salt, and pepper in a clean bowl.
2. Toss well to ensure it is coated.
3. Place the chicken pieces neatly on a lined baking dish, then place the dish under a preheated broiler, and broil for about 8 minutes.
4. Flip the chicken pieces, and broil for another 8 minutes.
5. Heat a pan containing butter on a medium-high heat source.
6. Pour the remaining hot sauce, salt, pepper, cayenne, and paprika, and stir gently.
7. Then cook the mixture for a couple of minutes.
8. Move the broiled chicken pieces to another clean bowl, then add the butter.
9. Add olive oil and cayenne pepper mixture over the broiled chicken pieces mixed with butter
10. Toss to ensure it is well coated.
11. Then serve.

Nutrition:
Calories: 610, Fat: 50, Fiber: 0.2, Carbs: 0.4, Protein: 40.7

Coconut Biscuits

Prep Time + Cook Time: 25 minutesServes: 6

Ingredients:
- Baking soda, ¼ tsp.
- Coconut flour, 6 tbsps.
- Black pepper
- Minced onion, ¼ cup
- Medium eggs, 2
- Salt
- Chopped parsley, 1tbsp.
- Coconut milk, 2 tbsps.
- Apple cider vinegar, ½ tsp.
- Coconut oil, 6 tbsps.
- Minced garlic cloves, 2

Directions:

1. Set a large mixing bowl on a working surface to combine the coconut milk, garlic, onion, parsley, and seasoning with coconut flour.
2. Mold the mixture into circles
3. Grease the baking tray with some butter
4. Set the oven for 15 minutes at 350°F, then allow to bake
5. Enjoy while still hot

Nutrition:
Calories: 213, Fat: 18.3, Fiber: 5.3, Carbs: 9.2, Protein: 4.1

Coconut Milk Soup

Prep Time + Cook Time: 40 minutes Servings: 2

Ingredients:
- chicken stock - 4 cups
- lime leaves - 3
- coconut milk - 1½ cups
- fried lemongrass - 1 tsp.
- fresh cilantro - 1 cup, chopped
- fresh ginger - 1–inch, peeled and grated
- Thai chilies - 4, dried and chopped
- Salt and ground black pepper, to taste
- Shrimp - 4 ounces, peeled and deveined
- Onion - 2 tbsps., chopped
- coconut oil - 1 tbsp.
- mushrooms - 2 tbsps., chopped
- fish sauce - 1 tbsp.
- fresh cilantro - 1 tbsp., chopped
- Juice from lime - 1

Directions:

1. Mix chicken stock with coconut milk, lime leaves, lemongrass, Thai chilies, 1 cup cilantro, ginger, salt, pepper in a pot, stir well.
2. Transfer it to a simmer over on medium heat. Cook for about 20 minutes, then strain and move it back to the pot.
3. Apply more heat to the soup again over medium heat. Add coconut oil, shrimp, fish sauce, mushrooms, onions, stir, and cook for about 10 minutes.
4. Pour lime juice and 1 tbsp. cilantro into the mixture, stir gently before ladling into bowls.
5. Then serve.

Nutrition:
Calories: 1673, Fat: 166.3, Fiber: 15, Carbs: 40.6, Protein: 30.3

Cold Apple Salad

Prep Time + Cook Time: 10 minutes Servings: 4

Ingredients:

- broccoli florets - 2 cups, chopped
- pecans - 2 ounces, chopped
- apple - 1, cored and grated
- green onion - 1, diced
- Salt and ground black pepper, to taste
- poppy seeds - 2 tsps.
- apple cider vinegar - 1 tsp.
- mayonnaise - ¼ cup
- lemon juice - ½ tsp.
- sour cream - ¼ cup

Directions:

1. Mix apple with broccoli, green onion, and pecans in a salad bowl, and stir gently.
2. Pour some poppy seeds, salt, and pepper into the mixture, and toss gently.
3. Mix mayonnaise with sour cream, vinegar, lemon juice, and whisk inside a bowl.
4. Spread the mixture over the salad
5. Toss to coat thoroughly, and ensure it is cold when served.

Nutrition:

Calories: 240, Fat: 18.9, Fiber: 4.3, Carbs: 17.5, Protein: 3.9

Creamy Eggs and Asparagus with Cayenne Pepper

Prep Time + Cook Time: 25 minutes Servings: 4

Ingredients:

- Butter: 2 ounces
- Coconut cream: 8 ounces
- Lemon juice: 1½ tbsp.
- Parmesan (grated): 3 ounces
- Salt and black pepper
- Eggs,(whisked): 4
- Green asparagus (trimmed & halved): 1½ pounds
- Cayenne pepper: a pinch
- Olive oil: 1 tbsp.

Directions:

1. Heat a pan with the butter over medium heat, put in the eggs and mix for 6-7 minutes.
2. Combine the Parmesan cheese, cream, salt, pepper, and cayenne pepper, stir, heat and spread on plates.
3. Heat a pan with the oil over medium heat, add asparagus, a pinch of cayenne pepper and lemon juice, cook on each side for 2-3 minutes, divide next to the scrambled eggs and serve for breakfast.
4. Dish and enjoy!

Nutrition: calories 212, fat 8, fiber 5, carbs 15, protein 7

Delicious Chicken Muffins

Prep Time + Cook Time:1 hour 10 minutes Servings: 3

Ingredients:

- Green onions (chopped)- 2 tbsps.
- Eggs- 6
- Tomato passata- 3 tbsps.
- Chicken breast (skinless and boneless) - 1 pound
- A Ground black pepper and a pinch Salt to taste
- Chili pepper - ½ tsp.
- Coconut oil (melted) - 2 tbsps.
- Garlic powder - ½ tsp.

Directions:

1. Place chicken breasts on a lined baking sheet in an orderly manner, sprinkle with salt and pepper and place in the oven at a temperature of 425° F, cook for 25 minutes.
2. Use two forks to Shred the meat, then place it in a bowl, also put tomato passata, chili pepper, and the ghee and toss it well.
3. In a separate bowl, mix the eggs with salt, pepper and green onions and stir carefully.
4. While the oven is set to a temperature of 425° F, divide the eggs mix into 6 muffin cups, divide the chicken meat as well, place them in the oven and cook for 30 minutes.
5. Serve for breakfast. enjoy!

Nutrition: calories 261, fat 3, fiber 7, carbs 16, protein 8

Easy Scrambled Eggs

Prep Time + Cook Time: 20 minutes Serves: 1

Ingredients:

- Coconut oil, 1 tbsp.
- Whisked eggs, 3
- Chopped ham slices, 2
- Black pepper
- Chopped bell mushrooms, 4
- Salt
- Chopped red bell pepper, ¼ cup
- Chopped spinach, ½ cup

Directions:

1. Set the pan over medium heat with a ½ tbsp. olive oil to fry the spinach, mushroom, bell pepper, and ham for four minutes.
2. Set another pan over medium heat with the remaining oil to scramble the eggs
3. Combine ham, veggies, and seasoning to cook for one minute then serve

Nutrition:
Calories: 430, Fat: 31.9, Fiber: 2.4, Carbs: 9, Protein: 29.5

Fried Asparagus with Sauce

Prep Time + Cook Time: 20 minutes Servings: 4

Ingredients:

- egg yolks - 2
- Salt and ground black pepper, to taste
- butter - ¼ cup
- lemon juice - 1 tbsp.
- A pinch of cayenne pepper
- asparagus spears - 40

Directions:

1. Whisk the egg yolks well in a clean bowl.
2. Move to a small pan put on a low heat source.
3. Then add lemon juice to the mixture, and whisk.
4. Add butter and whisk until it melts perfectly.
5. Pour some salt, pepper, cayenne pepper, and whisk once again.
6. Heat another clean pan over medium-high heat, then add asparagus spears, and fry this for about 5 minutes.
7. Divide the asparagus on different plates
8. Drizzle with sauce as topping.
9. You can serve now.

Nutrition:

Calories: 177, Fat: 14.1, Fiber: 5, Carbs: 9.6, Protein: 6.8

Hash Casserole

Prep Time + Cook Time: 26 minutes Serves: 2

Ingredients:

- Quartered radishes, 1 lb.
- Beef stock, ½ cup
- Salt
- Chopped corned beef, 2 cup
- Minced garlic cloves, 2
- Black pepper
- Chopped onion, 1
- Coconut oil, 1 tbsp.

Directions:

1. Set the pan over medium-high heat to fry the onions until tender.
2. Stir in the radishes to cook for 5 minutes then add garlic to cook for 1 minute as you stir gently
3. Mix in the beef, stock, and the seasoning. Allow to cook for 5 minutes
4. Serve and enjoy

Nutrition:

Calories: 316, Fat: 21.2, Fiber: 4.9, Carbs: 13.9, Protein: 18

Hemp Porridge

Prep Time + Cook Time: 6 minutes Serves: 1

Ingredients:

- Hemp hearts, 1 tbsp.
- Almond flour, ¼ cup
- Almond milk, 1 cup
- Flaxseeds, 2 tbsps.
- Hemp hearts, ½ cup
- Stevia, 1 tbsp.
- Chia seeds, 1 tbsp.
- Vanilla extract, ¾ tsp.
- Ground cinnamon, ½ tsp.

Directions:

1. Set the pan over medium heat to stir evenly almond milk with chia seeds, ½ cup hemp hearts, stevia, cinnamon, flaxseeds, and vanilla extract to cook for 2 minutes.
2. Remove from heat then stir in almond flour.
3. Set the porridge in a bowl
4. Serve topped with 1 tbsp. of hemp hearts.

Nutrition:
Calories: 1030, Fat: 91.6, Fiber: 18.5, Carbs: 32.7, Protein: 29.5

Her bed Frittata with Bacon

Prep Time + Cook Time: 40 minutes Servings: 4

Ingredients:

- Eggs (whisked): 12
- Yellow onion (chopped): 1
- Salt and black pepper
- Bacon slices (chopped): 8
- Tomatoes (chopped): 4
- Oregano (chopped): 1 tbsp.
- Basil (chopped): 1 tbsp.
- Parsley (chopped): 1 tbsp.

Directions:

1. Heat a pan over medium heat, add bacon, stir and cook for 5 minutes.
2. Add the onion, stir and continue to cook for 2-3 minutes.
3. Add tomatoes, salt, parsley, basil and oregano, pepper, stir and cook for 1 minute.
4. Add the beaten eggs, toss into the oven for 20 minutes at 350° F.
5. Dish, divide between plates and serve for breakfast.
6. Serve and enjoy!

Nutrition: calories 251, fiber 7, carbs 17, fat 3, protein 7

Hot Broccoli Soup

Prep Time + Cook Time: 40 minutes Servings: 4

Ingredients:

- white onion - 1, peeled and chopped
- butter - 1 tbsp.
- vegetable stock - 2 cups
- Salt and ground black pepper, to taste

- water - 2 cups
- garlic cloves - 2, peeled and minced
- heavy cream - 1 cup
- cheddar cheese - 8 ounces, grated
- broccoli florets - 12 ounces
- paprika - ½ tsp.

Directions:
1. Heat a saucepan containing butter over medium heat, then put some onions and garlic Stir gently, and cook for about 5 minutes.
2. Pour stock, cream, water, salt, pepper, paprika. Gently stir the resulting mixture, and move to a boil.
3. Pour broccoli, stir, and simmer the soup for 25 minutes.
4. Transfer the mixture to a food processor and ensure it perfectly blended.
5. After blending, add cheese. Then blend again.
6. Divide into different soup bowls.
7. Ensure the food is still hot when served.

Nutrition:
Calories: 400, Fat: 33.1, Fiber: 2.9, Carbs: 10.4, Protein: 17.6

Hot Green Bean Casserole

Prep Time + Cook Time: 45 minutes Servings: 8

Ingredients:
- green beans - 1 pound, halved
- Salt and ground black pepper, to taste
- almond flour - ½ cup
- butter - 2 tbsps.
- Mushrooms - 8 ounces, chopped
- Onion - 4 ounces, peeled and chopped
- Shallots - 2, peeled and chopped
- garlic cloves - 3, peeled and minced
- chicken stock - ½ cup
- heavy cream - ½ cup
- Parmesan cheese - ¼ cup, grated
- Avocado oil for frying

Directions:
1. Add some amount of water in a saucepan, add a pinch of salt to the water, and boil over medium-high heat
2. Add green beans to the mixture, and cook for about 5 minutes
3. Move to a bowl containing ice water; this would cool it down.
4. Drain well, and keep it aside for a while.
5. Mix the shallots with the onions, almond flour, salt, and pepper, in a bowl, and toss to coat.
6. Over medium-high heat, heat a frying pan containing some avocado oil.
7. Then add some onions, shallots mixture, fry until it shows a golden brown coloration.
8. Move into paper towels, and remove the grease by draining.

9. Heat the pan over medium heat, add butter and melt it.
10. Add garlic and mushrooms to the mixture, and gently stir. Cook for about 5 minutes.
11. Gently stir after adding stock and heavy cream. Pour into a pot to boil, and simmer until it becomes thick. Put some Parmesan cheese and green beans, toss to coat, and remove the heat.
12. Move the mixture to a baking dish, then sprinkle some crispy onions mixture all over it.
13. Place in an oven at 400°F, and bake for 15 minutes.
14. Make sure to serve when the food is still warm.

Nutrition:
Calories: 104, Fat: 7.1, Fiber: 2.7, Carbs: 8.6, Protein: 3.5

Keto Breakfast Burger

Prep Time + Cook Time: 25 minutes Servings: 4
Ingredients:
- Beef (ground): 1 pound
- Homemade mayonnaise: ¼ cup
- Mustard 1 tsp.
- Garlic powder: ½ tsp.
- Ghee: 2 tbsps.
- Onion powder: ½ tsp.
- Salt and black pepper
- Chili sauce: 1 tsp.

Directions:
1. Mix the meat in a bowl with mustard, onion and garlic powder, salt and pepper, stir and make 4 burgers from this mixture.
2. Heat a pan with the ghee over medium heat, add hamburger, cook on each side for 4-5 minutes, divide over the plates and serve with some chili sauce and mayo spread over and in keto bread.
3. Dish and Enjoy!

Nutrition:
calories 200, fat 7, fiber 8, carbs 16, protein 29

Keto Veggie Frittata

Prep Time + Cook Time: 45 minutes Servings: 4
Ingredients:
- Chopped yellow onion- 1
- 8 (Whisked) eggs
- Chopped bacon- ½ pound
- Chopped basil- ¼ cup
- Chopped carrot- 1
- Chopped mushroom- 5 ounces
- Chopped asparagus- 1 bunch
- A Ground black pepper and a pinch Salt to taste

Directions:
1. Set the oven to medium temperature, heat cooking pan over, add bacon, mix properly and cook for five minutes.

2. Put, mushrooms, onions, asparagus, and carrots, then mix thoroughly and cook for another five minutes.
3. While the Oven is set to a temperature of 350 ° F, put salt, pepper, eggs, and basil, toss it, mix properly and spread on cooking pan then place it inside the oven for 25 minutes.
4. Put off the oven.
5. Slice the frittata, spread over plates and serve for breakfast.
6. Delicious!

Nutrition:
calories 288, fat 3, fiber 6, carbs 18, protein 7

Mexican Casserole with Cilantro Topping

Prep Time + Cook Time: 45 minutes Servings: 6

Ingredients:
- chipotle peppers - 2, chopped
- Jalapeno - 2, chopped
- olive oil - 1 tbsp.
- heavy cream - ¼ cup
- small white onion - 1, peeled and chopped
- Salt and ground black pepper, to taste
- chicken thighs - 1 pound, skinless, boneless, and chopped
- tomato paste - 1 cup
- cream cheese - 4 ounces
- Vegetable oil cooking spray
- pepper jack cheese - 1 cup, shredded
- fresh cilantro: 2 tbsps., chopped
- homemade tortillas - 2

Directions:
1. Heat a pan containing oil over medium heat, then add the chipotle peppers and jalapeno peppers.
2. Gently stir the mixture, and cook for a few seconds.
3. Add onion to the mixture, stir, and cook for about 5 minutes.
4. Add cream cheese, heavy cream, and stir until the cheese melts.
5. Add chicken, salt, pepper, tomato paste, stir well, and remove the heat.
6. Use a cooking spray to grease a baking dish, then place tortillas on the bottom and spread the chicken mixture all over.
7. Sprinkle with shredded cheese.
8. Cover with aluminum foil, and transfer to an oven at a temperature of 350°F, and bake for about 15 minutes.
9. Discard the aluminum foil, and bake for about 15 minutes.
10. Sprinkle cilantro as topping and serve.

Nutrition:
Calories: 331, Fat: 19.7, Fiber: 2.4, Carbs: 11.7, Protein: 28.1

Minted Meatball Pilaf

Prep Time + Cook Time: 40 minutes Servings: 4

Ingredients:

- cauliflower florets - 12 ounces
- Salt and ground black pepper, to taste
- egg - 1
- ground lamb - 1 pound
- fennel seed - 1 tsp.
- paprika - 1 tsp.
- garlic powder - 1 tsp.
- Onion - 1, peeled and chopped
- garlic cloves - 2, peeled and minced
- coconut oil - 2 tbsps.
- fresh mint - 1 bunch, chopped
- lemon zest - 1 tbsp.
- goats cheese - 4 ounces, crumbled

Directions:

1. Place the cauliflower florets in a food processor, sprinkle some salt and pulse well.
2. Grease a frying pan with some coconut oil, and bring to medium heat.
3. Add cauliflower rice, cook for about 8 minutes.
4. Use salt and pepper as seasoning, then remove the heat and ensure that it stays warm.
5. Mix the lamb with salt, pepper, egg, paprika, garlic powder, fennel seed, and stir well inside a bowl.
6. Make 12 meatballs and put them on a plate.
7. Apply medium heat to a frying pan containing coconut oil, add onion, stir, and cook for about 6 minutes. Add garlic, stir, and cook for 1 minute.
8. Add the meatballs, make sure they are well cooked on all sides, and then remove the heat.
9. Divide cauliflower rice on different plates before adding the meatballs and onion mixture on top.
10. Sprinkle the mint, lemon zest, and goat cheese when you are done cooking.
11. Then serve.

Nutrition:

Calories: 345, Fat: 16.5, Fiber: 3.2, Carbs: 8.7, Protein: 35.6

Mixed Nuts Breakfast Bowl

Prep Time + Cook Time: 5 minutes Serves: 1

Ingredients:

- Raspberries, 2 tsps.
- Chopped walnuts, 1 tsp.
- Coconut milk, ½ cup
- Raw sunflower seeds, 1 tsp.
- Chopped almonds, 1 tsp.
- Raw pine nuts, 1 tsp.
- Stevia, 1 tsp.
- Chopped pistachios, 1 tsp.
- Chopped pecans, 1 tsp.
- Honey

Directions:

1. Set a mixing bowl in a clean working surface to combine honey with milk.
2. Mix in almonds, pine nuts, pecans, pistachios, sunflower seeds, and walnuts
3. Give the mixture a gentle stir then top with raspberries.
4. Enjoy

Nutrition:

Calories: 435, Fat: 44.2, Fiber: 5.2, Carbs: 10.8, Protein: 6.2

Mixed Veggie Breakfast Bread

Prep Time + Cook Time: 35 minutes Serves: 7

Ingredients:

- Black pepper
- Chopped parsley, ½ cup
- Torn spinach, 1 cup
- Ground pecans, ½ cup
- Cauliflower head, 1
- Medium eggs, 3
- Coconut oil, 1 tbsp.
- Minced garlic cloves, 2
- Salt
- Chopped onion, 1

Directions:

1. Set the blender in position to process cauliflower florets and a little bit of the seasonings.
2. Set the pan over medium heat to cook the onion, cauliflower, garlic, pepper, and salt for 10 minutes.
3. Meanwhile, combine the spinach, eggs, parsley, nuts, pepper, and salt in a bowl
4. Stir in the cauliflower then spread the mixture on a baking tray.
5. Set the oven for 15 minutes at 350°F, allow to bake
6. Enjoy while still warm

Nutrition:

Calories: 105, Fat: 8.2, Fiber: 2.2, Carbs: 5.2, Protein: 4.2

Mushroom Breakfast Bowl

Prep Time + Cook Time: 30 minutes Serves: 1

Ingredients:

- Sliced black olives, 12
- Chopped onion, 1
- Ground beef, 4 oz.
- Sliced mushrooms, 8
- Salt
- Ground beef, 4 oz.
- Black pepper
- Whisked eggs, 2
- Smoked paprika, ½ tsp.
- Chopped avocado, 1
- Coconut oil, 1 tbsp.

Directions:

1. Set the pan over medium heat to heat the coconut oil for frying onions, then mushrooms and season for 5 minutes
2. Stir in paprika and beef to cook for 10 minutes then reserve in a bowl
3. Return the pan on heat to fry seasoned eggs over medium heat until scrambled
4. Put the beef mixture back to the pan to cook for 1 minute with a gentle stir
5. Serve and enjoy

Nutrition:
Calories: 1002, Fat: 74.9, Fiber: 19.4, Carbs: 36.9, Protein: 55.6

Nutritious Breakfast Salad

Prep Time + Cook Time: 16 minutes Servings: 2

Ingredients:
- Kale (torn): 3 cups
- Cherry tomatoes (halved): 10
- Red vinegar: 1 tsp.
- Salt and black pepper
- Olive oil: 2 tsps.
- Eggs: 2
- Bacon (chopped): 4 strips
- Avocado (pitted, peeled and sliced): 2 ounces

Directions:
1. Pour water into a pan, bring to a boil over medium heat, add eggs, boil for 6 minutes, drain, rinse, cool, peel and slice.
2. Combine the kale in a salad bowl with vinegar, salt, pepper, oil, eggs, bacon, tomatoes, and avocado, toss well, divide between the plates and serve for breakfast.
3. Enjoy!

Nutrition:
calories 292, fat 14, fiber 7, carbs 18, protein 16

Oven baked Sausages and Eggs

Prep Time + Cook Time: 45 minutes Serves: 6

Ingredients:
- Chopped red bell pepper, 1
- Butter, 5 tbsps.
- Salt
- Chopped sausages, 2
- Black pepper
- Torn spinach, 1 oz.
- Ham slices, 12
- Medium eggs, 12
- Chopped onion, 1

Directions:
1. Melt one tbsp. butter in a pan to fry the onion and sausages for 5 minutes over medium heat.

2. Stir in the seasonings and bell pepper to cook for 3 minutes then reserve in a bowl.
3. Heat the remaining butter then divide into 12 cupcake molds
4. Top with a ham slice, then spinach, and then add sausage mixture
5. Crash the egg on top of each cupcake
6. Set the oven for 20 minutes at 425°F, then allow to bake
7. Allow cooling before serving

Nutrition:
Calories: 378, Fat: 28.4, Fiber: 1.5, Carbs: 6.2, Protein: 24.5

Oven-Baked Eggs and Sausage Mix

Prep Time + Cook Time: 50 minutes Serves: 6

Ingredients:
- Melted coconut oil, 1 tbsp.
- Chopped leek, 1
- Whisked eggs, 8
- Chopped asparagus stalks, 6
- Chopped dill, 1 tbsp.
- Salt
- Chopped sausage, 1 lb.
- Black pepper
- Garlic powder, ¼ tsp.
- Coconut milk, ¼ cup

Directions:
1. Set the pan over medium heat to let the sausages brown for a few minutes
2. Stir in the leek and asparagus then allow to cook for some minutes
3. Set a mixing bowl in position to combine garlic powder, seasoning, coconut milk, and dill
4. Grease the baking tray then pour on the mixture.
5. Set the oven for 40 minutes at 325°F, then allow to bake
6. Serve warm

Nutrition:
Calories: 397, Fat: 32, Fiber: 1, Carbs: 4, Protein: 23.1

Serrano Poached Eggs

Prep Time + Cook Time: 45 minutes Serves: 4

Ingredients:
- Medium eggs, 6
- Butter, 1 tbsp.
- Chopped white onion, 1
- Salt
- Minced garlic cloves, 3
- Black pepper
- Chopped tomatoes, 3
- Paprika, 1 tsp.
- Chopped cilantro, 1 tbsp.
- Cumin, 1 tsp.
- Chopped Serrano pepper, 1
- Chili powder, ¼ tsp.
- Chopped red bell pepper, 1

Directions:
1. Set the pan over medium heat to melt the butter for frying onions for 10 minutes

2. Stir in garlic and Serrano pepper to cook for one minute. Mix the red bell pepper to cook for 10 minutes as you stir
3. Mix in paprika, chili powder, seasonings, and cumin to cook for 10 minutes

4. Beat the eggs into the pan then sprinkle with some salt and pepper to cook for 6 minutes with the pan covered
5. Top with chopped cilantro and serve

Nutrition:
Calories: 180, Fat: 10.9, Fiber: 2.5, Carbs: 10.5, Protein: 11.7

Shrimp Pasta with Chopped Basil

Prep Time + Cook Time: 20 minutes Servings: 4

Ingredients:
- Shirataki noodles - 12 ounces
- olive oil - 2 tbsps.
- Salt and ground black pepper, to taste
- butter - 2 tbsps.
- garlic cloves - 4, peeled and minced
- shrimp - 1 pound, peeled and deveined
- lemon juice - ½
- paprika - ½ tsp.
- fresh basil - ½ cup, chopped

Directions:
1. Pour some water in a saucepan, add some salt, and transfer to a boil.
2. Add the Shiritaki noodles, and cook for about 2 minutes.

3. Remove the water by draining and move to a pan that has been preheated.
4. Toast the noodles for a few seconds before removing the heat, and keep them aside.
5. Heat a pan containing butter and olive oil over medium heat.
6. Add the garlic, and stir, until it turns brown for 1 minute.
7. Then add shrimp, lemon juice, and cook for about 3 minutes on each side.
8. Add the noodles, salt, pepper, and paprika, and stir gently.
9. Finally divide into different bowls.
10. You can serve with chopped basil on top.

Nutrition:
Calories: 262, Fat: 15.3, Fiber: 2.2, Carbs: 5.9, Protein: 26.7

Simple Sausage Muffins

Prep Time + Cook Time: 20 minutes Servings: 2

Ingredients:
- Chopped sausage - ¼ pound
- Eggs- 2
- Melted ghee - 2 tbsps.

- A Ground black pepper and a pinch Salt to taste

Directions:

1. Use half of the ghee to grease the muffin tin.
2. With medium-high heat, Pour the rest of the ghee over a pan and heat, add sausage, pepper, and salt, mix properly and allow to cook for 3 minutes.
3. Add eggs with the sausage in a bowl, whisk and place into the separate muffin tin.
4. Set the oven to a temperature of 425F, place the muffin tin in the oven and cook for 8 minutes.
5. Put off the heat and divide the muffins between plates and serve for breakfast.

Nutrition:
calories 200, fat 4, fiber 8, carbs 11, protein 8

Simple Spinach Frittata

Prep Time + Cook Time: 1 hour 10 minutesServes: 4

Ingredients:
- Shredded mozzarella cheese, 5 oz.
- Spinach, 9 oz.
- Medium eggs, 12
- Nutmeg, ¼ tsp.
- Minced garlic, 1 tsp.
- Salt
- Olive oil, 4 tbsps.
- Black pepper
- Grated Parmesan cheese, ½ cup
- Pepperoni, 1 oz.
- Ricotta cheese, ½ cup

Directions:
1. Press the spinach to drain all the liquid then reserve in a bowl
2. Whisk the seasonings, eggs, garlic, and nutmeg in another bowl
3. Mix in the parmesan cheese, spinach, and ricotta cheese. Whisk again
4. Pour the mixture in a baking tray topped with mozzarella cheese and pepperoni
5. Set the oven for 45 minutes at 375°F, then allow to bake.
6. Allow the frittata to cool before serving.
7. Enjoy.

Nutrition:
Calories: 525, Fat: 40.7, Fiber: 1.4, Carbs: 6.7, Protein: 35.9

Simple Tomato Soup with Topping

Prep Time + Cook Time: 15 minutes Servings: 4

Ingredients:
- canned tomato passata -1 quart
- butter -4 tbsps.
- olive oil -½ cup
- cayenne pepper powder -3 tbsp
- apple cider vinegar -2 tbsps.

- Salt and ground black pepper, to taste
- dried oregano -1 tsp.
- turmeric -2 tsps.
- bacon strips - 8, cooked and crumbled
- green onions - ½ cup, chopped
- fresh basil leaves - ½ cup, chopped

Directions:
1. Put the tomato passata in a saucepan using medium heat.
2. Mix olive oil, butter, cayenne pepper, vinegar, salt, pepper, turmeric, oregano, and stir the mixture.
3. Simmer for 5 minutes.
4. Remove the heat, divide the soup into different bowls.
5. Use some crumbled bacon, basil, and green onions as topping.

Nutrition:
Calories: 385, Fat: 41.4, Fiber: 0.8, Carbs: 3.5, Protein: 2.9

Smoked Salmon with Green sauce

Prep Time + Cook Time: 20 minutes Serves: 3

Ingredients:
- Avocado oil, ½ tsp.
- Chopped smoked salmon, 4 oz.
- Whisked eggs, 4

For the sauce:
- Lemon juice, 1 tbsp.
- Chopped green onions, ¼ cup
- Coconut milk, 1 cup
- Soaked cashews, ½ cup
- Salt
- Garlic powder, 1 tsp.
- Black pepper

Directions:
1. Set your blender in position to process garlic powder, cashews, lemon juice, and coconut milk
2. Mix in green onions and the seasoning to process again.
3. Pour the mixture in a bowl then refrigerate.
4. Set the pan over medium-low heat with oil to fry the whisked eggs until almost cooked.
5. Finish cooking the eggs in a pre-heated broiler.
6. Set the eggs on a plate topped with smoked salmon.
7. Enjoy with the green onion sauce

Nutrition:
Calories: 448, Fat: 37.3, Fiber: 2.7, Carbs: 13.1, Protein: 19.8

Spaghetti Casserole Italian style

Prep Time + Cook Time: 1 hour 5 minutes Serves: 4

Ingredients:
- Chopped parsley, ½ cup
- Halved spaghetti squash, 1
- Salt
- Italian seasoning, ½ tsp.

- Black pepper
- Chopped tomatoes, ½ cup
- Chopped onion, 1 cup
- Chopped Italian salami, 3 oz.
- Minced garlic cloves, 2
- Chopped Kalamata olives, ½ cup
- Butter, 4 tbsps.
- Medium eggs, 4

Directions:
1. Set the halved squash in a well-lined baking tray then add the seasonings with 1 tbsp. of butter spread on top.
2. Set the oven for 45 minutes at 400°F then allow to bake.
3. Set the pan over medium heat to heat the remaining butter for frying the onions, garlic and the seasoning for a few minutes

4. Stir in the tomatoes and salami to cook for 10 minutes, then add the olives to cook for a few minutes
5. Remove the halved squash from the oven then scoop the flesh using a fork to mix with the salami mixture to the pan
6. Mix then make 4 holes in the mixture, crash an egg in each then add some seasonings
7. Set the oven at 400°F to bake until the eggs are fully baked
8. Top with sprinkled parsley to serve

Nutrition:
Calories: 220, Fat: 18.1, Fiber: 1.7, Carbs: 9.4, Protein: 7

Spiced Avocado Muffins

Prep Time + Cook Time: 30 minutes Serves: 12

Ingredients:
- Coconut flour, ½ cup
- Chopped onion, 1
- Coconut milk, 1 cup
- Chopped avocado, 2
- Salt
- Medium eggs, 4
- Black pepper
- Chopped bacon slices, 6
- Baking soda, ½ tsp.

Directions:
1. Set the pan over medium heat to fry the onion and bacon for a few minutes
2. Meanwhile, set the mixing bowl in position to mash the avocado pieces as you whisk in the eggs.

3. Stir in the seasoning, coconut flour, and baking soda. Mix in the bacon mixture then give it a gentle stir.
4. Prepare the baking sheet with some greasing then set the eggs and avocado mixture on it
5. Set the oven for 20 minutes at 350°F, allow to bake
6. Serve

Nutrition:
Calories: 175, Fat: 15.1, Fiber: 2.6, Carbs: 4.8, Protein: 6.5

Spiced Lunch Curry

Prep Time + Cook Time: 1 hour 10 minutes Servings: 4

Ingredients:

- Tomatoes - 3, cored and chopped
- olive oil - 2 tbsps.
- chicken stock - 1 cup
- canned coconut milk - 14 ounces
- lime juice - 1 tbsp.
- Salt and ground black pepper, to taste
- chicken thighs - 2 pounds, boneless, skinless, and cubed
- garlic cloves - 2, peeled and minced
- Onion - 1 cup, peeled and chopped
- red chilies - 3, chopped
- Peanuts - 1 ounce, toasted
- water - 1 tbsp.
- fresh ginger - 1 tbsp., grated
- coriander - 2 tsps.
- ground cinnamon - 1 tsp.
- turmeric - 1 tsp.
- cumin - 1 tsp.
- ground black pepper - ½ tsp.
- ground fennel seeds - 1 tsp.

Directions:

1. Mix onion with garlic, peanuts, red chilies, water, ginger, coriander, cinnamon, turmeric, cumin, fennel, and black pepper in a food processor.
2. Blend the mixture until it turns into a paste. Keep it aside for a while.
3. Heat a frying pan containing olive oil over medium-high heat. Then add the spice paste you already made and stir gently. Apply some heat for a few seconds.
4. Put some chicken pieces, stir gently, and cook for about 2 minutes.
5. Then add some stock and tomatoes, stir gently.
6. Lower the heat, and cook for 30 more minutes.
7. Add coconut milk to the mixture, stir gently, and cook for about 20 minutes.
8. Add salt, pepper, lime juice, stir, divide into different bowls
9. Then serve.

Nutrition:

Calories: 804, Fat: 51.6, Fiber: 5.4, Carbs: 16.1, Protein: 71.5

Spinach Rolls with Mayonnaise

Prep Time + Cook Time: 35 minutes Servings: 16

Ingredients:

- coconut flour - 6 tbsps.
- almond flour - ½ cup
- mozzarella cheese - 2, and ½ cups, shredded
- eggs - 2
- A pinch of salt

For the filling:

- cream cheese - 4 ounces
- Spinach - 6 ounces, torn
- A drizzle of avocado oil
- A pinch of salt
- Parmesan cheese - ¼ cup, grated

- Mayonnaise, for serving

Directions:

1. Using medium heat, heat a frying a pan. Then add spinach, and cook for about 2 minutes.
2. Then add some Parmesan cheese, sprinkle a pinch of salt, add some cream cheese, and stir the resulting mixture properly.
3. Remove the heat, and keep it aside for a while.
4. Pour mozzarella cheese into a heatproof bowl and put inside a microwave for about 30 seconds. Then add some eggs, salt, coconut, almond flour, and stir gently.
5. Place dough on a lined cutting board put a parchment paper on top. Use a rolling pin to flatten the dough.
6. Separate the dough into 16 different rectangles, then put spinach mixture on each and spread.
7. Then roll each rectangle to a cigar shape.
8. Put all the rolls on a lined baking sheet, and place in an oven with a temperature at 350°F. Bake for about 15 minutes.
9. Leave the rolls to cool down for some minutes before serving them with some mayonnaise on top.

Nutrition:
Calories: 113, Fat: 7.3, Fiber: 2.6, Carbs: 5.1, Protein: 7.3

Steak Bowl served with Chipotle Adobo Sauce

Prep Time + Cook Time: 23 minutes Servings: 4

Ingredients:

- skirt steak - 16 ounces
- pepper jack cheese - 4 ounces, shredded
- sour cream - 1 cup
- Salt and ground black pepper, to taste
- fresh cilantro - ½ cup, chopped
- tomato paste - 1 tbsp
- cider vinegar - 1 tbsp
- chipotle powder - 1 tsp

For the guacamole:

- Onion - ¼ cup, chopped
- Avocados - 2, pitted and peeled
- Juice from lime - 1
- olive oil - 1 tbsp.
- cherry tomatoes - 6, cored and chopped
- garlic clove - 1, peeled and minced
- fresh cilantro - 1 tbsp., chopped
- Salt and ground black pepper, to taste

Directions:

1. Use a fork to mash some avocados in a bowl. Add tomatoes, onion, garlic, salt, pepper to the mesh, and stir properly.
2. Pour some olive oil, lime juice, and 1 tbsp. cilantro, stir again thoroughly. Keep it aside for a while.
3. Heat a frying pan using high heat, before adding steak. Use salt, pepper as

seasoning, and cook for 4 minutes on each side.

4. Move to a cutting board, then keep it aside to ensure that it cools, and cut into thin strips.

5. Mix tomato paste, cider vinegar, and chipotle powder in a bowl to make chipotle adobo sauce.

6. Separate the steak into 4 different bowls, then add cheese, sour cream, and guacamole on top.

7. Serve with a splash of chipotle adobo sauce.

Nutrition:
Calories: 743, Fat: 56.1, Fiber: 9.3, Carbs: 20, Protein: 43

Tasty Breakfast Muffins

Prep Time + Cook Time: 40 minutes Serves: 4

Ingredients:
- Chopped chives, ¼ cup
- Medium eggs, 6
- Black pepper
- Coconut oil, 1 tbsp.
- Salt
- Chopped kale, ¼ cup
- Prosciutto slices, 8
- Almond milk, ½ cup

Directions:
1. Set a mixing bowl in position to combine chives, seasonings, and kale with eggs
2. Prepare the muffin tray with melted coconut oil then line with prosciutto slices.
3. Transfer the egg mixture on the baking tray
4. Set the oven for 30 minutes at 350°F, allow to bake
5. Enjoy the muffins

Nutrition:
Calories: 257, Fat: 19.5, Fiber: 0.8, Carbs: 3.4, Protein: 18.1

Tasty Granola Breakfast

Prep Time + Cook Time: 10 minutes Serves: 2

Ingredients:
- Hulled strawberries, 7
- Chopped pecans, 2 tbsps.
- A splash of lemon juice
- Chopped chocolate, 2 tbsps.

Directions:
1. Set a large mixing bowl in a clean working surface to combine pecans, lemon juice, and the strawberries.
2. Give the mixture a gentle stir
3. Enjoy while cold

Nutrition:
Calories: 167, Fat: 13.2, Fiber: 2.7, Carbs: 11.5, Protein: 2.6

Zucchini Noodle Soup with Lime Wedges

Prep Time + Cook Time: 25 minutes Servings: 8

Ingredients:

- Onion - 1, peeled and chopped
- garlic cloves - 2, peeled and minced
- jalapeño pepper - 1, chopped
- coconut oil - 1 tbsp.
- curry paste - 1½ tbsps.
- chicken stock - 6 cups
- canned coconut milk - 15 ounces
- chicken breasts - 1 pound, boneless, skinless, and sliced
- red bell pepper - 1, seeded and sliced
- fish sauce - 2 tbsps.
- zucchini - 2, cut with a spiralizer
- fresh cilantro - ½ cup, chopped
- Lime wedges, for serving

Directions:

1. Heat a pot containing oil using medium heat, before adding some onions. Stir gently, and cook for 5 minutes.
2. Then add garlic, jalapeño, and curry paste, stir properly, and cook for 1 minute.
3. Add stock and coconut milk to the mixture. Move to a boil after stirring.
4. Add red bell pepper, chicken, fish sauce, stir, and simmer for 4 minutes.
5. Finally, add some cilantro to the mixture and stir well, cook for about 1 minute, and remove the heat.
6. Put the zucchini noodles into different soup bowls, and put some soup on top.
7. Then serve with lime wedges on the side.

Nutrition:

Calories: 343, Fat: 25.2, Fiber: 2.3, Carbs: 11, Protein: 19.9

Chapter 3 Ketogenic Vegetable Recipes

Arugula and Chorizo Salad Recipe

Prep Time + Cook Time: 18 minutes Servings: 4

Ingredients:

- Rosemary, chopped 1 tbsp.
- Garlic (minced): cloves
- Salt and black pepper
- Chorizo sausage (sliced): 1
- Arugula: 4 cups
- Olive oil: 1 tbsp.
- Green onions (chopped): 2

For the salad covering:

- Apple vinegar: 2 tbsps.
- Lemon juice: ½ tsp.
- Mustard: 2 tsps.
- Olive oil: 4 tbsps.

Directions:

1. Heat a pan with 1 tbsp. of oil over medium heat, add garlic, rosemary, salt, and pepper, stir and cook for 5 minutes
2. Add chorizo, stir, cook for 3 minutes, put everything in a salad bowl, add rocket and spring onions and dice.
3. Mix 4 tbsps. of oil with lemon juice, vinegar, mustard and black pepper in a bowl, beat well, add the salad, toss and serve.
4. Enjoy!

Nutrition:

fat 3, fiber 2, calories 170, carbs 5, protein 7

Avocado n Egg Salad

Prep Time + Cook Time: 21 minutes Servings: 3

Ingredients:

- Avocado-1 (pitted, peeled and cut into chunks)
- Homemade mayonnaise-1/4 cup
- Eggs-6
- Mustard-1 tsp.
- Lemon juice-1 tsp.
- Dill-1 tsp. (chopped)
- Parsley-1/2 tbsp. (chopped)
- Salt and black pepper-A pinch

Directions:

1. Beat in the eggs in a pot.
2. Cover them with water.
3. Bring to a simmer.
4. Cook them for 10 minutes.
5. Drain and rinse them with cold water.
6. Peel, chop and put them in a salad bowl.
7. Add mayonnaise, avocado, mustard, lemon juice, parsley, dill, salt and pepper.
8. Stir well and serve for lunch.
9. Enjoy!

Nutrition:

calories 200, fat 3, fiber 6, carbs 14, protein 6

Broccoli Stew with lemon flavor

Prep Time + Cook Time: 30 minutes Servings: 2

Ingredients:

- Two chopped tomatoes
- Chopped red onion - ½ cup
- lemon juice - 1 tsp.
- veggie stock - 2 cups
- Coriander (ground) - 1 tsp.
- Minced garlic cloves- Four
- Broccoli florets - 1 cup
- Cumin seeds - ½ tsp.
- Turmeric powder- ½ tsp.
- Seasoning- A pinch of salt and black pepper
- Olive oil - ½ tsp.

Directions:

1. Mix tomatoes with garlic, onion, salt, pepper, coriander, and turmeric in a blender and pulse really well.
2. With medium temperature, heat up a pan with the oil, add tomato, stir and sauté for ten minutes.
3. Put cumin, broccoli, stock, and lemon juice, mix well, cook for 10 minutes.
4. Divide into separate bowls and serve.
5. Enjoy!

Nutrition:

calories 199, fat 6, fiber 7, carbs 10, protein 8

Brussels Sprouts Soup with chicken stock

Prep Time + Cook Time: 30 minutes Servings: 4

Ingredients:

- Brussels sprouts (trimmed and halved): 2 pounds
- A pinch of salt and black pepper
- Yellow onion (chopped): 1
- Olive oil: 2 tbsps.
- Chicken stock: 4 cups
- Coconut cream: ¼ cup

Directions:

1. Heat a pan with the oil over medium heat, add the onion, stir and cook for 3 minutes.
2. Add Brussels sprouts, broth, salt, and pepper stir, simmer and cook for 20 minutes.
3. Use a hand blender to make your cream, add cream, stir, shovel into bowls and serve.

Nutrition:

calories 190, fiber 3, carbs 6, fat 11, protein 8

Buttered Asparagus

Prep Time + Cook Time: 25 minutes Serves: 4

Ingredients:

- Medium eggs, 4
- Butter, 5 oz.

- Avocado oil, 1 tbsp.
- Cayenne pepper, ¼ tsp.
- Sour cream, 8 tbsps.
- Salt
- Trimmed asparagus, 1½ lbs.
- Black pepper
- Grated Parmesan cheese, 3 oz.
- Lemon juice, 1 ½ tbsps.

Directions:
1. Set the pan over medium-high heat to melt 2 oz. butter.
2. Stir in the seasoning and eggs.
3. Set your blender in position, add in the eggs, sour cream, seasonings, parmesan cheese, and cayenne pepper. Blend until well combined.
4. Set the pan over medium-high heat to roast the asparagus with the seasonings. Reserve in a plate.
5. Set the same pan again over medium-high heat to brown the rest of butter
6. Remove from heat then stir in the lemon juice
7. Melt the butter again then set the asparagus to the pan to coat evenly
8. Heat then divide on plates topped with blended eggs

Nutrition:
Calories: 566, Fat: 43.9, Fiber: 13.3, Carbs: 26.5, Protein: 27.2

Butternut Squash Salad

Prep Time + Cook Time: 10 minutes Servings: 2
Ingredients:
- Walnuts (chopped): 1/3 cup
- Salt and black pepper
- Butternut squash (baked, peeled and cut into wedges): 10 oz
- Olive oil: 2 tbsps.
- White vinegar: 1 tbsp.
- Mustard: ½ tsp.
- Lettuce leaves (torn): 3 cups
- Cinnamon powder: ¼ tsp.

Directions:
1. Mix the pumpkin in a bowl with vinegar, walnuts, cinnamon, oil, mustard, lettuce, salt and pepper and serve.
2. Enjoy!

Nutrition:
calories 120, fat 3, carbs 5, fiber 4, protein 11

Cabbage and Brussels Sprouts Salad

Prep Time + Cook Time: 10 minutes Servings: 4
Ingredients:
- Red cabbage (chopped): 2 cup
- Brussels sprouts (shredded): 4 cups
- Salt and black pepper
- Walnuts (chopped): ¼ cup
- Lemon juice: 2 tbsps.

- Balsamic vinegar: 4 tbsps.
- Avocado mayonnaise: ¼ cup

Directions:

1. In a salad bowl, combine the cabbage with Brussels sprouts, walnuts, salt, pepper, vinegar, mayo and lemon juice, dice and serve.

Nutrition:

calories 90, fiber 1, fat 0, carbs 6, protein 7

Cabbage with Coconut aminos Salad

Prep Time + Cook Time: 10 minutes Servings: 4

Ingredients:

- Avocado mayonnaise: ½ cup
- Lime juice: 1 tsp.
- Salt and black pepper
- Stevia: 1 tsp.
- Fennel bulb (sliced): 1
- Coconut aminos: 1 and ½ tsps.
- Red cabbage head (sliced): 1
- Parsley (chopped): 1 bunch

Directions:

1. Mix the fennel in a salad bowl with cabbage, parsley, salt, and pepper.
2. Add coconut aminos, mayonnaise, lime juice, and stevia shake well and serve.

Nutrition: fat 3, fiber 2, carbs 7, calories 180, protein 11

Capers Eggplant Medley

Prep Time + Cook Time: 40 minutes Servings: 4

Ingredients:

- Eggplants; cut into medium chunks-2
- Red onion; chopped-1
- Oregano; dried-1 tsp.
- Olive oil-2 tbsps.
- Capers; chopped-2 tbsps.
- Garlic cloves; chopped-2
- Parsley; a chopped-1 bunch
- Green olives; pitted and sliced-1 handful
- Tomatoes; chopped-5
- Herb vinegar-3 tbsps.
- Salt and black pepper -to the taste

Directions:

1. Add a cooking pot with cooking oil on medium heat.
2. Toss in eggplants along with salt, pepper, and oregano.
3. Stir cook for 5 minutes then add parsley, onion, and garlic
4. Saute for 4 minutes then add tomatoes, vinegar, olives, and capers.
5. Cook for 15 minutes then adjust seasoning with salt and pepper.
6. Enjoy fresh.

Nutrition :

Calories: 200; Fat: 13g; Fiber: 3g; Carbs: 5g; Protein: 7g

Casserole Of Cauliflower

Prep Time + Cook Time: 23 minutes Servings: 5

Ingredients:

- Cauliflower florets-1 pound
- Chives2 tbsp. (chopped)
- Cheddar cheese-1 cup (grated)
- Bacon slices-2 (cooked and crumbled)
- Coconut cream-4 ounces
- Ghee-3 tbsp. (melted)
- Salt and black pepper-A pinch
- Garlic powder-1/4 tsp.

Directions:

1. Oil a baking dish with the ghee.
2. Spread cauliflower on the bottom; add chives, bacon, cream, garlic powder, salt and pepper.
3. Toss a bit, sprinkle cheese at the end.
4. Transfer the in the oven and cook at 370 °F for 15 minutes.
5. Slice and divide between plates.
6. Serve for lunch.
7. Enjoy!

Nutrition: calories 200, fat 12, fiber 3, carbs 7, protein 8

Celery and Walnuts Salad Recipe

Prep Time + Cook Time: 20 minutes Servings: 4

Ingredients:

- Celery (grated): 1 and ½ pounds
- Avocado mayonnaise ¼ cup
- Salt and black pepper
- Walnuts (chopped): ½ cup
- Garlic (minced): 2 cloves
- Parsley (chopped): ¼ cup

Directions:

1. Mix the celery in a salad bowl with walnuts, garlic, parsley, salt, pepper, and mayonnaise and serve cold.
2. Enjoy!

Nutrition:
fiber 3, calories 150, fat 4, carbs 6, protein 8

Chard Chicken Soup

Prep Time + Cook Time: 45 minutes Servings: 12

Ingredients:

- Swiss chard; chopped-4 cups
- Chicken breast; cooked and shredded -4 cups
- Water-2 cups
- Mushrooms; sliced-1 cup
- Onion; chopped-1/4 cup
- Chicken stock-8 cups
- Vinegar-2 tbsps.
- Basil; chopped-1/4 cup
- Garlic; minced-1 tbsp.
- Bacon slices; chopped-4

- Sun dried tomatoes; chopped-1/4 cup
- Yellow squash; chopped-2 cups
- Green beans; cut into medium pieces-1 cup
- Coconut oil; melted-1 tbsp.
- Salt and black pepper -to the taste

Directions:
1. Place a cooking pot with oil on medium-high heat.
2. Stir in bacon then saute for 2 minutes.
3. Toss in mushrooms, onion, tomatoes, and garlic

4. Saute for 5 minutes then add chicken, stock and water.
5. Cook for 15 minutes then stirs in salt, pepper, squash, swiss chard, and green beans.
6. Continue cooking for 10 minutes then add basil and vinegar.
7. Mix well then serve.
8. Enjoy warm.

Nutrition :
Calories: 140; Fat: 4g; Fiber: 2g; Carbs: 4g; Protein: 18 g

Cheesy Asparagus Fries

Prep Time + Cook Time: 20 minutes Serves: 2
Ingredients:
- Pork rinds, 2 oz.
- Large whisked egg, 1
- Trimmed asparagus spears, 16
- Onion powder, ½ tsp.
- Grated Parmesan cheese, ¼ cup

Directions:
1. Set the crushed pork rinds in a bowl
2. Stir in cheese and onion powder
3. Pass the asparagus spear in the egg, then pork rind mixture.

4. Line the baking tray to arrange the asparagus
5. Set the oven for 10 minutes at 425°F, then allow to bake
6. Serve with sour cream as a side

Nutrition:
Calories: 279, Fat: 15.6, Fiber: 4.1, Carbs: 8.6, Protein: 29.8

Cheesy Asparagus Frittata

Prep Time + Cook Time: 25 minutes Serves: 4
Ingredients:
- Grated cheddar cheese, 1 cup
- Olive oil
- Chopped onion, ¼ cup
- Asparagus spears, 1 lb.
- Black pepper

- Whisked eggs, 4
- Salt

Directions:
1. Set your pan over medium-high heat with oil to cook until tender

2. Stir in the asparagus to cook for 6 minutes.
3. Stir in the eggs to cook for 3 minutes
4. Add the seasonings then top with grated cheese.

5. Allow to bake in the oven for 3 minutes
6. Serve the frittata hot

Nutrition:
Calories: 202, Fat: 13.9, Fiber: 2.5, Carbs: 5.8, Protein: 15.1

Cheesy Eggplant Soup

Prep Time + Cook Time: 1 hour Serves: 4

Ingredients:
- Grated Parmesan cheese, 4 tbsps.
- Chopped basil, 2 tbsps.
- Minced garlic, 1 tsp.
- Salt
- Tomatoes, 4
- Black pepper
- Chopped onion, ¼
- Chicken stock, 2 cup
- Bay leaf, 1
- Chopped eggplant, 1
- Heavy cream, ½ cup
- Olive oil, 1 tbsp.

Directions:
1. Grease the baking sheet and arrange the eggplant pieces mixed with garlic, oil, and the seasonings.
2. Set the oven for 15 minutes at 400°F. Allow to bake
3. Set a saucepan with some water to boil over medium heat. Steam in the tomatoes then peel and chop.
4. Once the eggplant mixture is fully baked, move to a saucepan
5. Stir in the tomatoes, seasonings, bay leaf, and stock,
6. Let it boil for 30 minutes
7. Mix in the parmesan cheese, heavy cream, and basil to serve

Nutrition:
Calories: 164, Fat: 11.3, Fiber: 5.7, Carbs: 13.5, Protein: 5.3

Cheesy Poached Eggs with collard greens

Prep Time + Cook Time: 25 minutes Serves: 6

Ingredients:
- Chicken stock, ½ cup
- Medium eggs, 6
- Black pepper
- Butter, 3 tbsps.
- Minced garlic cloves, 2
- Mashed chipotle, 1 tbsp.
- Chopped bacon slices, 6
- Chopped collard greens, 3 bunches
- Salt
- Chopped onion, 1
- Lime juice, 1 tbsp.
- Grated Cheddar cheese

Directions:
1. Set the pan over medium-high heat to cook the bacon to a crispy texture.

2. Drain the excess grease and set aside
3. Using the same pan, fry the onion and garlic over medium heat for about 2 minutes
4. Cook the bacon again in a pan for about 3 minutes
5. Stir in pepper, chipotle, salt, and collard greens to cook for 10 minutes
6. Mix in the stock then lime juice with a gentle stir.
7. Make 6 holes in collard greens mixture, divide butter, crack an egg in each hole and cook until eggs are done with the pan covered.
8. Enjoy with sprinkled cheddar cheese

Nutrition:
Calories: 235, Fat: 18.4, Fiber: 1.4, Carbs: 4.4, Protein: 13.6

Cheesy Zucchini Cups

Prep Time + Cook Time: 55 minutes Servings: 2

Ingredients:
- Zucchini, halved lengthwise and insides scooped- 1
- Yellow onion, chopped- ½
- Sugar-free sausage, ground -½ lbs.
- Cheddar cheese, shredded- ½ cup
- Garlic, minced-½ tbsp
- Sweet paprika -½ tsp
- Red pepper flakes -¼ tsp
- Oregano, dried -½ tsp
- Chicken stock -¼ cup
- Salt and black pepper- to taste

Directions:
1. Sauté sausage in a preheated pan for 5 minutes.
2. Stir in paprika, onion, garlic, oregano, salt, pepper and pepper flakes.
3. Sauté for another 5 minutes then remove the mixture from the heat.
4. Place the zucchini halves in a greased baking dish with their skin side down.
5. Stuff the zucchini halves with sausage mixture and top it with cheese.
6. Bake the stuffed zucchinis for 30 minutes at 350 0F.
7. Serve fresh to enjoy.

Nutrition:
Calories: 251, Fat: 4, Fiber: 8, Carbs: 12, Protein: 7

Coconut Asparagus Soup

Prep Time + Cook Time: 30 minutes Servings: 10

Ingredients:
- Green asparagus, chopped-4 lbs.
- Olive oil -4 tbsp
- Chicken stock -10 cups
- Yellow onion, chopped-2
- Salt and black pepper- to taste
- Lemon juice -½ tsp
- Coconut cream -2 cups

Directions:

1. Place a pot with cooking oil over medium-high heat.
2. Toss in asparagus, salt, pepper and onion. Sauté for 5 minutes.
3. Pour in the stock and cover it.
4. Let it cook for 15 minutes on a simmer, after bringing it to a boil.
5. Puree this mixture using a hand held blender.
6. Add coconut cream and lemon juice.
7. Dish out and devour.
8. Enjoy.

Nutrition:
Calories: 250, Fat: 5, Fiber: 9, Carbs: 8, Protein: 7

Coconut Spring Greens Soup

Prep Time + Cook Time: 40 minutes Serves: 4

Ingredients:
- Coconut aminos, 2 tbsps.
- Vegetable stock, 3 quarts
- Grated fresh ginger, 2 tbsps.
- Chopped onion, 1
- Salt
- Chopped collard greens, 2 cup
- Black pepper

Directions:
1. Set the saucepan over medium-high heat then allow the stock to simmer
2. Stir in collard greens, seasonings, mustard, ginger, and coconut aminos.
3. Let it cook for 30 minutes with the pan covered
4. Set the blender in position to process the soup until smooth.
5. Return the soup on heat then adjust the seasoning

Nutrition:
Calories: 35, Fat: 0.4, Fiber: 2.8, Carbs: 7, Protein: 1.9

Collard Greens with Cherry Tomatoes

Prep Time + Cook Time: 22 minutes Serves: 5

Ingredients:
- Apple cider vinegar, 1 tbsp.
- Chopped bacon strips, 3
- Salt
- Halved cherry tomatoes, ¼ cup
- Chicken stock, 2 tbsps.
- Collard greens, 1 lb.
- Black pepper

Directions:
1. Set the pan over medium heat to cook the bacon to a brown color
2. Stir in vinegar, tomatoes, salt, collard greens, pepper, and stock to cook for 8 minutes
3. Adjust the seasoning as required
4. Stir and serve

Nutrition:
Calories: 63, Fat: 3.4, Fiber: 3.7, Carbs: 6.6, Protein: 3.3

Creamed Asparagus and cheese

Prep Time + Cook Time: 25 minutes Serves: 3

Ingredients:

- Cooked and crumbled bacon, 3 tbsps.
- Black pepper
- Grated Parmesan cheese, 2 tbsps.
- Asparagus spears, 10 oz.
- Shredded Monterey jack cheese, 1/3 cup
- Salt
- Mustard, 2 tbsps.
- Heavy cream, 1/3 cup
- Cream cheese, 2 oz.

Directions:

1. Set the pan over medium heat to stir together heavy cream, mustard, and cream cheese
2. Stir in the Monterey Jack cheese and Parmesan cheese until it melts away
3. Mix in the asparagus and half of the bacon and cook for 3 minutes
4. Mix in the remaining bacon, adjust the seasoning then cook for 5 minutes
5. Serve hot

Nutrition:

Calories: 346, Fat: 27.5, Fiber: 3.1, Carbs: 7.8, Protein: 18.8

Creamed Spinach Soup

Prep Time + Cook Time: 25 minutes Serves: 8

Ingredients:

- Chopped onion, 1
- Minced garlic, 1 tsp.
- Black pepper
- Butter, 2 tbsps.
- Chopped spinach, 20 oz.
- Chicken stock, 45 oz.
- Ground nutmeg, ½ tsp.
- Heavy cream, 2 cup
- Salt

Directions:

1. Set your pan in position to heat oil over medium heat then sauté the onions until tender, approximately 4 minutes
2. Stir in the garlic and cook for one more minute
3. Stir in the spinach o cook for five minutes
4. Set the food processor in position and blend the spinach to a smooth texture.
5. Cook the soup again for about 5 minutes
6. Stir in the seasonings, cream, and nutmeg

Nutrition:

Calories: 158, Fat: 14.7, Fiber: 1.9, Carbs: 5.4, Protein: 3.3

Creamy Broccoli Soup

Prep Time + Cook Time: 40 minutes Serves: 4

Ingredients:

- Grated cheddar cheese, 8 oz.
- Minced garlic cloves, 2.
- Heavy cream, 1 cup
- Black pepper.
- Broccoli florets, 12 oz.
- Veggie stock, 2 cup
- Paprika, ½ tsp.
- Water, 2 cup
- Ghee, 1 tbsp.
- Chopped white onion, 1.
- Salt.

Directions:

1. Set a pot over medium high heat. Add in ghee and heat. Stir in garlic and onion and allow to cook for about 5 minutes.
2. Stir in pepper, water, paprika, stock, salt and cream. Allow to boil.
3. Stir in broccoli and allow simmering of the soup for about 25 minutes.
4. Remove from heat source and set in a blender to process.
5. Add in cheese and process well until done.
6. Separate the soup and set into soup dishes and enjoy while hot.

Nutrition :

calories: 350, carbs: 7, fiber: 7, fat: 34, protein: 11

Creamy Cauliflower Soup

Prep Time + Cook Time: 43 minutes Servings: 8

Ingredients:

- Olive oil-4 tbsp
- Small yellow onion, chopped -2
- Cauliflower head, florets separated and chopped -2
- Veggie stock -6 cups
- Garlic, minced-2 tsp
- Salt and black pepper- to taste
- Cheddar cheese, shredded -2 cups
- Coconut milk -1 cup

Directions:

1. Place the cooking pot with cooking oil on medium-high heat.
2. Stir in onion and sauté for 3 minutes.
3. Toss in cauliflower, garlic, salt, pepper and then pour in the stock.
4. Let this mixture simmer for 30 minutes on medium heat.
5. Add cheese and milk, puree this soup using a hand held blender.
6. Serve warm.
7. Devour.

Nutrition:

Calories: 271, Fat: 4, Fiber: 4, Carbs: 11, Protein: 7

Creamy Eggplant Soup

Prep Time + Cook Time: 60 minutes Servings: 4

Ingredients:

- eggplant; chopped-1
- tomatoes-4
- garlic; minced-1 tsp.
- yellow onion; chopped-1/4
- basil; chopped-2 tbsps.
- parmesan; grated-4 tbsps.
- olive oil-1 tbsp.
- chicken stock-2 cups
- bay leaf-1
- heavy cream-1/2 cup
- Salt and black pepper - to the taste

Directions:

1. Place eggplant pieces on a baking sheet.
2. Toss these pieces with oil, garlic, onion, salt, and pepper.
3. Place the eggplant pieces in the oven and bake for 15 minutes at 400 0F.
4. Meanwhile, boil 2- 3 cups water in a large pot and place steamer basket over it.
5. Add tomatoes to the basket and steam them for 1 minute.
6. Peel and chop the steam tomatoes.
7. Add the eggplant to a cooking pot and stir in salt, pepper, bay leaf, stock, and tomatoes.
8. Let this mixture cook for 30 minutes.
9. Stir in basil, heavy cream and parmesan.
10. Mix well and serve right away.

Nutrition :

Calories: 180; Fat: 2g; Fiber: 3g; Carbs: 5g; Protein: 10g

Creamy Roasted Bell Peppers Soup

Prep Time + Cook Time: 25 minutesServes: 6

Ingredients:

- Grated Parmesan cheese, ¼ cup
- Heavy cream, 2/3 cup
- Olive oil, 2 tbsps.
- Minced garlic cloves, 2
- Canned chicken stock, 29 oz.
- Salt
- Chopped roasted bell 12 oz.
- Chopped onion, 1
- Black pepper
- Water, 7 oz.
- Chopped celery stalks, 2

Directions:

1. Set the saucepan over medium heat to melt the oil for frying the celery, onion, garlic and the seasoning for 8 minutes
2. Stir in water, bell peppers, and stock to simmer for 5 minutes while covered
3. Set the immersion blender in position to process the soup until smooth
4. Return the soup to heat to adjust the seasoning, add the cream then boil
5. Serve topped with sprinkled parmesan cheese.

Nutrition:

Calories: 15, Fat: 12, Fiber: 2, Carbs: 8.6, Protein: 4.7

Delicious Cauliflower Soup

Prep Time + Cook Time: 25 minutes Servings: 2

Ingredients:

- Veggie stock - 3 cups
- Minced garlic cloves- 3
- Cooked and Crumbled Bacon - ¾ cup
- Chopped Cilantro - 2 tbsps.
- olive oil - 2 tbsps.
- 1 cauliflower head, florets separated and chopped
- Chopped yellow onion- 1
- Seasoning- A pinch of salt and black pepper

Directions:

1. With medium temperature, heat the oil in a cooking pot, Put onion, mix well and cook for 5 minutes.
2. Put stock, cauliflower, garlic, salt, and pepper, mix well and cook slowly (brings to simmer) for 10 minutes.
3. Put cilantro, mix properly. Divide into bowls with a ladle, sprinkle bacon on top and serve.
4. Enjoy!

Nutrition:

calories 222, fat 3, fiber 2, carbs 9, protein 11

Fast Salad For Lunch

Prep Time + Cook Time: 8 minutes Servings: 5

Ingredients:

- Cauliflower florets-4 cups (steamed)
- Salami-2 ounces (cut into strips)
- Marinated mushrooms-1 cup (sliced)
- Cheddar cheese-2 ounces (shredded)
- Black olives-6 ounces (pitted and sliced)
- Canned roasted peppers-12 ounces (chopped)
- Capers-3 tbsps. (drained)
- Balsamic vinegar-1/4 cup
- Olive oil-1 tbsp.
- Lemon juice-2 tbsps.
- Caper juice-1 tbsp.
- Oregano-1/2 tsp. (dried)

Directions:

1. Take a large salad bowl.
2. Add the cauliflower with the salami, mushrooms, cheese, olives, peppers, capers, vinegar, oil, lemon juice, caper juice and oregano.
3. Toss well. Divide between plates.
4. Serve for lunch.

Nutrition:

calories 188, fat 3, fiber 6, carbs 10, protein 5

Garlic-Squash and Mushrooms Mix

Prep Time + Cook Time: 30 minutes Servings: 4

Ingredients:

- Veggie stock- 1 cup
- Butternut squash (chopped)- 4 cups
- Chopped mushrooms- 8 ounces
- Minced garlic cloves: 3
- Dried oregano - ¼ tsp.
- Seasoning - A pinch of salt and black pepper
- Coriander (ground)- ½ tsp.
- Yellow onion - ½ cup
- Olive oil - 1 tbsp.
- One handful Chopped parsley

Directions:

1. With medium temperature, heat up a pan with the oil, put onion, squash, and garlic, mix properly and cook for 5 minutes.
2. Put stock, mushrooms, salt, pepper, oregano, and coriander, mix well and cook for another 15 minutes.
3. Divide into separate plates then sprinkle parsley on top and serve.
4. Delicious!

Nutrition:

calories 201, fat 5, fiber 3, carbs 9, protein 8

Green Beans n Stock Saucy Casserole

Prep Time + Cook Time: 48 minutes Servings: 9

Ingredients:

- Green beans-1 pound (halved)
- Mushrooms-8 ounces (chopped)
- Onion-4 ounces (chopped)
- Shallots-2 (chopped)
- Garlic cloves-3 (minced)
- Heavy cream-1/2 cup
- Almond flour-1/2 cup
- Chicken stock-1/2 cup
- Parmesan-1/4 cup (grated)
- Avocado oil-For frying
- Ghee-2 tbsp.
- Salt and black pepper-To taste

Directions:

1. Take a pot and pour some water in it.
2. Add the salt and bring the water to a boil over medium high heat.
3. Add the green beans and leave it to cook for 5 minutes.
4. Shift that to a bowl filled with ice water and then cool it down.
5. Strain well. Leave aside for now. In a bowl, mix shallots with onions, almond flour, salt and pepper.
6. And toss them to coat. Warm up a pan with some avocado oil over medium high heat.
7. Add the onions and shallots mix. Fry until they are golden.
8. Transfer to paper towels and drain grease. Heat up the same pan over medium heat.

9. Put in the ghee and melt it. Add garlic and mushrooms. Stir and cook for 5 minutes.
10. Add stock and heavy cream. Stir to bring to a boil. Let it simmer until it thickens. Add the Parmesan and green beans.
11. Roll to coat and take it off from the heat. Slip this mix into a baking dish.
12. Sprinkle the crispy onions mix all over the dish. And introduce it in the oven at 400 0F. Bake for 15 minutes.
13. Serve warm.

Nutrition:
Calories:- 155, fat, 11; Fiber : 6; Carbs : 8; Protein : 5

Grilled Eggplant Onion Salad

Prep Time + Cook Time: 20 minutes Servings: 8
Ingredients:
- Eggplants, sliced-2
- Red onions, sliced- 2
- Olive oil-4 tsp
- Avocados, pitted and chopped-2
- Mustard-2 tsp
- Balsamic vinegar-2 tbsp
- Zest of 2 lemons, grated
- Salt and black pepper- to taste
- Fresh oregano, chopped-2 tbsp

Directions:
1. Brush the eggplant and onion pieces with 1 tsp cooking oil.
2. Preheat the grill over medium-high heat.
3. Place the vegetables over grilling grates of the grill. Cook them for 5 minutes per side over medium-high heat.
4. Transfer them to a cutting board and dice the grilled veggies.
5. Place these chopped vegetables to a bowl.
6. Toss in avocado, vinegar, mustard, lemon zest, mustard, oregano, remaining oil, salt, and pepper.
7. Devour.

Nutrition:
Calories: 250, Fat: 3, Fiber: 2, Carbs: 14, Protein: 8

Hot Arugula Keto Soup

Prep Time + Cook Time: 23 minutes Servings: 6
Ingredients:
- baby arugula - 10 ounces
- mixed mint - 1/4 cup; tarragon and parsley
- yellow onion - 1; chopped.
- olive oil - 1 tbsp.
- garlic cloves - 2; minced
- Chives - 2 tbsps.; chopped.
- coconut milk yogurt - 4 tbsps.

- chicken stock - 6 cups
- coconut milk - 1/2 cup
- Salt and black pepper to the taste.

Directions:
1. Place a pit containing oil over medium high heat source.
2. Then add some onion and garlic; stir gently and cook for 5 minutes
3. Add stock and milk; stir gently and bring to a simmer.
4. Follow this by adding arugula, tarragon, parsley and mint to the mix; and stir gently.
5. Cook everything for about 6 minutes
6. Add coconut yogurt, salt, pepper and chives; stir gently.
7. Cook for about 2 minutes.
8. Divide into different soup bowls and serve immediately.

Nutrition :
Calories:- 200; Fat : 4; Fiber : 2; Carbs : 6; Protein : 10

Hot Catalan Greens

Prep Time + Cook Time: 25 minutes Servings: 4
Ingredients:
- Apple - 1; cored and chopped.
- yellow onion - 1; sliced
- avocado oil - 3 tbsps.
- raisins - 1/4 cup
- garlic cloves - 6; chopped.
- pine nuts - 1/4 cup; toasted
- balsamic vinegar - 1/4 cup
- A pinch of nutmeg
- mixed spinach and chard - 5 cups
- Salt and black pepper to the taste.

Directions:
1. Heat up a pan with the oil over medium high heat; add onion; stir and cook for 3 minutes
2. Then apple; and stir gently and cook for another 4 minutes.
3. Add garlic; stir and cook for another minute. Add raisins, vinegar and mixed spinach and chard; stir gently and cook for 5 minutes
4. Add the nutmeg, salt and pepper to taste. Stir gently and cook for a few more seconds.
5. Divide into different plates
6. Serve immediately.

Nutrition :
Calories:- 120; Fat : 1; Fiber : 2; Carbs : 3; Protein : 6

Kale with Pumpkin seed Salad

Prep Time + Cook Time: 20 minutes Servings: 4
Ingredients:
- Lemon juice: 3 tbsps.
- Olive oil: 2 tbsps.
- Kale (chopped): 1 bunch
- Red onion (chopped): 1/3 cup
- Basil leaves (chopped): 2
- Pumpkin seeds: ¼ cup

- Garlic clove (minced): 1

Directions:

1. In a salad bowl, combine kale with pumpkin seeds, onions, oil, lemon juice, basil and garlic, dice and serve.

Nutrition:

calories 120, fiber 1, carbs 2, fat 1, protein 9

Lemony celery with parsley stew

Prep Time + Cook Time: 40 minutes Serves: 6

Ingredients:

- Celery bunch: chopped- 1
- Pricked dried Persian lemons- 3
- Water- 2 cups
- Olive oil- 4 tbsp.
- Chicken bouillon- 2 tsp.
- Onion: chopped: 1
- Fresh mint bunches: chopped- 2
- Green onion: chopped- 1 bunch
- Garlic cloves: minced- 4
- Fresh parsley bunch: chopped- 1
- Black pepper
- Salt

Directions:

1. Pour oil in a pan over medium-high and add in the onions, garlic and the green onions. Mix and let cook for 6 minutes.
2. Add in the lemons, water, celery, bouillon, pepper and salt.
3. Mix and let cook for 20 minutes on medium heat.
4. Mix in the mint and parsley and cook for 10 minutes.
5. Serve into bowls.

Nutrition:

Calories- 100, carbs- 4.4, protein- 0.9, fiber- 1.4, fats- 9.5

Lettuce and Tomato Salad Recipe

Prep Time + Cook Time: 20 minutes Servings: 4

Ingredients:

- Basil (chopped): 2 tbsps.
- Avocado mayonnaise: ½ cup
- Halved Cherry tomatoes: 1 cup
- Lemon juice: 1 tsp.
- A pinch of salt and black pepper
- Baby lettuce heads (chopped): 6
- Green onions (chopped): 2

Directions:

1. In a bowl mix basil with mayo, lemon juice, salt, and black pepper and mix.
2. Mix salad in a salad bowl with tomatoes and spring onions, mix, add basil, throw away fur and serve.

Nutrition:

carbs 4, calories 140, fat 3, fiber 2, protein 7

Mushroom Chops Stew

Prep Time + Cook Time: 40 minutes Servings: 2

Ingredients:

- Bacon slices, chopped-1.5
- Garlic cloves, minced -1.5
- Olive oil-½ tbsp
- Small yellow onion, chopped -½
- Mushrooms, sliced-4 oz.
- Pork chops, bone in-2
- Veggie stock-½ cup
- Thyme spring, chopped -½
- Coconut cream-5 oz.
- Parsley, chopped -½ tbsp

Directions:

1. Place a cooking pot over medium-high heat with cooking oil.
2. Add bacon and sauté it for 2 minutes.
3. Toss in mushrooms, onion, and garlic Stir cook for 3 minutes.
4. Add stock, garlic powder, pork chops, and thyme.
5. Stir gently and let this mixture simmer for 30 minutes.
6. Add cream and parsley. Mix well and cook for 10 minutes on a simmer.
7. Serve fresh and devour.

Nutrition:

Calories: 270, Fat: 8, Fiber: 7, Carbs: 12, Protein: 11

Oven-Baked Radishes

Prep Time + Cook Time: 45 minutes Serves: 2

Ingredients:

- Lemon zest, 1 tbsp.
- Black pepper
- Butter, 2 tbsps.
- Quartered radishes, 2 cup
- Chopped chives, 1 tbsp.
- Salt

Directions:

1. Line the baking tray well to arrange on the radishes
2. Add the seasonings, lemon zest, chives, and butter. Allow to coat evenly
3. Set the oven for 35 minutes at 375°F.Allow to bake
4. Serve and enjoy

Nutrition:

Calories: 123, Fat: 11.7, Fiber: 2.1, Carbs: 4.6, Protein: 1

Pan-fried Collard Greens and Ham

Prep Time + Cook Time: 1 hour 50 minutes Serves: 4

Ingredients:

- Apple cider vinegar, ¼ cup
- Stripped collard greens, 2 lbs.
- Red pepper flakes, 1 tsp.
- Black pepper

- Cooked chopped ham, 4 oz.
- Chicken stock, 2 cup
- Melted butter, ½ cup
- Chopped onion, 1
- Dry white wine, 4 oz.
- Salt
- Salt pork, 1 oz.
- Olive oil, 1 tbsp.

Directions:
1. Set your pan over medium-high heat to quick fry the ham and onion as you gently stir for 4 minutes
2. Stir in stock, salt pork, wine, collard greens, and vinegar. Allow to boil
3. Cover the pan and simmer then cook for 1 hour and 30 minutes as you stir frequently
4. Remove the salt park then add in butter with a gentle stir
5. Allow to cook for about 10 minutes
6. Enjoy

Nutrition:
Calories: 430, Fat: 35.6, Fiber: 8.4, Carbs: 17.4, Protein: 11.2

Parmesan Fennel Soup

Prep Time + Cook Time: 35 minutes Servings: 6

Ingredients:
- Fennel bulbs, chopped -6
- Veggie stock -4 cups
- Olive oil -2 tbsp
- Salt and black pepper -to taste
- Parmesan cheese, grated-4 tsp

Directions:
1. Add oil to a pot and place it over medium-high heat.
2. Toss in chopped fennel and sauté for 5 minutes.
3. Pour in the stock, salt, and pepper.
4. Let it simmer for 20 minutes then add cheese.
5. Serve right away.

Nutrition:
Calories: 206, Fat: 3, Fiber: 7, Carbs: 12, Protein: 5

Pork With Cinnamon

Prep Time + Cook Time: 20 minutes Servings: 5

Ingredients:
- Ghee-2 tbsps.
- Salt and black pepper-A pinch
- Pork chops-4 (boneless)
- Stevia-2 tbsp.
- Nutmeg-A pinch (ground)
- Apple cider vinegar-1 tbsp.
- Cinnamon powder-1 tsp.

Directions:
1. Warm up a pan. Add the ghee over medium-high heat. Combine pork chops and cook them for 5 minutes.
2. Flip over the chops. Season them with salt, pepper, stevia, nutmeg and cinnamon.

3. Add the vinegar and cook for 5 minutes more.
4. Divide the chops between plates.
5. Serve for lunch.

Nutrition:

calories 261, fat 4, fiber 7, carbs 15, protein 7

Pumpkin Soup (Keto)

Prep Time + Cook Time: 34 minutes Servings: 7

Ingredients:

- Pumpkin puree-2 cups
- Heavy cream-1/2 cup
- Yellow onion-1/2 cup (chopped)
- Chicken stock-32 ounces
- Garlic clove-1 (minced)
- Cumin-1 tsp. (ground)
- Corriander-1 tsp. (ground)
- Vinegar-2 tsps.
- Stevia-2 tsps.
- Olive oil-2 tbsps.
- Chipotles in adobo sauce-1 tbsp.
- Allspice-A pinch
- Salt and black pepper-To taste

Directions:

1. Warm up a pot with the oil over medium heat.
2. Add onions and garlic, Stir and cook for 4 minutes.
3. Mix stevia, cumin, coriander, chipotles and cumin. Toss and cook for 2 minutes.
4. Combine stock and pumpkin puree.
5. Whisk and cook for 5 minutes.
6. Blend soup well using an immersion blender.
7. Then mix with salt, pepper, heavy cream and vinegar.
8. Stir to cook for another 5 minutes.
9. And divide into bowls.
10. Serve right away.

Nutrition :

Calories:- 140; Fat : 12; Fiber : 3; Carbs : 6; Protein : 2

Pureed creamy celery soup

Prep Time + Cook Time: 50 minutes Serves: 4

Ingredients:

- Celery: chopped- 1 bunch
- Chicken stock- 4 cups
- Bay leaves- 3
- Heavy cream- ¾ cup
- ½ garlic head: chopped
- Butter- 2 tbsp.
- Onions: chopped- 2
- Salt
- Black pepper

Directions:

1. Put butter, onions, pepper and salt in a saucepan over medium-high and let cook for 5 minutes.
2. Mix in celery, bay leaves and garlic

and cook for 15 minutes.

3. Pour in the stock and season with salt and pepper. Reduce the heat and cover the pan to cook for 20 minutes.
4. Mix in cream and puree with a dipping blender.
5. Ladle and serve.

Nutrition:
Calories- 191, carbs- 12.9, protein- 3.1, fiber- 2.8, fat- 15

Pureed Pumpkin Soup

Prep Time + Cook Time: 30 minutes Servings: 3

Ingredients:

- Yellow onion, chopped-¼ cup
- Olive oil-1 tbsp
- Garlic clove, minced-1/2
- Cumin, ground-½ tsp
- Coriander, ground-½ tsp
- Pumpkin puree -½ cup
- Salt and black pepper -to taste
- Chicken stock -16 oz.
- Coconut cream -¼ cup

Directions:
1. Add cooking oil to a pot and place it over medium heat.
2. Toss in garlic and onions to sauté for 4 minutes.
3. Stir in coriander and cumin, continue cooking for 1 minute.
4. Pour in pureed pumpkin and stock.
5. Stir gently and continue cooking for 5 mins then add cream, salt, and pepper.
6. Blend this soup using a hand held blender.
7. Cook for another 10 minutes then dish out.
8. Serve warm.

Nutrition:
Calories: 270, Fat: 12, Fiber: 6, Carbs: 14, Protein: 5

Roasted Bell Peppers Soup Recipe with Parmesan

Prep Time + Cook Time: 25 minutes Servings: 6

Ingredients:

- roasted bell peppers - 12 ounces; chopped.
- canned chicken stock - 29 ounces
- olive oil - 2 tbsps.
- Celery stalks - 2; chopped.
- water - 7 ounces
- heavy cream - 2/3 cup
- 1 yellow onion; chopped.
- garlic cloves - 2; minced
- Parmesan - 1/4 cup; grated
- Salt and black pepper to the taste.

Directions:
1. Add heat to a pan containing oil medium heat.
2. Then add onions, garlic, celery, some salt and pepper.
3. Stir gently and cook for about 8 minutes
4. Add the bell peppers, water and stock.
5. Stir gently and, bring to a boil, cover.
6. Follow this by reducing heat and simmer for 5 minutes

7. Use an immersion blender to puree the soup, then sprinkle some more salt, pepper as well as cream. Stir gently, bring to a boil and take off remove the heat.

8. Ladle into bowls, sprinkle parmesan and serve

Nutrition :

Calories:- 176; Fat : 13; Fiber : 1; Carbs : 4; Protein : 6

Roasted Lemon Asparagus

Prep Time + Cook Time: 20 minutes Serves: 3

Ingredients:

- Chopped oregano, 1 tbsp.
- Salt
- Avocado oil, 3 tsps.
- Trimmed asparagus 1 bunch
- Lemon juice
- Black pepper

Directions:

1. Season the asparagus then align in a baking tray. Sprinkle with olive oil, oregano, and lemon juice. Toss to coat evenly
2. Set the oven for 10 minutes at 450°F then allow to bake
3. Serve hot

Nutrition:

Calories: 14, Fat: 0.6, Fiber: 1, Carbs: 1.8, Protein: 0.9

Roasted Tomato Cream

Prep Time + Cook Time: 1 hour 10 minutes Serves: 8

Ingredients:

- Olive oil, ¼ cup
- Chopped jalapeño pepper, 1
- Halved cherry tomatoes, 2 lbs.
- Minced garlic cloves, 4
- Dried oregano, ½ tsp.
- Quartered onion, 1
- Salt
- Grated Parmesan cheese, ½ cup
- Black pepper
- Chicken stock, 4 cup
- Chopped basil, ¼ cup

Directions:

1. Prepare your baking sheet then spread on it the onions and tomatoes
2. Mix in chili pepper, garlic, oregano, seasonings then sprinkle the oil. Mix to coat evenly
3. Set the oven for 30 minutes at 425oF. Allow to bake
4. Once fully baked, move the mixture to a saucepan, stir in the stock to heat over medium-high heat.
5. Let the mixture simmer for 20 minutes
6. Set the immersion blender in position to blend the mixture.
7. Adjust the seasonings and serve topped with sprinkled parmesan

Nutrition:

Calories: 133, Fat: 9.9, Fiber: 1.8, Carbs: 7.2, Protein: 6.1

Seasoned Keto Cabbage Soup

Prep Time + Cook Time: 55 minutes Servings: 8

Ingredients:

- Beef - 2 pounds; ground
- garlic clove - 1; minced
- yellow onion - 1; chopped.
- cumin - 1 tsp.
- bouillon cubes - 4
- Cabbage head - 1; chopped.
- canned tomatoes and green chilies - 10 ounces
- water - 4 cups
- Salt and black pepper to the taste.

Directions:

1. Place a pan over medium heat and add beef.
2. Then stir gently and brown for a few minutes
3. Add onion; stir, cook for 4 extra minutes.
4. Move to a pot.
5. Heat up, add cabbage, cumin, garlic, bouillon cubes, tomatoes and chilies and water.
6. Stir gently, and bring to a boil over high heat.
7. Cover the top and reduce temperature and cook for about 40 minutes
8. Season with salt and pepper to taste.
9. Stir gently, ladle into soup bowls
10. Serve immediately.

Nutrition :

Calories:- 200; Fat : 3; Fiber : 2; Carbs : 6; Protein : 8

Sesame Alfalfa Sprouts Salad

Prep Time + Cook Time: 10 minutes Serves: 4

Ingredients:

- Coconut milk yogurt, ¼ cup
- Alfalfa sprouts, 4 cup
- Salt
- Dark sesame oil, 1 ½ tsps.
- Black pepper
- Grape seed oil, 1 ½ tsps.

Directions:

1. Set a large mixing bowl in a clean working surface.
2. Combine all the ingredients, toss to coat evenly.
3. Serve immediately

Nutrition:

Calories: 83, Fat: 7.6, Fiber: 1.8, Carbs: 3.4, Protein: 1.6

Sesame Mustard Greens

Prep Time + Cook Time: 20 minutes Serves: 4

Ingredients:

- Dark sesame oil, ¼ tsp.
- Torn mustard greens, 1 lb.
- Black pepper
- Olive oil, 1 tbsp.
- Sliced onion, ½ cup
- Minced garlic cloves, 2
- Salt
- Vegetable stock, 3 tbsps.

Directions:

1. Set the pan over medium heat then heat the oil to fry the onion until browned evenly. About 1 minute
2. Stir in garlic to cook until soft.
3. Toss in the seasonings and sesame oil to coat evenly.
4. Serve and enjoy

Nutrition:
Calories: 70, Fat: 4, Fiber: 4.1, Carbs: 7.5, Protein: 3.3

Sliced Swiss Chard Pie

Prep Time + Cook Time: 55 minutes Servings: 12

Ingredients:

- Swiss chard - 8 cups; chopped.
- Onion - 1/2 cup; chopped.
- Parmesan - 1/4 cup; grated
- Sausage - 1 pound; chopped.
- eggs - 3
- ricotta cheese - 2 cups
- olive oil - 1 tbsp.
- garlic clove - 1; minced
- A pinch of nutmeg
- Mozzarella - 1 cup; shredded
- Salt and black pepper to the taste.

Directions:

1. Heat up a pan containing some oil over medium-high heat.
2. Add some onions and garlic; stir gently and cook for 3 minutes
3. Add the Swiss chard; stir and cook for 5 minutes more
4. Add salt, pepper and nutmeg; stir, take off heat and leave aside for a few minutes
5. Whisk some eggs with mozzarella, parmesan and ricotta in a clean bowl and stir well.
6. Add Swiss chard mix and stir properly.
7. Spread sausage meat on the bottom of a pie pan and press well.
8. Add Swiss chard and eggs mix,
9. Spread well, and move to an oven at 350 0F and bake for 35 minutes
10. Leave the pie aside to cool down.
11. Slice and serve it.

Nutrition :
Calories:- 332; Fat : 23; Fiber : 3; Carbs : 4; Protein : 23

Slow cooked Mixed Vegetable Soup

Prep Time + Cook Time: 2 hours 20minutesServes: 7

Ingredients:

- Chopped onion, 1
- Chopped zucchini, 1
- Chopped green bell pepper, 1
- Salt
- Chopped Swiss chard, 1 bunch
- Black pepper

- Chopped butternut squash, 8 oz.
- Chopped tomatoes, 4 cup
- Chopped cauliflower florets, 1 cup
- Chicken stock, 6 cup
- Canned tomato paste, 7 oz.
- Chopped summer squash, 1
- Water, 2 cup
- Chopped sausage, 1 lb.
- Chopped green beans, 1 cup
- Minced garlic cloves, 2
- Grated Parmesan cheese
- Chopped thyme, 2 tbsps.
- Dried rosemary, 1 tsp.
- Minced fennel, 1 tbsp.
- Red pepper flakes, ½ tsp.

Directions:

1. Set the pan over medium-high heat to cook the sausages and garlic to attain the brown color the move to a slow cooker
2. Stir in the Swiss chard, onion, summer squash, zucchini, bell pepper, butternut squash, cauliflower, tomatoes, stock, green beans, tomato paste, water, seasonings, thyme, rosemary, fennel, and pepper flakes.
3. Cook for 2 hours while covered
4. Open slow cooker and mix the soup
5. Serve on soup plates topped with sprinkled parmesan cheese

Nutrition:

Calories: 324, Fat: 19.6, Fiber: 5.7, Carbs: 22.4, Protein: 17.7

Sour cream and celery soup

Prep Time + Cook Time: 35 minutes Serves: 8

Ingredients:

- Celery leaves and stalks: chopped-26 oz.
- Fenugreek powder- 3 tsp.
- Sour cream- 10 oz.
- Dried onion flakes- 1 tbsp.
- Vegetable stock powder- 3 tsp.
- Salt
- Black pepper

Directions:

1. Pour water and celery into a pan and add stock powder, onion flakes, pepper, fenugreek powder and salt. Mix well and boil for 20 minutes over medium heat.
2. Puree with a dipping blender and add the sour cream, more pepper and salt and blend again.
3. Heat soup to warm and serve.

Nutrition:

Calories- 99, carbs- 5.8, protein 2.1, fiber- 1.9, fats- 7.9

Spiced Collard Greens and Butternut Soup

Prep Time + Cook Time: 50 minutes Serves: 12

Ingredients:

- Chopped butternut squash, 10 oz.
- Water, 10 cup
- Avocado oil, 1 tbsp.
- Herb seasoning, 1 tbsp.
- Smoked paprika, tsps.
- Cumin, 1 tsp.
- Chopped onion, 1
- Red pepper flakes, ¼ tsp.
- Chopped celery stalks, 3
- Tamari sauce, 2 tbsps.
- Sugar-free tomato passata, 6 oz.
- Diced sugar-free tomatoes, 15 oz.
- Lemon juice, 2 tbsps.
- Salt
- Chili powder, 1 tsp.
- Black pepper
- Collard greens, 6 cup
- Swerve, 1 tbsp.
- Dried garlic, 1 tsp.

Directions:

1. Set your pot over medium-high heat then stir in pepper flakes, cumin, chili powder, and paprika
2. Mix in the squash, onion, and celery to cook for 10 minutes as you stir
3. Mix in the seasoning, water, tamari sauce, herb seasoning, tomato passata, swerve, tomatoes, collard greens, lemon juice, and garlic granules.
4. Allow boil and cook for 30 minutes while covered.
5. Give the mixture a gentle stir then serve

Nutrition:
Calories: 384, Fat: 6.8, Fiber: 2.2, Carbs: 7.1, Protein: 16.6

Spicy Cabbage Soup

Prep Time + Cook Time: 55 minutes Serves: 8

Ingredients:

- Chopped cabbage head, 1
- Canned tomatoes, and green chilies, 10 oz.
- Black pepper
- Onion, 1
- Cumin, 1 tsp.
- Minced garlic clove, 1
- Ground beef, 2 lbs.
- Bouillon cubes, 4
- Salt
- Water, 4 cup

Directions:

1. Set the pan on fire to brown the beef over medium heat.
2. Stir in the onions to cook for four minutes then set on a saucepan.
3. Put the saucepan on fire then add garlic, chilies, cabbage, cumin, bouillon cubes, tomatoes, and water.
4. Allow to a boil as you stir occasionally over high heat for 40 minutes while covered
5. Adjust the seasoning then serve.
6. Enjoy.

Nutrition:
Calories: 251 ,Fat: 7.5 ,Fiber: 3 ,Carbs: 8.5 ,Protein: 36.4

Spinach and Mustard Greens Soup

Prep Time + Cook Time: 25 minutes Serves: 6

Ingredients:

- Chopped jalapeno, 1 tbsp.
- Coconut milk, 3 cup
- Cumin seeds, 1tsp.
- Coriander seeds, 1 tsp.
- Chopped onion, 1
- Salt
- Minced garlic, 1 tbsp.
- Avocado oil, 1 tsps.
- Grated fresh ginger, 1 tbsp.
- Turmeric, ½ tsp.
- Fenugreek seeds, ½ tsp.
- Paprika, ½ tsp.
- Chopped mustard greens, 5 cup
- Torn spinach, 5 cup
- Black pepper
- Butter, 2 tsps.

Directions:

1. Set your pan over medium-high heat to heat the oil.
2. Fry the fenugreek, cumin seeds, and coriander to a brown color, for about 2 minutes
3. Stir in the onion and cook for 3 more minutes
4. Stir in half of the garlic, ginger, jalapeno, and turmeric and cook for 3 minutes
5. Gently stir in spinach and mustard greens to sauté for 10 minutes
6. Add the seasonings and milk.
7. Set the blender in position and blend the soup until fine.
8. Set the pan over medium heat to melt the butter.
9. Stir in paprika, and garlic
10. Return the soup over medium heat.
11. Adjust the seasonings and enjoy

Nutrition:

Calories: 324, Fat: 30.6, Fiber: 5.6, Carbs: 13.4, Protein: 5.3

Spinach Stew Recipe

Prep Time + Cook Time: 30 minutes Servings: 4

Ingredients:

- Ga ram masala - ½ tsp.
- Chopped tomatoes- 2
- Torn Spinach- 8 ounces
- Seasoning- A pinch of salt and black pepper
- Minced garlic cloves- four
- Olive oil - 1 tsp.
- Grated ginger - 1 tsp.
- One green chili pepper (chopped)
- Cinnamon powder - ¼ tsp.
- Turmeric powder - ½ tsp.
- Water - 1 cup

Directions:

1. With medium or moderate temperature, heat up a pan with the oil, pepper add chili, ginger, and

garlic, mix well and cook for 3 minutes.

2. Put tomatoes, salt, pepper, cinnamon, turmeric, and garam masala, mix well and cook for another 3-4 minutes more.

3. Put the water and spinach, mix well, cook for another 10 minutes. Divide into separate bowls and serve.

4. Enjoy!

Nutrition:

calories 199, fat 3, fiber 1, carbs 12, protein 10

Spinach, Broccoli and Cauliflower Soup

Prep Time + Cook Time: 35 minutes Servings: 6

Ingredients:

- Seasoning- A pinch of salt and black pepper
- Two broccoli heads, florets separated
- Chopped spinach- Two handfuls
- Veggie stock -8 cups
- Chopped parsley: One handful
- Coconut cream - 1 tbsp.
- Melted ghee - 2 tbsps.
- Chopped celery sticks- four
- Chopped leeks- 2
- One small cauliflower head, florets separated

Directions:

1. With medium-high, heat up the ghee in a cooking pot, put leeks, mix well and cook for 3 minutes.

2. Put celery, broccoli, cauliflower, and stock mix carefully and cook for another 15 minutes.

3. Put salt, pepper, cream, parsley, and spinach, grind using an immersion blender.

4. Divide into bowls with a ladle and serve

5. Enjoy!

Nutrition:

calories 213, fat 4, fiber 3, carbs 10, protein 6

Stewed Eggplant

Prep Time + Cook Time: 40 minutes Serves: 4

Ingredients:

- Chopped capers, 2 tbsps.
- Chopped onion, 1
- Chopped parsley, 1 bunch
- Salt

- Herb vinegar, 3 tbsps.
- Black pepper
- Dried oregano, 1 tsp.
- Cubed eggplants, 2

- Chopped garlic cloves, 2
- Olive oil, 2 tbsps.
- Sliced green olives, 12
- Chopped tomatoes, 5

Directions:

1. Set the saucepan over medium heat to heat some oil to fry eggplant, seasonings, and oregano to cook for five minutes
2. Stir in the parsley, garlic, and onion to cook for four minutes
3. Mix in the vinegar, capers, tomatoes, olives, to cook for 15 minutes
4. Adjust the seasonings then serve

Nutrition:

Calories: 280, Fat: 17.9, Fiber: 14, Carbs: 28.9, Protein: 5.4

Stir-Fried Mustard Greens

Prep Time + Cook Time: 30 minutes Serves: 4

Ingredients:

- Lemon juice, 1 tsp.
- Olive oil, 1 tbsp.
- Salt
- Chopped collard greens, 1½ lbs.
- Minced garlic cloves, 2
- Butter, 1 tbsp.
- Black pepper

Directions:

1. Have some water in a saucepan to simmer with salt
2. Add the greens to cook for 15 minutes while covered
3. Remove all the liquid in the greens then reserve in a bowl
4. Set the pan over medium heat to heat the oil to fry the greens.
5. Add the seasonings and garlic
6. Gently stir as you cook for 5 minutes
7. Adjust the seasoning as you sprinkle with lemon juice.
8. Serve and enjoy

Nutrition:

Calories: 385, Fat: 14.7, Fiber: 39.3, Carbs: 66, Protein: 26.3

Stress-free Cheesy Tacos

Prep Time + Cook Time: 35 minutes Serves: 3

Ingredients:

- Chopped tomatoes, ¼ cup
- Black pepper.
- Cooked favorite taco meat, 1 cup
- Grated cheddar cheese, 2 cup
- Cooking spray
- Salt.
- Sriracha sauce, 2 tsps.
- Chopped and pitted small avocado, 1.

Directions:

1. Ensure your baking dish is lined. Spray the baking sheet with cooking oil. Spread over the cheddar cheese and set in an oven preheated to 400 0F. Bake the mixture for about 15 minutes.
2. Over the cheese, lay out the taco meat and continue baking for another 10 minutes.
3. In a separate bowl, stir in salt, tomatoes, pepper, sriracha sauce and avocado. Mix well to obtain the desired consistency. Spread over the baked taco.
4. Remove from oven and let cool. Slice and enjoy your lunch.

Nutrition:

calories: 400, fiber: 0, fat: 23, carbs: 2, protein: 37

Sweet Coconut Cauliflower Mix

Prep Time + Cook Time: 25 minutes Servings: 4

Ingredients:

- Coconut cream - 1 tbsp.
- Seasoning- A pinch of salt and black pepper
- Cauliflower florets - 3 cups
- Coconut milk - 14 ounces

Directions:

1. Put the cauliflower with coconut milk, coconut cream, salt, and pepper in a cooking pot, mix well and cook for 15 minutes.
2. Divide into separate bowls and serve.
3. Share and Enjoy!

Nutrition:

calories 201, fat 5, fiber 4, carbs 6, protein 12

Sweet Mushroom Cream

Prep Time + Cook Time: 35 minutes Servings: 4

Ingredients:

- Chopped garlic cloves- 3
- Brown mushrooms (chopped): 14
- Seasoning- A pinch of salt and black pepper
- Dijon mustard - ½ tsp.
- Grated lemon zest - 1 tsp.
- lemon juice - 1 tbsp.
- Ghee - 2 tbsps.
- Chopped thyme - 1 tbsp.
- Olive oil - 2 tbsps.
- Chopped celery stick- One
- Veggie stock - 3 cups

Directions:

1. With medium or moderate temperature, heat the oil in a cooking pot, put celery, mushrooms, thyme, and garlic, mix well and cook for 10 minutes.
2. Put stock, mustard, salt, black pepper, and lemon zest, mix well, cover the pot and cook slowly (brings to

simmer) over medium heat for another 15 minutes.
3. With an immersion blender, blend the mixture, put lemon juice and ghee, mix well.

4. Divide into bowls with a ladle and serve
5. Enjoy!

Nutrition:
calories 200, fat 2, fiber 3, carbs 8, protein 7

Swiss Vegetable Soup

Prep Time + Cook Time: 2 hours 20 minutes Servings: 4

Ingredients:
- Red onion; chopped-1
- Swiss chard; a chopped-1 bunch
- Yellow squash; chopped-1
- Zucchini; chopped-1
- Green bell pepper; chopped-1
- Sausage; chopped-1 pound
- Garlic cloves; minced-2
- Cauliflower florets; chopped-1 cup
- Green beans; chopped-1 cup
- Chicken stock-6 cups
- Canned tomato paste-7 ounces
- Water-2 cups
- Thyme; chopped-2 tsps.
- Rosemary; dried-1 tsp.
- Fennel; minced-1 tbsp.
- Red pepper flakes-1/2 tsp.
- Some grated parmesan for serving
- Carrots; chopped-6
- Tomatoes; chopped-4 cups
- Salt and black pepper -to the taste

Directions:
1. Place a skillet over medium-high heat.
2. Add garlic and sausage, saute until brown then transfer to a slow cooker.
3. Add squash, onion, bell pepper, Swiss chard, carrots, tomatoes, green beans, zucchini, cauliflower, water, stock, tomato paste, fennel, rosemary, salt, pepper, and pepper flakes.
4. Cover the mixture in the slow cooker and cook on High for 2 hours.
5. Remove the lid from the cooker and mix well.
6. Drizzle parmesan cheese and serve right away.

Nutrition:
Calories: 150; Fat: 8g; Fiber: 2g; Carbs: 4g; Protein: 9g

Tangy Poblano Soup

Prep Time + Cook Time:1 hour 10 minutes Servings: 3

Ingredients:
- Poblano peppers -5
- Ghee, melted -½ tbsp
- Yellow onion, chopped -½
- Garlic cloves, minced -2
- Cilantro, chopped -½ cup
- Salt and black pepper- to taste
- Veggie stock -23.5 oz.
- Cumin, ground -½ tsp

- Mexican cheese, grated -7 oz.

Directions:

1. Spread all the peppers in a baking sheet, lined with wax paper.
2. Bake them for 20 minutes at 450 0F in a preheated oven.
3. Once done, allow the peppers to cool down, peel and chop them.
4. Take ghee in a cooking pot and place it over medium heat to heat up.
5. Add cumin, garlic, cilantro, salt, onions, and pepper. Sauté them for 6 minutes.
6. Pour in the stock and continue cooking for 20 minutes with occasional stirring.
7. Stir in cheese then blend the soup using a handheld blender.
8. Serve warm and fresh.

Nutrition:

Calories: 261, Fat: 4, Fiber: 7, Carbs: 11, Protein: 6

Tasty Onion and Tomato Soup

Prep Time + Cook Time:3 hours 10 minutes Servings: 4

Ingredients:

- Seasoning- A pinch of salt and black pepper
- Chicken stock - 5 cups
- Olive oil - 2 tbsps.
- halved and sliced yellow onions- 2
- Three Thyme springs
- Tomato paste - 2 tbsp.

Directions:

1. With medium-high, heat the oil in a cooking pot, put onions and thyme, mix it well, gradually reduce the heat to low, cover with the lid and cook for 30 minutes.
2. Remove the lid and cook onions for another 1 hour and 30 minutes.
3. Put tomato paste and stock, cook slowly (brings to simmer) for another 1 hour.
4. Divide into bowls with a ladle
5. Enjoy!

Nutrition:

calories 210, fat 4, fiber 4, carbs 7, protein 8

Tomato Soup (Keto)

Prep Time + Cook Time: 18 minutes Servings: 5

Ingredients:

- Bacon strips-8 (cooked and crumbled)
- Ghee-4 tbsps.
- Olive oil-1/4 cup
- Red hot sauce-1/4 cup
- Basil leaves-A handful of (chopped)
- Tomato soup-1 quart (canned)
- Oregano-1 tsp. (dried)
- Turmeric-1 tsp. (ground)

- Green onions-A handful of (chopped)
- Apple cider vinegar-2 tbsps.
- Salt and black pepper-To taste

Directions:

1. Pour the tomato soup in a pot.
2. Over the medium heat, boil the soup.
3. Mix the olive oil, ghee, hot sauce, vinegar, salt, pepper, turmeric and oregano.

4. Combine and simmer for 5 minutes.
5. Put off the heat.
6. Equally put the soup into bowls.
7. Top them with bacon crumbles, basil and green onions.

Nutrition :

Calories:- 400; Fat : 34; Fiber : 7; Carbs : 10; Protein : 12

Vegetable Lunch Pate

Prep Time + Cook Time: 10 minutes Serves: 1

Ingredients:

- Salt
- Sliced radishes, 3
- Sautéed chicken livers; 4 oz.
- Chopped mixed thyme; sage and oregano, 1 tsp.
- Crusted bread slices for serving
- Butter, 3 tbsps.
- Black pepper.

Directions:

1. Combine chicken livers with sage, thyme, butter, oregano, pepper, and salt then blend until done.
2. Rub the mixture on crusted bread slices then top with radishes slices
3. Serve immediately.

Nutrition:

calories: 380, fat: 40, carbs: 1, fiber: 5, protein: 17

Watermelon Radish Salad

Prep Time + Cook Time: 14 minutes Servings: 4

Ingredients:

- Green onions (chopped): 4
- Olive oil: 2 tbsps.
- Radishes, sliced: 4 ounces
- Watermelon radish (thinly sliced): 4 ounces
- Fennel bulb (chopped): ½ cup
- lemon juice: 2 tbsps.
- Salt and black pepper
- Mint (chopped): ¼ cup
- Avocado mayonnaise: 2 tbsps.

Directions:

1. In a salad bowl, mix the radishes with fennel, spring onions, lemon juice, mint, mayo, oil, salt and pepper, dice and serve.
2. Enjoy!

Nutrition:

calories 200, fat 3, carbs 6, fiber 3, protein 9

Wraps Filled with Tomato, Avocado & Turkey

Prep Time + Cook Time: 11 minutes Servings: 3

Ingredients:

- Lettuce leaves-4 big
- Deli turkey slices-4 (cooked)
- Bacon slices-4 (cooked)
- Avocado-1 (peeled, pitted and sliced)
- Tomato-1 (sliced)
- Homemade mayonnaise-1/2 cup
- Basil leaves-6 (torn)
- Lemon juice-1 tsp.
- Salt and black pepper-A pinch
- Garlic clove-1 (minced)

Directions:

1. Take a mixing bowl.
2. Combine the mayo with basil, garlic, salt, pepper and lemon juice
3. Whisk well.
4. Layer out 2 lettuce leaves on a cutting board.
5. Add 1 turkey slice and spread some mayo mix.
6. Layer the second slice of turkey.
7. Then add a bacon slice, some avocado and tomato slices.
8. Fold and wrap like a burrito.
9. Repeat with the rest of the ingredients and 2 more lettuce leaves.
10. Serve them for lunch.

Nutrition:

calories 265, fat 4, fiber 7, carbs 14, protein 6

Zucchini And Hot Avocado Soup

Prep Time + Cook Time: 25 minutesServings: 4

Ingredients:

- Big avocado - 1; pitted, peeled and chopped.
- Zucchinis - 2; chopped.
- water - 1 cup
- lemon juice - 1 tbsp.
- Red bell pepper - 1; chopped.
- garlic clove - 1; minced
- veggie stock - 29 ounces
- Scallions - 4; chopped.
- Ginger - 1 tsp.; grated
- avocado oil - 2 tbsps.
- Salt and black pepper to the taste.

Directions:

1. Place a pot containing oil over medium-high heat source.
2. Then add some onions; stir gently and cook for 3 minutes
3. Follow this by adding garlic and ginger; stir gently, then cook for about a minute.
4. Add zucchini, salt, pepper, water and stock to the mix; stir again, and bring to a boil.
5. Cover the pot and cook for about 10 minutes
6. Remove the heat; keep the soup aside for a while and add avocado.
7. Stir gently, and blend everything using an immersion blender
8. Then heat up again
9. Add more salt and pepper, bell pepper and lemon juice.
10. Stir gently, and heat up the soup again.
11. Ladle into different soup bowls
12. Serve immediately.

Nutrition :

Calories:- 154; Fat : 12; Fiber : 3; Carbs : 5; Protein : 4

Chapter 4 Ketogenic Snacks and Appetizers Recipes

Almond Broccoli Biscuits

Prep Time + Cook Time: 35 minutes Serves: 12

Ingredients:

- Baking soda, ½ tsp.
- Almond flour, 1½ cup
- Sweet paprika, 1 tsp.
- Apple cider vinegar, ½ tsp.
- Salt
- Olive oil, ¼ cup
- Grated cheddar cheese, 2 cup
- Black pepper
- Garlic powder, 1 tsp.
- Medium eggs, 2
- Broccoli florets, 4 cup

Directions:

1. Set the blender in position and switch on.
2. Add the broccoli with some pepper and salt, process until smooth then reserve in a bowl
3. Stir in all the remaining ingredients then mold into 12 patties
4. Arrange the patties in a well-greased baking tray
5. Set the oven for 20 minutes at 375°F, allow to bake
6. Serve on the platter and enjoys as a snack

Nutrition:

Calories: 183, Fat: 12, Fiber: 2, Carbs: 8, Protein: 4

Almond Flaxseed Muffins

Prep Time + Cook Time: 30 minutes Serves: 20

Ingredients:

- Baking powder, ¼ tsp.
- Flaxseed meal, ½ cup
- Swerve, 3 tbsps.
- Coconut milk, ¼ cupHot dogs, 4Psyllium powder, 1 tbsp.
- Salt
- Vegetable oil cooking
- Large egg, 1
- Almond flour, ½ cup
- Sour cream, 1/3 cup

Directions:

1. Mix swerve, flaxseed meal, salt, flour, and baking powder as you gently stir in a medium bowl.
2. Whisk in coconut milk, sour cream, and the egg.
3. Prepare the muffin tray by greasing with oil.
4. Divide the mixture each with a hot dog piece in the middle
5. Set the oven for 12 minutes at 350°F. Let it bake.

6. Meanwhile, preheat the broiler
7. Once the timer is over, allow to broil for about 3 minutes then enjoy

Nutrition:
Calories: 65, Fat: 3.4, Fiber: 0.9, Carbs: 7.1, Protein: 1.7

Artichoke, Tomato and Mozzarella Appetizer

Prep Time + Cook Time: 10 minutes Servings 10

Ingredients:

- Marinated artichoke hearts, drained: 15 ounces
- Artichoke marinade: ½ cup
- Red vinegar: 2 tbsps.
- Olive oil: 2 tbsps.
- Plum tomatoes, sliced: 6
- Mozzarella cheese, sliced: 1 pound
- Chopped basil: 2 cups
- Ground black pepper: ¼ tsp.

Directions:

1. Scatter artichoke hearts on a serving platter, top with tomatoes and mozzarella cheese and then sprinkle with basil.
2. Place artichoke marinade in a bowl, add black pepper, oil, and vinegar and whisk well until combined.
3. Pour this mixture over artichokes and toss until coated.
4. Serve straight away as an appetizer.

Nutrition:
calories: 200, fat: 7, fiber: 1, carbs: 6, protein: 7

Asian Mint Chutney: Side Dish

Prep Time + Cook Time: 10 minutes Servings: 8

Ingredients:

- big bunch cilantro - 1
- tamarind juice - 1 tbsp.
- green chili pepper - 1, seedless
- mint leaves - 1½ cup
- yellow onion - 1, cut into medium chunks
- water - 1/4 cup
- Salt and black pepper to the taste.

Directions:

1. Blend a mixture of mint and coriander leaves inside a food processor
2. Add chili pepper, salt, black pepper, onion and tamarind paste and blend again.
3. Add some water to the resulting mixture, then blend some more until you obtain cream.
4. Move to a clean bowl
5. Serve as a side for a tasty keto steak.

Nutrition :
Calories:- 100; Fat : 1; Fiber : 1; Carbs : 0.4; Protein : 6

Baked Chia Seeds

Prep Time + Cook Time: 45 minutes Serves: 36

Ingredients:

- Salt
- Ice water, 1 ¼ cup
- Sweet paprika, ¼ tsp. Ground chia seeds, ½ cup
- Xanthan gum, ¼ tsp.
- Olive oil, 2 tbsps.
- Psyllium husk powder, 2 tbsps.
- Grated cheddar, 3 oz.
- Dried oregano, ¼ tsp.
- Onion powder, ¼ tsp.
- Black pepper
- Garlic powder, ¼ tsp.

Directions:

1. Combine xanthan gum, paprika, oregano, chia seeds, psyllium powder, pepper, and onion powder in a medium bowl as you gently stir.
2. Stir in oil then add ice water. Mix to attain a firm dough
3. Align the mixture on a greased baking sheet.
4. Set your oven for 35 minutes at 350°F. Let it bake.
5. Once fully baked, allow to cool down before serving

Nutrition:

Calories: 11, Fat: 1, Fiber: 0, Carbs: 0.1, Protein: 0.6

Balsamic Zucchini Chips

Prep Time + Cook Time: 3 hours 10 minutes Serves: 8

Ingredients:

- Balsamic vinegar, 2 tbsps.
- Salt
- Olive oil, 2 tbsps.
- Black pepper
- Sliced zucchinis, 3

Directions:

1. Add the seasonings, oil, and vinegar then whisk well
2. Toss in the zucchini slices to coat evenly
3. Line up the baking tray then arrange the zucchini slices on it.
4. Set the oven for 3 hours at 200°F, allow to bake
5. Let the chips to cool down before serving as a snack

Nutrition:

Calories: 100, Fat: 3, Fiber: 3, Carbs: 7, Protein: 7

Beef Spicy Shots

Prep Time + Cook Time: 1 hours Servings: 28

Ingredients:

- Ground beef-1 pound
- Cheddar cheese-2 cups (shredded)
- Water-1/4 cup
- Salt and black pepper-to taste (ground)
- Cumin-2 tbsps.
- Chili powder-2 tbsps.
- Pico de gallo-for serving

Directions:

1. Distribute a spoonful of cheddar cheese on a lined baking sheet.
2. Keep the sheet in an oven at 350°F.
3. Let it bake for 7 minutes.
4. Allow the cheese to cool down for 1 minute.
5. Then shift them to mini cupcake molds.
6. Take a pan over medium-high heat.
7. When heated, stir beef in it and cook until it browns.
8. Cook for 5 minutes by adding water, salt, pepper, cumin, and chili powder.
9. Equally, shape the mixture into cheese cups.
10. Top the cups with pico de gallo.
11. Shift the cups to display on a platter to serve.

Nutrition:

Calories: 58, Fat: 3.4, Fiber: 0, Carbs: 0.1, Protein: 6.5

Blueberry, Jalapeno and Pepper Salad

Prep Time + Cook Time: 5 minutes Servings 4

Ingredients:

- Whole blueberries: 1 cup
- Blueberries, chopped: 2 cups
- Chopped cilantro: 3 tbsps.
- Lemon juice: ¼ cup
- Jalapeno pepper, chopped: 2
- White onion, chopped: ¼ cup
- Red bell pepper, chopped: ¼ cup
- Salt: ¼ tsp.

Directions:

1. Place all the ingredients for the salad in a medium bowl and stir until combined.
2. Serve straight away as an appetizer.

Nutrition:

calories: 90, fat: 1, fiber: 2, carbs: 7, protein: 8

Braised Eggplant Dish: Side Dish

Prep Time + Cook Time: 25 minutes Servings: 4

Ingredients:

- big Asian eggplant - 1, cut into medium pieces
- vegetable oil - 2 tbsp.
- garlic - 2 tsps., minced
- Vietnamese sauce - 1/2 cup
- yellow onion - 1, thinly sliced
- chili paste - 2 tsps.
- coconut milk - 1/4 cup
- green onions - 4, chopped.
- water - 1/2 cup

For the Vietnamese sauce:

- chicken stock - 1/2 cup
- palm sugar - 1 tsp.
- fish sauce - 2 tbsps.

Directions:

1. Put stock in a pan and place on medium-high heat source.
2. Then add sugar and fish sauce; stir well and keep it aside for a while.
3. Add heat to a pan placed on medium high heat source.
4. Add eggplant pieces, and leaving it for about 2 minutes until they become brown.
5. Then move to a plate
6. Add more heat to the pan still containing the oil using medium high heat.
7. Follow this by adding yellow onion and garlic; stir and cook for 2 minutes
8. Return the eggplant pieces and cook for 2 minutes
9. Pour some water, the Vietnamese sauce you already made, chili paste and coconut milk; stir gently and cook for 5 minutes
10. Add green onions; stir, cook for another minute.
11. Move to clean plates
12. Now you can serve as a side dish.

Nutrition :

Calories:- 142; Fat : 7; Fiber : 4; Carbs : 5; Protein : 3

Broccoli and Cheddar Biscuits

Prep Time + Cook Time: 35 minutes Serves: 12

Ingredients:

- Medium eggs, 2
- Almond flour, 1 ½ cup
- Baking soda, ½ tsp. Paprika, 1 tsp.
- Salt
- Broccoli florets, 4 cup
- Black pepper
- Coconut oil, ¼ cup
- Garlic powder, 1 tsp.
- Grated cheddar cheese, 2 cup
- Apple cider vinegar, ½ tsp.

Directions:

1. Have your blender in position then add broccoli florets with seasoning to process evenly

2. Meanwhile, stir together pepper, almond flour, garlic powder, salt, baking soda, and paprika in a medium bowl.
3. Again stir in coconut oil, cheddar cheese, broccoli, vinegar, and eggs.
4. Molt the mixture into 12 patties.
5. Set the oven for 20 minutes at 375ºF then allow to bake.
6. Once done, switch the oven to broiler then broil for 5 minutes.
7. Enjoy the biscuits

Nutrition:
Calories: 210, Fat: 18.1, Fiber: 2.3, Carbs: 5.3, Protein: 9.3

Brussels sprouts with Bacon and Cream Cheese

Prep Time + Cook Time: 1 hour Servings 20
Ingredients:
- Slices of bacon: 6
- Brussels sprouts, halved: 20
- Medium white onion, chopped: 1
- Minced garlic: 1 tsp.
- Salt: ½ tsp.
- Ground black pepper: ½ tsp.
- Red chili powder: 1 tsp.
- Stevia: 2 tbsps.
- White vinegar: 2 tbsps.
- 2 tbsps. unsalted butter, melted
- Cream cheese, cut into squares: 7 ounces
- Olive oil: 2 tbsps.

Directions:
1. Set oven to 375 0F and let preheat.
2. In the meantime, place a medium skillet pan over medium-high heat, add butter and when hot, add the onion.
3. Cook onion for 8 minutes or until sauté, then add garlic, season with a ¼ tsp. each of salt, black pepper, chili powder, and stevia and stir in vinegar until combined and cook for 10 to 12 minutes.
4. Then remove the pan from heat, set aside until required.
5. Place Brussel sprouts on a baking sheet lined with parchment sheet in a single layer, season with remaining salt and black pepper, then drizzle with oil.
6. Toss sprouts well, then place the baking sheet into the oven and bake for 20 minutes or until cooked through.
7. Meanwhile, place another skillet pan over medium-high heat, add bacon slices and cook for 8 minutes or until crispy.
8. Then drain grease from the pan, transfer bacon to a cutting board and cut into squares.
9. Working on one Brussels sprout at a time, first tip a sprout half with a piece of bacon, then top with a cheese piece, cover with other sprout half and secure with a toothpick.
10. Prepare remaining sprouts, in the same manner, using all the bacon and cheese pieces.
11. Serve straightaway.

Nutrition:
calories: 188, fat: 2, fiber: 3, carbs: 9, protein: 6

Cauliflower with Side Salad

Prep Time + Cook Time: 15 minutes Servings: 10

Ingredients:

- Cauliflower - 21 ounces, florets separated
- Eggs - 4, hard-boiled, peeled and chopped.
- red onion - 1 cup, chopped.
- Celery - 1 cup, chopped.
- cider vinegar - 2 tbsps.
- mayonnaise - 1 cup
- water - 1 tbsp.
- splenda - 1 tsp.
- Salt and black pepper to the taste.

Directions:

1. Add some cauliflower florets in a heatproof bowl, before adding water.
2. Place the lid on the top and cook in your microwave for 5 minutes
3. Keep it aside for extra minutes before moving to a salad bowl.
4. Add celery, eggs and onions and stir gently.
5. Mix mayo with salt, pepper, splenda and vinegar in a clean bowl and whisk well.
6. Add this to salad, toss to ensure it is well coated.
7. Serve immediately with a side salad.

Nutrition :

Calories:- 211; Fat : 20; Fiber : 2; Carbs : 3; Protein : 4

Cheesy and Olives Bombs

Prep Time + Cook Time: 10 minutes Serves: 6

Ingredients:

- Cream cheese, 4 oz.
- Salt
- Chopped pepperoni slices, 14
- Black pepper
- Basil pesto, 2 tbsps.
- Chopped black olives, 8

Directions:

1. With the bowl set in position, combine all the ingredients
2. Mold the mixture into balls
3. Set on a serving platter to serve

Nutrition:

Calories: 140, Fat: 4, Fiber: 4, Carbs: 14, Protein: 3

Cheesy Bread sticks

Prep Time + Cook Time: 25 minutes Serves: 24

Ingredients:

- Italian seasoning, 2 tbsps.
- Salt
- Grated cheddar cheese, 3 oz.
- Psyllium powder, 1 tbsp.

- Softened cream cheese, 3 tsps.
- Almond flour, ¾ cup
- Onion powder, 1 tsp.
- Melted mozzarella cheese, 2 cup
- Baking powder, 1 tsp.
- Large egg, 1
- Black pepper

Directions:

1. Set up the mixing bowl in a clean working table.
2. Whisk in almond flour, psyllium powder, pepper, baking powder, and salt.
3. Mix in melted mozzarella cheese, cream cheese, and egg to form a dough.
4. Grease the baking tray and place the dough as you divide into 24 sticks.
5. Top with onion powder and Italian seasoning then cheddar cheese.
6. Set your oven for 15 minutes at 350°F

Nutrition:

Calories: 35, Fat: 2.7, Fiber: 0.4, Carbs: 0.9, Protein: 2.1

Cheesy Snack Italian Style

Prep Time + Cook Time: 1 hour 10 minutes Serves: 12

Ingredients:

- Minced garlic clove, 1
- Black pepper
- Halved mozzarella cheese strings, 8
- Salt
- Grated parmesan, 1 cup
- Olive oil, ½ cup
- Whisked eggs, 2
- Italian seasoning, 1 tbsp.

Directions:

1. Set a mixing bowl in a clean working surface to stir together the parmesan cheese, Italian seasoning, pepper, garlic, and salt
2. Set the whisked eggs in another bowl
3. Pass the mozzarella sticks in the egg mixture followed by the cheese mixture.
4. Dip them in the eggs again then in the parmesan mixture
5. Allow to refrigerate for one hour.
6. Set up the pan over medium-high heat with oil to fry the coated sticks
7. Set on a platter to enjoy as a snack

Nutrition:

Calories: 140, Fat: 5, Fiber: 1, Carbs: 3, Protein: 4

Cider and Cashew Hummus

Prep Time + Cook Time: 10 minutes Servings 4

Ingredients:

- Cashews, soaked for 12 hours: 5 tbsps.
- Apple cider vinegar: 1 tsp.
- Vegetable stock: 1 cup

- Water: 1 tbsp.

Directions:

1. Place all the ingredients for hummus in a blender and pulse for 1 to 2 minutes or until smooth.

2. Tip hummus in a bowl and serve as an appetizer.

Nutrition:

calories: 201, fat: 6, fiber: 5, carbs: 9, protein: 8

Coconut Almond Bars

Prep Time + Cook Time: 2 hours 2 minutes Serves: 12

Ingredients:

- Melted coconut oil, 2 tbsps.
- Almond butter, 1¾ cup
- Shredded coconut, ¾ cup
- Chopped dark chocolate, 4 oz.
- Stevia, ¾ cup

Directions:

1. Combine stevia, almond flour, and coconut in a medium mixing bowl

2. Set the pan with 1 cup of almond butter and coconut oil over medium-low heat and whisk well

3. Stir the mixture to the almond flour

4. Set the mixture on the baking tray and press. Set up another pan over medium-high heat to whisk together chocolate and the remaining almond butter

5. Pour the mixture on top of almond mix to spread evenly. Allow to refrigerate for 2 hours then divide into 12 bars

6. Enjoy this awesome snack

Nutrition:

Calories: 160, Fat: 2, Fiber: 3, Carbs: 8, Protein: 4

Coconut Avocado Dip

Prep Time + Cook Time: 3 hours 20 minutes Serves: 4

Ingredients:

- Coconut milk, 1 cup Stevia, ¼ tsp.
- Chopped cilantro, ½ cup
- Avocados slices, 2
- Erythritol powder, ¼ cup
- Juice, and zest of 2 limes

Directions:

1. Line the baking sheet then align the avocado slices.

2. Sprinkle with the lime juice over the avocados then freeze for 3 hours

3. Meanwhile, heat the coconut milk over medium heat

4. Mix in the lime zest then allow to boil.

5. Stir in erythritol powder then reserve to cool

6. Place the avocado in a blender then add cilantro and lime juice to pulse evenly.

7. Blend in stevia and coconut milk.

8. Enjoy the dip.

Nutrition:

Calories: 352, Fat: 33.9, Fiber: 8.1, Carbs: 17.3, Protein: 3.3

Creamy Smoked Salmon and Dill Spread

Prep Time + Cook Time: 10 minutes Servings 10

Ingredients:

- Smoked salmon, flaked: 4 ounces
- Salt: ½ tsp.
- Ground black pepper: ½ tsp.
- Chopped dill: 1 tbsp.
- Creole seasoning: ¼ tsp.
- Lemon juice: 1 tbsp.
- Cream cheese: 16 ounces

Directions:

1. Place all the ingredients for the dip in a blender and pulse for 1 to 2 minutes or until smooth.
2. Divide dip evenly between small bowls and serve as a party dip.

Nutrition:

calories: 100, fat: 8, fiber: 2, carbs: 2, protein: 4

Creamy Spinach and Onion Dip

Prep Time + Cook Time: 10 minutes Servings 10

Ingredients:

- Spinach, chopped: 10 ounces
- White onion, peeled and chopped: ¼ cup
- Dried basil: 1 tsp.
- Dried oregano: ½ tsp.
- Ranch dressing, low-carb: 1 ounce
- Coconut cream: 2 cups

Directions:

1. Place all the ingredients for the dip in a medium bowl and stir until combined.
2. Divide dip evenly between small bowls and serve as a party dip.

Nutrition:

calories: 161, fat: 6, fiber: 2, carbs: 17, protein: 5

Creamy Spinach Dip with Garlic

Prep Time + Cook Time: 45 minutes Serves: 6

Ingredients:

- Minced garlic, 1 tbsp. Black pepper
- Sour cream, ½ cup
- Softened cream cheese, 8 oz.
- Bacon slices, 6
- Chopped parsley, 1½ tbsps.
- Spinach, 5 oz.
- Grated Parmesan cheese, 2 ½ oz.
- Salt

Directions:

1. Quick fry the bacon in a pan over medium heat to attain a crispy texture.

2. Let the excess oil be drained with a paper towel
3. Reserve in a bowl.
4. Again, fry the spinach on the pan with bacon oil until soft then set on a plate
5. Meanwhile, stir together sour cream, cream cheese, parsley, pepper, garlic, bacon, and salt in a medium bowl.
6. Stir in the spinach, lemon juice, and the Parmesan cheese.
7. Set the mixture into ramekins
8. Set your oven for 25 minutes at 350°F then allow to bake
9. Once the timer clicks, set the oven to broil and broil for 4 minutes.
10. Enjoy with crackers

Nutrition:
Calories: 358, Fat: 30.3, Fiber: 0.6, Carbs: 4, Protein: 18.9

Delicious Caramelized Bell Peppers: Side Dish

Prep Time + Cook Time: 42 minutes Servings: 4

Ingredients:
- red bell peppers - 2, cut into thin strips
- red onions - 2, cut into thin strips
- ghee - 1 tsp.
- basil - 1 tsp., dried
- olive oil - 1 tbsp.
- Salt and black pepper to the taste.

Directions:
1. Place a pan containing ghee and oil on a medium-high heat source.
2. Then add onion and bell peppers; stir gently and cook for 2 minutes
3. Decrease the temperature and cook for another 30 minutes while stirring frequently.
4. Then sprinkle some salt, pepper and basil; stir again.
5. Remove the heat and serve as a keto side dish.

Nutrition :
Calories:- 97; Fat : 4; Fiber : 2; Carbs : 6; Protein : 2

Dessert With Bacon

Prep Time + Cook Time:1 hour and 45 minutes Servings: 18

Ingredients:
- Ground cinnamon-1/2 tsp.
- Erythritol-2 tbsps.
- Bacon slices-16
- Coconut oil-1 tbsp.
- Dark chocolate-3 ounces
- Maple extract-1 tbsp.

Directions:
1. Combine cinnamon with the erythritol in a bowl.
2. Mix well and layer bacon slices on a lined baking sheet.

3. Sprinkle some cinnamon mixture over the slices and flip to cover the other side as well.
4. After the mixture is well coated, in an oven settle the dish at 275°F.
5. Bake the dish for an hour.
6. Warm oil in a pot over medium heat.
7. Spread chocolate, and stir until it melts.
8. Drizzle maple extract; toss in to take off from heat.
9. Set the prepared slices aside to cool.
10. Let them cool down after taking it out of the oven.
11. Dip each of the slices in chocolate mixture.
12. Settle them on a parchment paper to let them cool down completely.
13. Serve when cold.

Nutrition:
Calories: 139, Fat: 10.4, Fiber: 0.2, Carbs: 3.5, Protein: 7.5

Easy Cheese Sauce: Side Dish

Prep Time + Cook Time: 22 minutes Servings: 8

Ingredients:
- cream cheese - 1/4 cup, soft
- whipping cream - 1/4 cup
- onion powder - 1/2 tsp.
- garlic powder - 1/2 tsp.
- cheddar cheese - 1/4 cup, grated
- ghee - 2 tbsps.
- water - 2 tbsps.
- cayenne pepper - 1/4 tsp.
- sweet paprika - 1/2 tsp.
- parsley - 4 tbsps., chopped.
- A pinch of salt

Directions:
1. Heat up a pan containing ghee over medium-high heat.
2. Then add whipping cream and stir properly.
3. Also, add cream cheese; stir gently and bring to a simmer.
4. Remove the heat; add cheddar cheese; stir gently before returning to medium-high heat and cook for 3-4 minutes
5. Pour some water in the mixture, sprinkle a pinch of salt, cayenne pepper, and add onion and garlic powder, paprika and parsley; stir properly.
6. Remove the heat and serve on top of meat or fish based meals

Nutrition :
Calories:- 200; Fat : 13; Fiber : 0; Carbs : 1; Protein : 6

Easy Tuna Cakes

Prep Time + Cook Time: 18 minutes Serves: 12

Ingredients:

- A drizzle of olive oil
- Medium eggs, 3
- Dried parsley, 1 tsp.
- Garlic powder, 1 tsp.
- Salt
- Chopped red onion, ½ cup
- Black pepper
- Canned tuna, 15 oz.

Directions:

1. Set a mixing bowl in position to stir together parsley, seasonings, eggs, garlic powder, and onion then mold the mixture into patties.
2. Set a pan on fife with the oil to cook the cakes evenly over medium-high heat.
3. Set the patties on a serving platter and enjoy as an appetizer

Nutrition:

Calories: 160, Fat: 2, Fiber: 4, Carbs: 6, Protein: 6

Eggplant, Olives and Basil Salad

Prep Time + Cook Time: 15 minutes Servings 4

Ingredients:

- Tomatoes, chopped: 1 ½ cups
- Eggplant, cubed: 3 cups
- Capers: 2 tsps.
- Green olives, pitted and sliced: 6 ounces
- Minced garlic: 2 tsps.
- Salt: ½ tsp.
- Ground black pepper: ¼ tsp.
- Chopped basil: 1 tbsp.
- Olive oil: 2 tsps.
- Balsamic vinegar: 2 tsps.

Directions:

1. Place a medium skillet pan over medium-high heat, add oil and when hot, add eggplant pieces and cook for 5 minutes.
2. Then add remaining ingredients, stir well and cook for 5 minutes.
3. When done, remove the pan from heat and let cool for 5 minutes.
4. Then divide salad evenly between small cups and serve as an appetizer.

Nutrition:

calories: 199, fat: 6, fiber: 5, carbs: 7, protein: 7

Fresh Tomato, Onion and Jalapeno Pepper Salsa

Prep Time + Cook Time: 5 minutes Servings 4

Ingredients:

- Cherry tomatoes, halved: 2 cups
- Red onion, peeled and chopped: ¼ cup
- Jalapeno pepper, chopped: 1
- Minced garlic: ½ tsp.
- Chopped cilantro: 2 tbsps.
- Salt: ¼ tsp.
- Ground black pepper: ¼ tsp.
- Lime juice: 2 tbsps.

Directions:

1. Place all the ingredients for salsa in a medium bowl and stir until combined.
2. Serve straight away as a snack.

Nutrition:

calories: 87, fat: 1, fiber: 2, carbs: 7, protein: 5

Fresh Veggie Bars

Prep Time + Cook Time: 40 minutes Servings: 18

Ingredients:

- Egg-1
- Broccoli florets-2 cups
- Cheddar cheese-1/3 cup (grated)
- Onion-¼ cup (peeled and chopped)
- Cauliflower rice-½ cup
- Fresh parsley-2 tbsps. (chopped)
- Olive oil-A drizzle (for greasing)
- Salt and black pepper-to taste (ground)

Directions:

1. Warm up a saucepan with water over medium heat
2. Stir into the broccoli and let it simmer for a minute.
3. Strain and finely chop it to put into a bowl.
4. Mix in the egg, cheddar cheese, cauliflower rice, salt, pepper, parsley, and mix.
5. Give them the shape of bars by using the mixture on your hands.
6. Put them on a greased baking sheet.
7. Keep it in an oven at 400°F and bake for 20 minutes.
8. Settle the prepared dish on a platter to serve.

Nutrition:

Calories: 19, Fat: 1, Fiber: 0.3, Carbs: 1.3, Protein: 1.3

Green Beans And Avocado with Chopped Cilantro

Prep Time + Cook Time: 15 minutes Servings: 4

Ingredients:

- Avocados: 2; pitted and peeled
- green beans - 2/3 pound, trimmed
- scallions - 5, chopped.
- olive oil - 3 tbsps.
- A handful cilantro, chopped.
- Salt and black pepper to the taste.

Directions:

1. Heat up a pan containing oil on a medium-high heat source; then add green beans and stir gently. Cook this mixture for about 4 minutes
2. Add salt and pepper to the pan; and stir gently, then remove the heat and move to a clean bowl.
3. Mix the avocados with salt and pepper and mash with a fork inside a clean bowl.
4. Then add onions and stir properly.
5. Add this over green beans, then toss to ensure it is well coated.
6. Finally, serve with some chopped cilantro on top.

Nutrition :

Calories:- 200; Fat : 5; Fiber : 3; Carbs : 4; Protein : 6

Italian Pizza Dip

Prep Time + Cook Time: 30 minutes Serves: 4

Ingredients:

- Italian seasoning, ½ tsp.
- Black pepper
- Mozzarella cheese, ½ cup
- Chopped green bell pepper, 1 tbsp.
- Sour cream, ¼ cup
- Salt
- Grated Parmesan cheese, ¼ cup
- Tomato sauce, ½ cup
- Mayonnaise, ¼ cup
- Softened cream cheese, 4 oz.
- Chopped pepperoni slices, 6
- Chopped black olives, 4

Directions:

1. Gently stir together pepper, sour cream, cream cheese, mayonnaise, mozzarella cheese, and salt in a big bowl
2. Put the mixture into four ramekins then top with tomato sauce, parmesan cheese, then bell pepper, pepperoni, Italian seasoning, and black olives
3. Set your oven for 20 minutes at 3500F
4. Allow to bake . Enjoy the meal warm.

Nutrition:

Calories: 284, Fat: 24.4, Fiber: 1, Carbs: 9.5, Protein: 8.6

Jalapeno Cheesy Balls

Prep Time + Cook Time: 10 minutes Serves: 2

Ingredients:

- Cream cheese, 3 oz.
- Garlic powder, ¼ tsp.
- Onion powder, ¼ tsp.
- Black pepper
- Chopped jalapeno peppers, 2
- Salt
- Dried parsley, ½ tsp.
- Cooked and crumbled bacon slices, 3

Directions:

1. Set the mixing bowl in position to combine garlic powder, bacon, seasonings, parsley, and onion with the jalapeno peppers
2. Shape the mixture into balls
3. Set the balls on a flat plate to take as a cold appetizer

Nutrition:

Calories: 200, Fat: 5, Fiber: 4, Carbs: 12, Protein: 6

Keto Veggie Noodles: Side Dish

Prep Time + Cook Time: 30 minutes Servings: 6

Ingredients:

- Zucchini - 1, cut with a spiralizer
- summer squash - 1, cut with a spiralizer
- yellow, orange and red bell peppers - 6 ounces; cut into thin strips
- bacon fat - 4 tbsps.
- garlic cloves - 3, minced
- carrot - 1, cut with a spiralizer
- sweet potato - 1, cut with a spiralizer
- red onion - 4 ounces, chopped.
- Salt and black pepper to the taste.

Directions:

1. Arrange zucchini noodles neatly on a lined baking sheet.
2. Then add squash, carrot, sweet potato, onion and all bell peppers
3. Sprinkle a pinch of salt, pepper and garlic and toss to coat.
4. Then add bacon fat, toss again all noodles.
5. Move to an oven set at a temperature of 400 0F and bake for about 20 minutes
6. Move to clean plates
7. Serve immediately as a keto side dish.

Nutrition :

Calories:- 50; Fat : 1; Fiber : 1; Carbs : 6; Protein : 2

Minty Zucchini Rolls

Prep Time + Cook Time: 20 minutes Serves: 24

Ingredients:

- Chopped basil, ¼ cup
- Sliced zucchinis, 3
- Ricotta cheese, 1 1/3 cup
- Salt
- Chopped mint, 2 tbsps.
- Black pepper
- Basil leaves, 24
- Olive oil, 2 tbsps.

Directions:

1. Prepare the baking tray by lining well.
2. Add the zucchini slices then splash the oil and the seasonings on it
3. Set the oven for 10 minutes at 375°F, allow to bake
4. Meanwhile, set the mixing bowl in position to stir together chopped basil, ricotta, seasonings, and mint.
5. Divide the mixture on the zucchini slices as you roll
6. Set the rolls on a flat plate
7. Enjoy

Nutrition:
Calories: 172, Fat: 3, Fiber: 4, Carbs: 9, Protein: 4

Mushrooms Stuffed with shrimp mixture.

Prep Time + Cook Time: 30 minutes Serves: 5

Ingredients:

- Cooked shrimp, 1 cup
- Garlic powder, 1 tsp.
- Salt
- Chopped onion, 1
- Chopped white mushroom caps, 24 oz.
- Black pepper
- Softened cream cheese, 4 oz.
- Mayonnaise, ¼ cup
- Sour cream, ¼ cup
- Curry powder, 1 tsp.
- Queso blanco or Monterey Jack cheese, ½ cup

Directions:

1. Set the mixing bowl in a working surface.
2. Whisk in onion, mayonnaise, shrimp, curry powder, Mexican cheese, Pepper, cream cheese, garlic powder, salt, and sour cream.
3. Fill the mushrooms with the combination and set on a baking tray
4. Set your oven for 20 minutes at 350°F, allow too bake
5. Enjoy the meal once fully baked

Nutrition:
Calories: 259, Fat: 16.8, Fiber: 1.9, Carbs: 10.7, Protein: 17.6

Oven-baked Crackers

Prep Time + Cook Time: 25 minutes Serves: 6

Ingredients:

- Ghee, 3 tbsps.
- Salt
- Minced garlic clove, 1
- Black pepper
- Dried basil, ¼ tsp.
- Baking powder, ½ tsp.
- Basil pesto, 2 tbsps.
- Almond flour, 1¼ cup

Directions:

1. Set the mixing bowl in position to combine the almond flour, seasonings, basil pesto, baking powder, ghee, and the garlic to make a dough
2. Line the baking tray then set the dough on it.
3. Set the oven for 17 minutes at 325°F, allow to bake
4. Slice into medium crackers the moment they are cold then serve them as a snack.

Nutrition:

Calories: 200, Fat: 20, Fiber: 1, Carbs: 4, Protein: 7

Pan-Fried Cheesy Sticks

Prep Time + Cook Time: 1 hour 30 minutes Serves: 16

Ingredients:

- Black pepper
- Mozzarella string cheese pieces, 8
- Whisked eggs, 2
- Italian seasoning, 1 tbsp.
- Olive oil, ½ cup
- Grated Parmesan cheese, 1 cup
- Minced garlic clove, 1
- Salt

Directions:

1. Set a medium mixing bowl on a clean working area.
2. Stir together salt, Italian seasoning, parmesan cheese, pepper, and garlic
3. In another mixing bowl, place the whisked eggs then coat the mozzarella sticks in egg mixture then cheese mixture.
4. Repeat the process twice to coat well then freeze for an hour.
5. After one hour, heat the oil in a pan over medium-high heat to fry the sticks to a golden color evenly
6. Set on a platter and enjoy

Nutrition:

Calories: 116, Fat: 10.4, Fiber: 0, Carbs: 0.8, Protein: 5.8

Pan-fried Italian Meatballs

Prep Time + Cook Time: 16 minutes Serves: 16

Ingredients:

- Chopped basil, 2 tbsps.
- Salt
- Chopped sundried tomatoes, 2 tbsps.
- Black pepper
- Almond flour, ¼ cup
- Large egg, 1Ground turkey, 1 lb.
- Shredded mozzarella cheese, ½ cup
- Garlic powder, ½ tsp.
- Olive oil, 2 tbsps.

Directions:

1. Set your medium size mixing bowl in a clean working surface

2. Stir together the egg, ground turkey, garlic powder, pepper, basil, salt, mozzarella, almond flour, and sun-dried tomatoes

3. Mold the mixture into12 even meatballs

4. Set the pan over medium-high heat to melt the oil

5. Fry the meatballs in the oil until browned

Nutrition:

Calories: 81, Fat: 5.5, Fiber: 0.1, Carbs: 0.5, Protein: 8.5

Parmesan Basil Dip

Prep Time + Cook Time: 5 minutes Servings 10

Ingredients:

- Chopped basil: 1 tbsp.
- Minced garlic: ½ tsp.
- Lemon juice: 1 tsp.
- Basil pesto: 2 tbsps.
- Avocado mayonnaise: 1 cup
- Grated parmesan cheese: 1 tbsp.

Directions:

1. Place all the ingredients for the dip in a medium bowl and stir until combined.

2. Divide dip evenly between small bowls and serve.

Nutrition:

calories: 100, fat: 4, fiber: 2, carbs: 5, protein: 3

Parmesan Chicken Wings

Prep Time + Cook Time: 34 minutes Serves: 6

Ingredients:

- Medium egg, 1 Black pepper
- Italian seasoning, ½ tsp.

- Butter, 2 tbsps.
- Salt

- Halved chicken wings, 6 lbs.
- Grated Parmesan cheese, ½ cup
- Red pepper flakes, ¼ tsp.
- Garlic powder, 1 tsp.

Directions:
1. Line the baking tray well and arrange the wings.
2. Set the oven for 17 minutes at 425ºF. Allow to bake.
3. Meanwhile, plug in and set the food processor in position.
4. Add in the Italian seasoning, butter, salt, garlic powder, cheese, red pepper flakes, egg, and pepper. Blend to mix well
5. Once the oven timer beeps, remove the wings and turn them.
6. Set the oven to broil
7. Allow the chicken wings to broil for 5 minutes
8. Remove the wings to coat with sauce over
9. Broil again for one minute.
10. Enjoy.

Nutrition:
Calories: 677, Fat: 50.1, Fiber: 0, Carbs: 0.1, Protein: 54.2

Parmesan Spinach Balls

Prep Time + Cook Time: 22 minutes Serves: 30

Ingredients:
- Whipping cream, 3 tbsps.
- Grated Parmesan cheese, 1/3 cup
- Medium eggs, 2
- Crumbled feta cheese, 1/3 c
- Almond flour, 1 cup
- Spinach, 16 oz.
- Salt
- Melted butter, 4 tbsps.
- Ground nutmeg, ¼ tsp.
- Black pepper
- Onion powder, 1 tbsp.
- Garlic powder, 1 tsp.

Directions:
1. Plug in and set your food processor in position
2. Add in feta cheese, spinach, nutmeg, eggs, whipping cream, garlic powder, almond flour, pepper, butter, onion, and salt.
3. Process until smooth.
4. Pour the mixture in a bowl to refrigerate in the freezer for 10 minutes.
5. Mold into 30 spinach balls and set them on a well-greased baking tray.
6. Set your oven for 12 minutes at 350ºF, allow to bake thoroughly.
7. Allow the balls to cool and enjoy

Nutrition:
Calories: 40, Fat: 3.5, Fiber: 0.5, Carbs: 1, Protein: 1.7

Pecan with Maple syrup Bars

Prep Time + Cook Time: 35 minutes Serves: 12

Ingredients:

- Maple syrup, ¼ cup
- Stevia, ¼ tsp.
- Crushed pecans, toasted, 2 cup
- Almond flour, 1 cup
- Coconut oil, ½ cup
- Flaxseed meal, ½ cup
- Shredded coconut, ½ cup

For the maple syrup:

- Vanilla extract, ½ tsp.Coconut oil, 2 ¼ tbsp.
- Xanthan gum, ¼ tsp.
- Erythritol, ¼ cup
- Water, ¾ cup
- Maple extract, 2 tsps.
- Butter, 1 tbsp.

Directions:

1. Microwave 2¼ tsp. coconut oil, butter, xanthan gum, in a heatproof bowl for about one minute.
2. Mix in maple, erythritol, vanilla extract, and water as you stir gently.
3. Microwave again for another one minute.
4. Meanwhile, combine coconut flour, flaxseed meal, and almond flour in another bowl as you stir gently.
5. Stir in the pecans then add coconut oil, ¼ cup maple syrup, and stevia.
6. Set the mixture in a baking sheet
7. Set your oven for 25 minutes at 350°F then allow to bake.
8. Allow cooling before slicing and serving.

Nutrition:

Calories: 313, Fat: 31.1, Fiber: 3, Carbs: 11.8, Protein: 2.7

Plum and Jalapeno Salad with Basil

Prep Time + Cook Time: 10 minutes Servings 6

Ingredients:

- Plums, chopped: 1 cup
- Chopped basil: 2 tbsps.
- Jalapeno pepper, chopped: 1
- Red onion, peeled and chopped: 2 tbsps.
- Lime juice: 2 tsps.
- Salt: ½ tsp.
- Ground black pepper: ¼ tsp.
- Stevia: 2 tbsps.
- Ground cumin: ½ tsp.
- Olive oil: 1 tsp.

Directions:

1. Place all the ingredients for the salad in a medium bowl and stir until combined.
2. Place salad bowl in a refrigerator for 1 hour or until chilled and then serve as an appetizer.

Nutrition:

calories: 137, fat: 2, fiber: 2, carbs: 7, protein: 5

Seasoned Easy Fried Cabbage

Prep Time + Cook Time: 25 minutes Servings: 4

Ingredients:

- green cabbage - 1½ pound, shredded
- ghee - 3.5 ounces
- A pinch of sweet paprika
- Salt and black pepper to the taste.

Directions:

1. Add heat to a pan containing ghee over medium-high heat source.
2. Then pour some cabbage to the pan and cook for 15 minutes stirring frequently.
3. Then sprinkle a pinch of salt, pepper and paprika.
4. Stir gently, cook for another minute
5. Divide into different plates
6. Now you can serve

Nutrition :

Calories:- 200; Fat : 4; Fiber : 2; Carbs : 3; Protein : 7

Sesame Zucchini Spread

Prep Time + Cook Time: 16 minutes Serves: 4

Ingredients:

- Lemon juice, ½ cup
- Veggie stock, 3 tbsps.
- Olive oil, ¼ cup
- Salt
- Chopped zucchinis, 4 cup
- Black pepper
- Minced garlic cloves, 4
- Sesame seeds paste, ¾ cup

Directions:

1. Set your pan over medium-high heat with half of the oil to cook the garlic and zucchini for two minutes
2. Stir in the seasonings and stock to cook for four minutes
3. Move the zucchinis to the blender with the remaining oil, lemon juice, and sesame seeds paste to process until smooth.
4. Set the mixture in bowls to serve
5. Enjoy.

Nutrition:

Calories: 140, Fat: 5, Fiber: 3, Carbs: 6, Protein: 7

Shrimp Salad with Tomato and Radish

Prep Time + Cook Time: 10 minutes Servings 8

Ingredients:

- Shrimp, cooked, peeled and deveined: 1 pound
- Medium white onion, chopped: ¼ cup
- Tomato, cubed: 1
- Radishes, chopped: 4
- Minced jalapeno: 1 ½ tsp.
- Salt: ¼ tsp.
- Ground black pepper: ¼ tsp.
- Lime juice: 2 tbsps.
- Chopped cilantro: ¼ cup

Directions:

1. Place all the ingredients for the salad in a medium bowl and stir until combined.
2. Serve salad straightaway as an appetizer.

Nutrition:
calories: 90, fat: 1, fiber: 1, carbs: 2, protein: 6

Shrimp wrapped with prosciutto

Prep Time + Cook Time: 30 minutes Serves: 16

Ingredients:

- Red wine, 1/3 cup Chopped mint, 1 tbsp.
- Erythritol, 2 tbsps.
- Cooked shrimp, 10 oz.
- Olive oil, 2 tbsps.
- Blackberries, 1/3 cup
- Sliced prosciutto 11

Directions:

1. Have the shrimp well wrapped with prosciutto slices.
2. Arrange the wrapped shrimp in a baking sheet then sprinkle with olive oil
3. Set the oven for 15 minutes at 425°F then allow to bake.
4. In the meantime, heat the mashed blackberries over medium heat.
5. Stir in erythritol, mint, and wine.
6. Set the shrimp on a serving plate, top the blackberries sauce and enjoy.

Nutrition:
Calories: 89, Fat: 5.5, Fiber: 0.2, Carbs: 1.1, Protein: 10.1

Simple Tomato Tarts

Prep Time + Cook Time: 1 hour 20 minutes Serves: 12

Ingredients:

- Salt
- Olive oil, ¼ cup
- Black pepper
- Sliced tomatoes, 2

For the base:

- Coconut flour, 2 tbsps.

- Psyllium husk, 1 tbsp.
- Butter, 5 tbsps.
- Almond flour, ½ cup
- Salt

For the filling:
- Sliced onion, 1Chopped thyme, 3 tsps.
- Olive oil, 2 tbsps.
- Minced garlic, 2 tbsps.
- Crumbled goats cheese, 3 oz.

Directions:
1. Season the tomato slices then align on a baking sheet then dazzle some olive oil. Set your oven for 40 minutes at 425°F.
2. Allow to bake. On the other hand, combine cold butter, coconut flour, pepper, almond flour, salt, psyllium husk in a food processor to achieve a dough.
3. Divide dough into silicone cupcake molds, press.
4. Set the oven for 20 minutes at 350°F then allow to bake.
5. Once fully baked, remove from oven and reserve.
6. Remove the tomato slices from the oven and allow them to cool
7. Top the tomato slices on the cupcakes
8. Meanwhile, quick fry the onions in a pan over medium-high heat, for about four minutes.
9. Stir in thyme and garlic, for about one minute. Spread mixture on top of tomato slices.
10. Sprinkle the goat cheese on top.
11. Set your oven for 5 minutes at 350°F
12. Bake until the cheese melts away

Nutrition:
Calories: 125, Fat: 11.7, Fiber: 3.1, Carbs: 5.1, Protein: 0.9

Special Tomato And Bocconcini: Side Dish

Prep Time + Cook Time: 6 minutes Servings: 4

Ingredients:
- baby bocconcini - 8 ounces, drain and torn
- basil leaves - 1 cup, roughly chopped.
- Tomatoes - 20 ounces, cut in wedges
- stevia - 1 tsp.
- garlic clove - 1, finely minced
- extra virgin olive oil - 2 tbsps.
- balsamic vinegar - 1½ tbsps.
- Salt and black pepper to the taste.

Directions:
1. Mix stevia with vinegar, garlic, oil, salt and pepper in a bowl and whisk very well.
2. Add bocconcini with tomato and basil to a clean salad and mix.
3. Add dressing, toss to keep well coated
4. Serve immediately as a keto side dish.

Nutrition :
Calories:- 100; Fat : 2; Fiber : 2; Carbs : 1; Protein : 9

Stir-Fried Queso

Prep Time + Cook Time: 20 minutes Serves: 6

Ingredients:

- Olive oil, 1 ½ tbsps.Cubed queso blanco, 5 oz.
- Chopped olives, 2 oz.
- Red pepper flakes

Directions:

1. Set up the pan to heat the oil over medium-high heat to cook the queso cubes
2. Turn the queso cubes using a spatula then sprinkle with olives
3. Allow the cubes to cook more for 5 minutes then turn again to sprinkle with red pepper flake.
4. Allow to cook to a crispy texture.
5. Turn the cubes again to cook on the other side
6. Once cooked, set on the chopping board then slice into small pieces
7. Enjoy.

Nutrition:

Calories: 152, Fat: 15.8, Fiber: 0.3, Carbs: 0.6, Protein: 3.2

Tasty Avocado Spread

Prep Time + Cook Time: 1 minute Serves: 4

Ingredients:

- Stevia, ¼ tsp.
- Halved avocados, 2
- Juice of 2 limes
- Coconut milk, 1 cup
- Chopped cilantro, ½ cup
- Zest of 2 limes

Directions:

1. Plug and switch on the blender in position.
2. Add in the stevia, avocados, lime juice, coconut milk, and cilantro, and lime zest to process until smooth.
3. Set into serving bowls to enjoy

Nutrition:

Calories: 190, Fat: 6, Fiber: 2, Carbs: 9, Protein: 6

Chapter 5 Seafood & Fish Recipes

Arugula Cod

Prep Time + Cook Time: 32 minutes Servings: 1

Ingredients:

- Cod fillets-2
- Olive oil-1 tbsp.
- Salt and ground black pepper-to taste
- Lemon-1 (juiced)
- Arugula-3 cups
- Black olives-1/2 cup (pitted and sliced)
- Capers-2 tbsps.
- Garlic clove-1 (peeled and chopped)

Directions:

1. Set the fish fillets in a heatproof dish, season with salt, pepper.
2. Pour the oil and lemon juice, toss to coat, place in an oven at 450°F.
3. Bake for 20 minutes.
4. In a food processor, add the arugula with salt, pepper, capers, olives, garlic
5. Blend well.
6. Settle the fish on plates, top with arugula tapenade, and serve.

Nutrition:
Calories: 294, Fat: 12.9, Fiber: 2.3, Carbs: 5.8, Protein: 41.4

Baked Calamari Mix with Sauce

Prep Time + Cook Time: 30 minutes Servings: 1

Ingredients:

- Calamari - 16 ounces, cut into medium rings
- egg - 1
- coconut flour - 3 tbsps.
- olive oil - 1 tbsp.
- avocado - 2 tbsps., chopped
- tomato paste - 1 tsp.
- avocado mayonnaise - 1 tbsp.
- lemon juice - 1 tsp.
- Salt and black pepper to the taste
- turmeric powder - ½ tsp.

Directions:

1. Whisk the egg using the oil in a clean bowl.
2. Then add calamari rings and toss to make it well coated.
3. Mix the flour with salt, pepper, and turmeric in another bowl and stir gently.
4. Dredge calamari rings into the mix.
5. Then place them on a lined baking sheet, and transfer to an oven at 400 0F.
6. Bake for about 10 minutes, then flip to the other side and bake for another 10 minutes.
7. Get another bowl and mix avocado with mayo, tomato paste, lemon juice,

salt, and pepper together. Stir gently and well.

8. Divide the baked calamari into different plates

9. Then serve with the sauce as topping.

Nutrition:

calories: 268, fat: 13, fiber: 3, carbs: 10, protein: 15

Baked Eggplant, Sardines and Artichokes Salad

Prep Time + Cook Time: 30 minutes Servings: 4

Ingredients:

- canned sardines - 7 ounces, drained and cut into chunks
- olive oil - 4 tbsps.
- eggplant - 1, cubed
- A pinch of salt and black pepper
- canned artichoke hearts - 2 ounces, drained
- baby spinach - 4 ounces
- cherry tomatoes - 10, halved
- capers - 2 tbsps.
- balsamic vinegar - 1 tbsp.

Directions:

1. Spread the eggplant on a lined baking sheet.

2. Drizzle 1/2 of the oil over the eggplant.
3. Use salt and pepper as seasoning.
4. Then move to an oven set at a temperature of 400 0F for about 20 minutes.
5. Mix the sardines with the baked eggplant, the rest of the oil, artichokes, spinach, tomatoes, capers and vinegar in a clean bowl.
6. Toss to make sure it is coated.
7. Now you can serve.

Nutrition:

calories: 231, fat: 4, fiber: 7, carbs: 15, protein: 9

Baked Fish with Mushrooms

Prep Time + Cook Time: 40 minutes Servings: 2

Ingredients:

- yellow onions - 2, chopped
- medium cod fillets - 2, boneless
- Parsley - 1 tbsp., chopped
- white mushrooms - 8 ounces, sliced
- thyme - 1 tsp., dried
- olive oil - 1 tbsp.
- A pinch of salt and black pepper

Directions:

1. Place the fish in a clean baking dish.

2. Follow this by adding onions, parsley, mushrooms, thyme, oil, salt, and pepper.
3. Toss to ensure it is properly coated.
4. Move to an oven set at 375 0F.
5. Time the oven at 30 minutes.
6. Cut into different plates and serve.

Nutrition:

calories: 280, fat: 3, fiber: 1, carbs: 4, protein: 17

Balsamic Calamari Salad

Prep Time + Cook Time: 19 minutes Servings: 8

Ingredients:

- 2 long red chilies, diced
- 2 small red chilies, diced
- 2 garlic cloves, peeled and minced
- 3 green onions, chopped
- 1 tbsp. balsamic vinegar
- Salt and black pepper ground, to taste
- Juice of 1 lemon
- 6 lbs. calamari hoods, tentacles set aside
- 3. 5 oz. olive oil
- 3 oz. arugula, to serve

Directions:

1. Toss green onions with vinegar, red chilies, salt, pepper, lemon juice, garlic, and half of the olive oil in a bowl.

2. Mix tentacles and calamari in another bowl and toss them with salt, pepper and remaining olive oil.
3. Grill the seasoned seafood in a preheated grill on medium high heat for 2 minutes per side.
4. Add the grilled seafood to the green onions mixture and set them aside for 30 minutes.
5. To serve, divide the arugula on the serving plates.
6. Top it with grilled seafood and serve fresh.

Nutrition:

Calories: 1288, Fat: 72.5g, Fiber: 4.8g, Carbs: 78.5g, Protein: 73g

Butter Glazed Mussels

Prep Time + Cook Time: 10 minutes Servings: 4

Ingredients:

- 1 tbsp. butter
- A splash of lemon juice
- 2 lb. mussels, debearded and scrubbed
- 2 garlic cloves, peeled and minced

Directions:

1. To cook mussels, first, pour water into a medium-sized cooking pot.
2. Place mussels in the water and let them cook for 5 minutes.

3. Remove the mussels from the water and place them in a suitable bowl.
4. Discard any of the unopened mussels.
5. Mix melted butter with lemon juice and minced garlic in a small bowl.
6. Pour this butter mixture over the cooked mussels.
7. Serve right away.

Nutrition:

Calories: 224, Fat: 8g, Fiber: 0.1, Carbs: 9g, Protein: 27.2g

Cake up Tuna

Prep Time + Cook Time: 24 minutes Servings: 11

Ingredients:

- Canned tuna-15 ounces (drained well and flaked)
- Eggs-3
- Dried dill-1/2 tsp.
- Dried parsley-1 tsp.
- Onion-1/2 cup (chopped)
- Garlic powder-1 Tsp.
- Salt and ground black pepper to taste
- Oil-for frying

Directions:

1. Combine tuna with salt, pepper, dill, parsley, onion, garlic powder, and eggs.
2. Shake well and make the tuna cakes shape.
3. Keep them on a plate after preparation.
4. Warm up a pan with oil over medium-high heat.
5. Toss in the tuna cakes.
6. Cook for 5 minutes on each side.
7. Distribute on plates and serve.

Nutrition:

Calories: 84, Fat: 4, Fiber: 0.1, Carbs: 0.6, Protein: 10.8

Caper Sauce Salmon

Prep Time + Cook Time: 26 minutes Servings: 4

Ingredients:

- Salmon fillets-3
- Salt and ground black pepper-to taste
- Olive oil-1 tbsp.
- Italian seasoning-1 tbsp.
- Capers-2 tbsps.
- Lemon juice-3 tbsps.
- Garlic cloves-4 (peeled and minced)
- Butter-2 tbsps.

Directions:

1. Warm a pan with olive oil over medium heat.
2. Mix the fish fillets skin side up, season with salt, pepper, and Italian seasoning, cook for 2 minutes, flip, and cook for 2 minutes.
3. Then gradually put off heat, cover pan, and set aside for 15 minutes.
4. Slide in the fish to a plate, and leave them aside.
5. Warm up the same pan over medium heat, add capers, lemon juice, and garlic, stir, and cook for 2 minutes.
6. Keeping the pan off the heat, add the butter, and stir well.
7. Again shift the fish to pan, and toss to coat with the sauce.
8. Present on plates and serve.

Nutrition:

Calories: 369, Fat: 24.9, Fiber: 0.3, Carbs: 2.4, Protein: 35.

Catfish with Okra Mix

Prep Time + Cook Time: 40 minutes Servings: 4

Ingredients:

- Okra - 2 cups, sliced
- olive oil - 3 tbsps.
- yellow onion - 1, chopped
- catfish fillets - 1 pound, boneless
- Cajun seasoning - 2 tsps.
- A pinch of salt and black pepper

Directions:

1. Spread the okra and onion on a lined baking sheet, then season with a pinch of salt and pepper.
2. Follow this by drizzling about 1 tbsp. olive oil and sprinkle 1 tsp. Cajun seasoning.
3. Then toss gently to ensure it is coated.
4. Place in the oven set at 450 0F and bake for 20 minutes.
5. Season the fish with salt, pepper, and the remaining Cajun seasoning and drizzle the rest of the oil.
6. Place a pan over medium-high heat source, then add the fish to the pan, and cook for 5 minutes. Cook each side of the fish.
7. Then divide into different plates.
8. Serve with side okra mix.

Nutrition:

calories: 231, fat: 4, fiber: 7, carbs: 11, protein: 8

Citrus Rich Octopus Salad

Prep Time + Cook Time: 50 minutes Servings: 2

Ingredients:

- 3 oz. olive oil
- Juice of 1 lemon
- 21 oz. octopus, rinsed
- 4 celery stalks, roughly chopped
- Salt and black pepper ground, to taste
- 4 tbsp. fresh parsley, roughly chopped

Directions:

1. Place the octopus in a medium to a large pot and pour in enough water to cover it.
2. Cover the octopus with a lid and let it boil then cook for 40 minutes on medium heat.
3. Drain the octopus and keep it aside to cool down.
4. Slice the octopus into pieces then transfer it to a salad bowl.
5. Add parsley, celery stalks, lemon juice, and oil.
6. Mix well and adjust seasoning with salt and pepper.
7. Serve fresh and devour.

Nutrition:

Calories: 839, Fat: 46g, Fiber: 1.1g, Carbs: 15.6g, Protein: 89.3g

Cod La Pan–roasted

Prep Time + Cook Time: 30 minutes Servings: 3

Ingredients:

- Cod-1 pound (cut into medium–sized pieces)
- Salt and ground black pepper-to taste
- Green onions-2 (chopped)
- Garlic cloves-3 (peeled and minced)
- Soy sauce-3 Tbsp.
- Fish stock-1 cup
- Balsamic vinegar-1 Tbsp.
- Fresh ginger-1 Tbsp. (grated)
- Red chili flakes-1/2 Tsp.

Directions:

1. Warm up a pan over medium-high heat, add fish pieces.
2. Brown on each side.
3. Mix in the garlic, green onions, salt, pepper, soy sauce, fish stock, vinegar, chili pepper, ginger, and stir.
4. Cover, reduce heat and cook for 20 minutes.
5. Distribute on plates and serve.

Nutrition:

Calories: 131, Fat: 1, Fiber: 0.4, Carbs: 2.2, Protein: 26.9

Coriander Shrimp with Salad

Prep Time + Cook Time: 21 minutes Servings: 4

Ingredients:

- Shrimp - 2 pounds, peeled and deveined
- olive oil - 4 tbsps.
- Onions - 4, chopped
- A pinch of salt and black pepper
- Coriander - 2 tsp., ground
- curry powder - 1 tsp.
- Juice of lemon - 1

Directions:

1. Heat up a pan containing oil over medium-high heat source.
2. Pour some onions and the coriander into the pan, and stir gently.
3. Cook for about 5 minutes.
4. Finally add salt, pepper, curry, lemon juice and shrimp to the mixture.
5. Stir gently, then cook for 6 more minutes.
6. Divide into different plates
7. Serve with side salad.

Nutrition:

calories: 221, fat: 4, fiber: 1, carbs: 11, protein: 15

Crab Cakes with Sauce

Prep Time + Cook Time: 17 minutes Servings: 8

Ingredients:

- crab meat - 1 cup
- parsley - 2 tbsps., chopped
- Italian seasoning - 2 tbsps.
- mustard - 2 tsps.
- egg - 1, whisked
- lemon juice - 1 tbsps.
- olive oil - 2 tbsps.
- coconut flour - 1 and ½ tbsps.

For the sauce:

- olive oil - 1 tbsps.
- roasted red peppers - ¼ cup, chopped
- lemon juice - 1 tbsp.

Directions:

1. Mix crabmeat with the seasoning, parsley, mustard, egg, 1 tbsp. lemon juice and coconut flour in a clean bowl and stir gently.
2. Then proceed by shaping medium cakes out of this mix.
3. Place a pan containing 2 tbsps. of oil on a medium-high heat source.
4. Then add crab cakes, cook for about 3 minutes on each side and divide into different plates.
5. Mix olive oil with red pepper and 1 tbsp. lemon juice in a food processor.
6. Then blend and spread over the crab cakes. Now you can serve.

Nutrition:

calories: 230, fat: 4, fiber: 3, carbs: 5, protein: 14

Cream Cheese Salmon Sushi

Prep Time + Cook Time: 10 minutes Servings: 12

Ingredients:

- 6 oz. smoked salmon, sliced
- 4 oz. cream cheese
- 2 nori sheets
- 1 small avocado, pitted, peeled, and diced
- 1 tsp. wasabi paste
- 1 cucumber, sliced
- Pickled ginger, to serve

Directions:

1. Spread both the nori sheets on the bamboo mat.
2. Place half of the salmon, cucumber, and avocado at the center of each nori sheet.
3. Mix wasabi pasta with cream cheese and mix well until combined.
4. Divide this mixture over the salmon stuffing.
5. Roll each of the nori sheets into a sushi roll.
6. Slice them into 6 equal size pieces.
7. Serve fresh with ginger pickle.

Nutrition:

Calories: 89, Fat: 7.2g, Fiber: 1.4g, Carbs: 2.6g, Protein: 4g

Creamy Clam Chowder Luncheon

Prep Time + Cook Time: 12 minutes Servings: 4

Ingredients:

- 2 cups chicken stock
- 1 tsp. ground thyme
- 14 oz. canned baby clams
- 1 cup celery stalks, roughly chopped
- 2 cups heavy cream
- Salt and black pepper ground, to taste
- 1 cup onion, peeled and roughly chopped
- 12 bacon slices, roughly chopped

Directions:

1. Add bacon slices to a heated skillet and sauté until crispy and brown.
2. Transfer the sautéed bacon to the bowl while leaving the bacon greased in the skillet.
3. Add onion and celery to the same skillet and stir cook for 5 minutes.
4. Transfer this mixture to a slow cooker along with all the remaining ingredients.
5. Cover the slow cooker and set the cooking time to 2 hours with high temperature.
6. Once cooked, serve warm.

Nutrition:
Calories: 583, Fat: 46.6g, Fiber: 1.4g, Carbs: 17.2g, Protein: 23.8g

Creamy Salmon With Tinge

Prep Time + Cook Time: 25 minutes Servings: 3

Ingredients:

- Salmon fillets-4
- Olive oil-A drizzle
- Salt and ground black pepper to taste
- Parmesan cheese-1/3 cup (grated)
- Mustard-1 1/2 tsp.
- Sour cream-1/2 cup

Directions:

1. Keep the salmon on a lined baking sheet.
2. Season with salt, and pepper.
3. Pour the oil.
4. Take a bowl, mix sour cream with Parmesan cheese, mustard, salt, pepper, and stir well.
5. Place the sour cream mixture over the salmon.
6. Settle in an oven at 350°F, and bake for 15 minutes.
7. Divide on plates and serve.

Nutrition:
Calories: 319, Fat: 18.5, Fiber: 0, Carbs: 1.5, Protein: 37.7

Crispy Calamari Rings

Prep Time + Cook Time: 30 minutes Servings: 2

Ingredients:

- 1 egg, whisked
- 2 tbsp. coconut flour
- 1 squid, cut into medium rings
- A pinch of cayenne pepper
- Salt and black pepper ground, to taste
- Coconut oil for frying
- 1 tbsp. lemon juice
- 4 tbsp. mayonnaise
- 1 tsp. sriracha sauce

Directions:

1. Toss the squid rings with salt, cayenne pepper and black pepper in a large bowl.
2. Whisk egg with coconut flour, salt, and pepper in another bowl.
3. Add coconut oil to a pan for frying and let it heat on medium heat.
4. Take one ring at a time and coat it well with the flour batter.
5. Place the coated rings in the hot oil and cook until golden brown from both sides.
6. Layer a plate with a paper towel and place the fried rings over it.
7. Mix mayonnaise with sriracha and lemon juice in a serving bowl.
8. Serve the fried squid rings with the mayo sauce.
9. Enjoy fresh.

Nutrition:

Calories: 620, Fat: 42.9g, Fiber: 0.3g, Carbs: 15.7g, Protein: 42.9g

Crusted Coconut Salmon Nuggets

Prep Time + Cook Time: 30 minutes Servings: 6

Ingredients:

- 1 egg
- 1 tbsp. water
- 3 tbsp. coconut oil
- 1¼ cups coconut, desiccated, and unsweetened
- Salt and black pepper ground, to taste
- 1 lb. salmon, skinless and cubed
- ⅓ cup coconut flour

Sauce:

- ¼ cup balsamic vinegar
- ¾ cup of water
- ¼ tsp. agar
- ½ cup stevia
- 4 red chili peppers, finely chopped
- 3 garlic cloves, peeled and finely chopped
- A pinch of salt

Directions:

1. Whisk egg with 1 tbsp. water in one bowl and mix flour with salt and pepper in another.
2. Spread the coconut shred in another shallow bowl.

3. Add coconut oil to a shallow pan and heat it over medium heat.

4. First, dredge each of the salmon cubes through the flour mixture.

5. Then dip the cubes in the egg and finally coat with the coconut shreds.

6. Sear these coated salmon chunks in the heated oil for 3 minutes per side.

7. Transfer the chunks to a plate lined with a paper towel to absorb excess oil.

8. Add about a ¾ cup of water to a saucepan and heat it.

9. Drizzle agar in the water and let it cook to a boil.

10. Allow the agar to cook for 3 minutes then turn off the heat.

11. Blend garlic with stevia, salt, vinegar and chilies in a blender until smooth.

12. Pour this sauce into the small size pan and let it heat on medium heat.

13. Gently stir the agar mixture and stir cook for 3 minutes.

14. Pour this sauce over the seared salmon bites.

15. Enjoy with chili sauce.

Nutrition:

Calories: 342, Fat: 25.8g, Fiber: 6.8g, Carbs: 11.7g, Protein: 18.3g

Delicious Cod Salad

Prep Time + Cook Time: 2 hours 30 minutes Servings: 8

Ingredients:

- Salt cod - 2 pounds.
- Jarred pimiento peppers; chopped - 2 cups.
- Parsley; chopped - 1 cup.
- kalamata olives; pitted and chopped - 1 cup.
- Garlic cloves; minced - 4
- Celery ribs; chopped - 2
- Capers - 6 tbsps..
- Olive oil - ¾ cup.
- Lemon juice - 2 lemons.
- Red chili flakes - ½ tsp..
- Escarole head; leaves separated - 1
- Salt and black pepper to the taste.

Directions:

1. In a pot, add cod and water to cover and bring it to a boil over medium-high heat.

2. Let it boil for 20 minutes and drain the water. Cut cod in fine chunks.

3. Take a bowl and put cod in it.

4. Toss it well to coat by adding peppers, parsley, olives, capers, celery, garlic, lemon juice, salt, pepper, olive oil and chilli flakes.

5. Arrange escarole leaves on a platter and place cod salad on it and serve.

Nutrition :

Calories:- 240; Fat : 4; Fiber : 2; Carbs : 6; Protein : 9

Delicious Monk fish with Sauce

Prep Time + Cook Time: 30 minutes Servings: 4

Ingredients:

- Monk fish fillets - 1 and ½ pounds, boneless
- ghee - ¾ cup, melted
- veggie stock - 3 tbsps.
- lemon juice - 2 tsps.
- A pinch of salt and black pepper
- Parsley - ½ tsp., dried

Directions:

1. Mix the melted ghee with the stock, lemon juice, salt, pepper, and parsley in a bowl and whisk well.
2. Place the monk fish fillets in a baking dish.
3. Make sure to drizzle the ghee mix all over, then proceed by rubbing for a while.
4. Move them to a preheated broiler over medium-high heat and bake for about 20 minutes.
5. Divide the fish into different plates.
6. Finally, drizzle the already made sauce from the dish all over.
7. Now you can serve
8. Enjoy!

Nutrition:

calories: 300, fat: 12, fiber: 1, carbs: 4, protein: 18

Fish Ginger Soup

Prep Time + Cook Time: 46 minutes Servings: 2

Ingredients:

- Yellow onion, chopped-½
- White fish, skinless, boneless and roughly cubed -½ lb.
- Veggie stock -5 cups
- Olive oil -½ tbsp
- Salt and black pepper -to taste
- Ginger, grated -1 tbsp

Directions:

1. Add oil to a pot and place it over medium heat.
2. Toss in onion and sauté for 6 minutes.
3. Stir in ginger, salt, water, stock, and pepper.
4. Cook this mixture for 20 minutes on a simmer.
5. Place the fish in the pot and cook for another 10 minutes.
6. Serve warm.
7. Enjoy.

Nutrition:

Calories: 200, Fat: 6, Fiber: 6, Carbs: 9, Protein: 11

Flounder with Shrimp Etouffee

Prep Time + Cook Time: 35 minutes Servings: 4

Ingredients:

Seasoning:

- 1 tsp. dried oregano
- A pinch of cinnamon ground
- ¼ tsp. ground nutmeg
- ½ tsp. allspice
- ¼ tsp. ground cloves

Etouffee:

- 2 cups chicken stock
- 2 tbsp. coconut flour
- 1 tbsp. butter
- 8 oz. bacon, sliced
- 1 green bell pepper, seeded and diced
- 1 celery stalk, diced
- 1 tomato, cored and diced
- 2 shallots, peeled and roughly chopped
- 8 oz. shrimp, peeled, deveined, and diced
- 4 garlic cloves, peeled and minced
- 1 tbsp. coconut milk
- ½ cup fresh parsley, finely chopped

Flounder:

- 2 tbsp. butter
- 4 flounder fillets

Directions:

1. Add and mix all the seasoning ingredients in a small bowl.
2. Keep 2 tbsps. of this mixture aside and rub the rest on the flounder.
3. Preheat a pan and sauté bacon in it for 6 minutes.
4. Stir in bell pepper, celery, 1 tbsp. butter, and shallots.
5. Sauté for 4 minutes then add garlic and tomato.
6. Stir cook for another 4 minutes.
7. Add coconut flour and the reserved spice mixture.
8. Cook this mixture for 2 minutes then pour in chicken stock.
9. Allow the stock mixture to simmer on medium heat.
10. Add 2 tbsp. of butter to a skillet and set it over medium heat.
11. Place the seasoned fish in the melted butter.
12. Sear the fish for 2 minutes per side.
13. Transfer the cooked fish to the serving plates.
14. Add shrimp, salt, pepper, parsley and coconut milk to the stock mixture.
15. Allow the shrimp to cook for another 2 minutes then pour this sauce over the fish.
16. Enjoy.

Nutrition:

Calories: 623, Fat: 31.9g, Fiber: 3.6g, Carbs: 13.2g, Protein: 67.3g

Fresh Catfish Mix with Pineapple Salsa

Prep Time + Cook Time: 20 minutes Servings: 4

Ingredients:

- Scallions - ¼ cup, chopped
- Cilantro - 2 tbsps., chopped
- A pinch of salt and black pepper
- lime juice - 3 tbsps.
- jalapeno - 2 tbsps., chopped
- olive oil - 2 tbsps.
- catfish fillets - 1 pound, boneless

Directions:

1. Mix the scallions with the cilantro, salt, pepper, jalapeno, lime juice and half of the oil in a clean bowl and toss.
2. Rub the catfish with the remaining oil and sprinkle some salt and pepper as seasoning.
3. Add heat to a pan using medium-high source, then add the fish fillets, and cook them for 5 minutes on each side.
4. Divide into different plates
5. Finally, serve with the pineapple salsa.

Nutrition:

calories: 231, fat: 3, fiber: 7, carbs: 13, protein: 8

Freshly Made Calamari Salad

Prep Time + Cook Time: 34 minutes Servings: 4

Ingredients:

- Calamari hoods; tentacles reserved - 6 pounds.
- Long red chilies; chopped - 2
- Green onions; chopped - 3
- Small red chilies; chopped - 2
- Garlic cloves; minced - 2
- Balsamic vinegar - 1 tbsp..
- Lemon juice - 1 lemon.
- Olive oil - 5 ounces.
- Rocket for serving - 3 ounces.
- Salt and black pepper to the taste.

Directions:

1. Add long red chillies with small red chillies, green onions, vinegar, half of the oil, garlic, salt, pepper and lemon juice in a bowl and stir well.
2. Season calamari and tentacle with some salt and pepper in a bowl and drizzle it with rest of the oil and give it a toss.
3. Put this on preheated grill over medium-high heat and let it cook for 2 minutes on each side.
4. Once cooked, transfer to the bowl of chilli marinade.
5. Massage calamari and tentacle with the marinade extremely well and leave it aside for 30 minutes.
6. On different plates, place rocket and top it with calamari and its marinade and serve immediately.

Nutrition :

Calories:- 200; Fat : 4; Fiber : 2; Carbs : 2; Protein : 7

Greek Sardine Mix Salad

Prep Time + Cook Time: 10 minutes Servings: 3

Ingredients:

- canned sardines - 7 ounces; drained and cut into chunks
- black olives - 1 tbsp., pitted and sliced
- cherry tomatoes - 1 cup, halved
- feta cheese - 1 tbsp., cubed
- small cucumber - 1, sliced
- white vinegar - 1 tsp.
- A pinch of salt and black pepper
- olive oil - 2 tbsps.

Directions:

1. Mix the sardines with the black olives, cherry tomatoes, cheese, cucumber, vinegar.
2. Also add salt, pepper and the oil in a bowl.
3. Then toss to make sure it is well coated.
4. Now you can serve.

Nutrition:

calories: 200, fat: 4, fiber: 4, carbs: 11, protein: 8

Grilled Lemon Catfish

Prep Time + Cook Time: 30 minutes Servings: 4

Ingredients:

- catfish fillets - 4, boneless
- black peppercorns - 2 tsps., crushed
- lemon - 1, cut into wedges
- olive oil - 2 tbsps.
- lemon juice - 2 tbsps.
- A pinch of salt and black pepper

Directions:

1. Mix the lemon juice with the peppercorns, oil, salt, and pepper in a clean big bowl and whisk well.
2. Then add the fish fillets and toss to make sure it is coated.
3. Cover the top and put in the fridge. Keep in the fridge for about 10 minutes.
4. Place the fish in a pee-heated grill and cook them for 10 minutes on each side.
5. Divide into different plates, then serve with some side lemon wedges.

Nutrition:

calories: 214, fat: 4, fiber: 4, carbs: 12, protein: 9

Halibut With Simple Baking

Prep Time + Cook Time: 22 minutes Servings: 3

Ingredients:

- Parmesan cheese-1/2 (grated)
- Butter-1/4 cup
- Mayonnaise-1/4 cup
- Green onions-2 tbsps. (chopped)
- Garlic cloves-6 (peeled and minced)
- Tabasco sauce-A dash
- Halibut fillets-4
- Salt and ground black pepper-to taste
- Lemon-1/2 (juice)

Directions:

1. Marinate halibut with salt, pepper, and some of the lemon juice.
2. Keep it in a baking dish and cook in the oven at 450°F for 6 minutes.
3. Warm up a pan with butter over medium heat.
4. Mix in the Parmesan cheese, mayonnaise, green onions, Tabasco sauce, garlic, remaining lemon juice, and stir well.
5. Take out the fish from the oven, drizzle cheese sauce all over.
6. Flip the oven to broil and broil the fish for 3 minutes.
7. Divide on plates and serve.

Nutrition:

Calories: 530, Fat: 26.2, Fiber: 0.2, Carbs: 5.7, Protein: 65.6

Her bed Catfish with Salad

Prep Time + Cook Time: 25 minutes Servings: 2

Ingredients:

- catfish fillets - 2, boneless
- lemon juice - 1 tsp.
- hot paprika - 1 and ½ tsps.
- olive oil - 1 tsp.
- tarragon - ½ tsp., dried
- basil - ½ tsp., dried
- A pinch of salt and black pepper

Directions:

1. Place the catfish in a baking dish neatly, then drizzle the lemon juice and the olive oil.
2. Continue by rubbing the fillets.
3. Sprinkle a pinch of salt, pepper, paprika, tarragon, and basil as seasoning.
4. Then move to an oven set at 350 0F for about 15 minutes.
5. Divide the fish into different plates
6. Serve with side salad.

Nutrition:

calories: 261, fat: 12, fiber: 2, carbs: 4, protein: 17

Hot Balsamic Salmon Mix

Prep Time + Cook Time: 30 minutes Servings: 2

Ingredients:

- Ginger - ½ tsp., grated
- onion powder - 1 tsp.
- A pinch of salt and black pepper
- balsamic vinegar - 1 tbsp.
- medium salmon fillets - 2, boneless

Directions:

1. Use salmon with garlic powder as seasoning. Add onion powder and black pepper too and rub well.
2. Put the salmon fillets in a baking dish.
3. Then add ginger, onion powder, salt, pepper, and vinegar,
4. Toss them for a little while and move them into an oven set at 375 °F, bake for about 20 minutes.
5. Divide into different plates and serve.

Nutrition:
calories: 240, fat: 3, fiber: 3, carbs: 7, protein: 18

Hot Cod Pie

Prep Time + Cook Time: 30 minutes Servings: 4

Ingredients:

- cod fillets - 1 pound; skinless, boneless and cubed
- parsley - 2 tbsps., chopped
- lemon juice - 2 tsps.
- eggs - 2, whisked
- flax meal - ¼ cup
- ghee - 2 ounces, melted
- almond milk - ½ pint
- A pinch of salt and black pepper

Directions:

1. Mix fish with flax meal, lemon juice, parsley and pepper in a clean bowl and stir well.
2. Place a pan containing the ghee with them on a medium-high heat source and stir gently.
3. Cook for about 2-3 minutes, then move to a bowl and mix with the egg and fish.
4. Toss to ensure it is well coated.
5. Empty the entire content into a greased ramekin.
6. Transfer to an oven and cook at 425 °F for about 15 minutes.

Nutrition:
calories: 227, fat: 4, fiber: 7, carbs: 11, protein: 14

Hot Sardine Soup

Prep Time + Cook Time: 30 minutes Servings: 4

Ingredients:

- chicken stock - ½ quart
- Kaffir lime leaves - 3
- shallots - 3, chopped
- chili flakes - ½ tsp.
- lemongrass stalks - 2, crushed
- Lime juice: 2
- canned tomatoes - 12 ounces, chopped
- A handful mint, chopped

- canned sardines - 14 ounces, drained

Directions:

1. Add the stock to a pot, then add lime leaves, shallots, chili flakes, and lemongrass, and stir gently.
2. Move to a boil over medium heat and cook for about 15 minutes.
3. Remove the lime leaves and lemongrass, then add lime juice, tomatoes, sardines, and mint.
4. Stir the mixture gently and cook for another 5 minutes.
5. Then divide into different bowls and serve.

Nutrition:

calories: 201, fat: 3, fiber: 6, carbs: 14, protein: 9

Hot Shrimp with Pepper Mix

Prep Time + Cook Time: 40 minutes Servings: 4

Ingredients:

- Shrimp - 1 pound, peeled and deveined
- garlic powder - 1 tbsp.
- red bell peppers - 1 cup, chopped
- A pinch of salt and black pepper

Directions:

1. Place the shrimp in a baking dish, and add bell peppers, garlic powder, as well as salt and pepper.
2. Toss well to make sure it is coated, place in the oven set at 375 °F for 30 minutes.
3. Divide them to different plates
4. Serve when the food is still warm.
5. Enjoy!

Nutrition:

calories: 192, fat: 5, fiber: 1, carbs: 6, protein: 17

Italian Style Clams Delight

Prep Time + Cook Time: 20 minutes Servings: 6

Ingredients:

- Clams; scrubbed - 36
- Ghee - ½ cup.
- Garlic cloves; minced - 5
- Red pepper flakes; crushed - 1 tsp..
- Oregano; dried - 1 tbsp..
- White wine - 2 cups.
- Parsley; chopped - 1 tsp..

Directions:

1. Take a pan and heat some ghee over medium high heat and stir fry garlic for 1 minute.
2. Add parsley, oregano, wine and pepper flakes to the pan and stir well.
3. Finally, add clams and give it a stir. Cover the pan and cook for 10 minutes.
4. Discard any unopened clams and scoop out clams and their mix into a bowl and serve immediately.

Nutrition :

Calories:- 224; Fat : 15; Fiber : 2; Carbs : 3; Protein : 4

Juicy Salmon Skewers

Prep Time + Cook Time: 20 minutes Servings: 2

Ingredients:

- ¼ cup balsamic vinegar
- 2 lemons, sliced
- 1 lb. wild salmon, skinless and cubed
- 1 tsp. coconut oil
- ¼ cup lemon juice
- ⅓ cup sugar-free lemon marmalade

Directions:

1. Place a cooking pot on medium heat.
2. Add marmalade, vinegar, and lemon juice to the pot. Let this mixture cook for 1 minute on low temperature.
3. Once the mixture starts to thickens remove it from the heat.
4. Thread the salmon cubes and lemon slices on the skewers alternatively.
5. Brush each of the pieces with prepare lemon glaze.
6. Preheat a cooking grill and grease it grilling grates with coconut oil.
7. Place the salmon skewers in the grill and cook them for 4 minutes per side.
8. Keep basting the skewers with the remaining lemon glaze.
9. Devour.

Nutrition:

Calories: 332, Fat: 13.3g, Fiber: 2.5g, Carbs: 21.3g, Protein: 34.1g

Kale and Salmon Salad

Prep Time + Cook Time: 20 minutes Serves: 4

Ingredients:

- Skinless canned salmon, 12 oz.
- Water, ½ cup
- Trimmed beets, 4
- Apple vinegar, 2/3 cup + 2 tbsps.
- Olive oil, 2 tbsps.
- Black pepper
- Sliced red onion, 1/3 cup
- Stemmed kale, 6 cup
- Salt

Directions:

1. Set the pan on fire with water and 2/3 cup vinegar.
2. Allow to boil over medium heat, add the onion to cook for one minute
3. Set aside for 10 minutes then drain
4. Set a medium mixing bowl in a clean working surface to mix the kale with marinated onion and salmon.
5. Set another bowl in place to whisk together the remaining vinegar with seasonings and vinegar.
6. Pour the mixture over the salad to coat then serve.

Nutrition:

Calories: 230, Fat: 3, Fiber: 5, Carbs: 6, Protein: 12

Lobster with Avocado Mix

Prep Time + Cook Time: 10 minutes Servings: 4

Ingredients:

- Avocado - 2 cup, peeled, pitted and cubed
- Cucumber - 1 cup, chopped
- lobster tail - 2 cups, cooked and chopped
- parsley - 2 tsps., chopped
- lime juice - 1 tbsp.
- olive oil - 1 tbsp.
- A pinch of salt and black pepper

Directions:

1. Mix lobster tails with avocado, cucumber, parsley, salt, pepper, oil and lime juice in a clean bowl.
2. Toss a bit. Then serve.

Nutrition:

calories: 200, fat: 5, fiber: 4, carbs: 6, protein: 11

Luscious Herbed Clams

Prep Time + Cook Time: 20 minutes Servings: 6

Ingredients:

- 1 tbsp. dried oregano
- ½ cup butter
- 2 cups white wine
- 1 tsp. red pepper flakes
- 1 tsp. fresh parsley, roughly chopped
- 36 clams, scrubbed
- 5 garlic cloves, peeled and minced

Directions:

1. Let the butter melt in a skillet over medium heat.
2. Add garlic and stir cook it for 1 minute.
3. Stir in pepper flakes, wine, parsley, and oregano.
4. Mix well then place the clams in the pan.
5. Let them cook for 10 minutes. Discard any of the unopened clams.
6. Serve right away.

Nutrition:

Calories: 287, Fat: 15.8g, Fiber: 1g, Carbs: 21.6g, Protein: 1.5g

Mackerel with Sauce

Prep Time + Cook Time: 30 minutes Servings: 4

Ingredients:

- mackerel fillets: 4; skinless and boneless
- spring onions - 4, chopped
- olive oil - 1 tsp.
- ginger piece - 1-inch, grated
- A pinch of salt and black pepper

- Juice of orange - 1
- veggie stock - 1 cup
- Zest of orange - 1, grated

Directions:
1. Sprinkle a pinch of salt and pepper on the fish and rub with the oil.
2. Place the pan over medium-high heat source, then add mackerel.
3. Cook for about 5-6 minutes on each side and divide into different plates.
4. Add stock, ginger, orange juice, orange zest and onions inside a pan, then heat over a medium-high heat.
5. Cook the mixture for about 10 minutes.
6. Finally, drizzle over the fish.
7. Then you can serve.
8. Enjoy your delicious meal!

Nutrition:
calories: 210, fat: 4, fiber: 9, carbs: 11, protein: 12

Maple Glazed Salmon Fillet

Prep Time + Cook Time: 30 minutes Servings: 1

Ingredients:
- 1 tbsp. coconut oil
- 1 salmon fillet
- 2 tbsp. mustard
- 1 tbsp. maple syrup (sugar-free)
- Salt and black pepper ground, to taste

Directions:
1. Whisk maple syrup with mustard in a small bowl.
2. First season the salmon fillet with salt and pepper then brush it with half of the maple mixture.
3. Add oil to a pan and set it over medium-high heat.
4. Place the seasoned fillet in the pan with its flesh side down.
5. Let it cook for 5 minutes then brush the top with rest of the maple mixture.
6. Transfer the cooking pan to the oven and bake the fish for 15 minutes at 425 °F.
7. Serve warm.

Nutrition:
Calories: 465, Fat: 31g, Fiber: 3.3g, Carbs: 9.6g, Protein: 40.1g

Mediterranean Cod Salad

Prep Time + Cook Time: 2 hrs. 30 minutes Servings: 8

Ingredients:
- 1 escarole head, leaves separated
- 6 tbsp. capers
- 2 lbs. salt cod
- ¾ cup olive oil
- 1 cup fresh parsley, roughly chopped

- 2 cups jarred pimiento peppers, chopped
- 1 cup olives (Kalamata), pitted and roughly chopped
- Salt and black pepper ground, to taste
- ½ tsp. red chili flakes
- Juice from 2 lemons
- 4 garlic cloves, peeled and minced
- 2 celery stalks, roughly chopped

Directions:

1. Place cod in a saucepan and pour enough water to cover the fish.

2. Cook the fish for 20 minutes on medium heat then transfer the cooked fillets to the cutting board.

3. Once cooled, dice the fish into medium sized chunks.
4. Transfer these chunks to a salad bowl.
5. Add parsley, peppers, capers, olives, lemon juice, black pepper, salt, olive oil, chili flakes, garlic, and celery.
6. Toss them gently with the fish using a spatula.
7. Spread the escarole leaves in the serving plates.
8. Divide the salmon mixture into the escarole leaves.

Nutrition:
Calories: 342, Fat: 22.1g, Fiber: 2.2g, Carbs: 3.6g, Protein: 33.1g

Mix of Kimchi

Prep Time + Cook Time: 10 minutes Servings: 4

Ingredients:
- Sushi grade tuna-1 pound (cubed)
- Sesame oil-1/2 tsp.
- Coconut aminos-1 tbsp.
- Homemade mayonnaise-1/4 cup
- Avocado-1 (pitted, peeled and cubed)
- Kimchi-1/2 cup
- Green onions-1 tbsp. (chopped)

Directions:

1. In a mixing bowl, add the tuna cubes with the oil, a mines, mayo, avocado, Kimchi and green onions.
2. Mix well.
3. Serve for lunch.

Nutrition:
calories 200, fat 3, fiber 4, carbs 11, protein 6

Mixed Fish with Cauliflower Pie

Prep Time + Cook Time: 50 minutes Servings: 6

Ingredients:
- yellow onion - 1, chopped
- salmon fillets - 3, skinless, cut into medium pieces
- mackerel fillets - 3, skinless, cut into medium pieces

- Ghee - ¼ cup; melted and heated up
- cauliflower head - 1, riced
- eggs: 4; boiled, peeled and cubed
- coconut cream - 1 cup
- water - ½ cup
- cheddar cheese - 1 and ½ cup, shredded
- Salt and black pepper to the taste
- Chives - 4 tbsps., chopped

Directions:
1. Pour the cream and the water in a pan, then add fish, salt and pepper to the mixture.
2. Toss well to keep it coated and heat up on a medium-high heat source.
3. This is followed by adding onions, then move to a boil, and simmer for 10 minutes.
4. Move the fish to a baking dish and keep it aside for a while.
5. Put the egg on top of the fish, before adding coconut cream from the pan. Also add cheese mixed with melted ghee, cauliflower rice, sprinkle chives on top.
6. Transfer to an oven set at a temperature of 400 °F and cook for 30 minutes.
7. Slice and serve immediately.

Nutrition:
calories: 300, fat: 14, fiber: 3, carbs: 8, protein: 16

Monk fish and Tomato-Garlic Sauce

Prep Time + Cook Time: 45 minutes Servings: 8

Ingredients:
- olive oil - ¼ cup +3 tbsps.
- garlic heads: 2; peeled and chopped
- sweet paprika - 1 tbsp.
- canned tomatoes - 1 cup, crushed
- A pinch of salt and black pepper
- Monk fish fillets - 8, boneless
- water - 2 cups

Directions:
1. Put a pan containing about ¼-cup of oil over medium-high heat source. Then add the garlic to the pan and stir gently. Cook this for about 15 minutes.
2. Then add the paprika, tomatoes and the water, and slowly stir. Cook the sauce for another 10 minutes.
3. Get another pan and pour the remaining oil in it. Then place the pan over medium-high heat before adding the fish fillets.
4. Make sure they are brown for 2 minutes on each side.
5. Transfer to the oven and bake at a temperature of 400 °F for 15 minutes.
6. Divide the fish into different plates.
7. Use tomato and garlic sauce as topping and serve.

Nutrition:
calories: 273, fat: 4, fiber: 7, carbs: 6, protein: 7

Oysters with Plain Grilling

Prep Time + Cook Time: 29 minutes Servings: 2

Ingredients:

- Oysters-6 (shucked)
- Garlic cloves-3 (peeled and minced)
- Lemon-1 (cut in wedges)
- Parsley-1 tbsp.
- Sweet paprika-A pinch
- Butter-2 tbsp. (melted)

Directions:

1. Layer each oyster with melted butter, parsley, paprika, and butter on top.
2. Keep on preheated grill pan over medium-high heat.
3. Bake for 8 minutes.
4. Serve them with lemon wedges on the side.

Nutrition:

Calories: 272, Fat: 15.7, Fiber: 0.1, Carbs: 13, Protein: 20.3

Parmesan Shrimp Skewers

Prep Time + Cook Time: 30 minutes Servings: 4

Ingredients:

- 1 tbsp. lemon juice
- 1 lb. shrimp, peeled and deveined
- 1 garlic clove, peeled and minced
- 1 tbsp. pine nuts, toasted
- ½ cup fresh basil leaves
- 2 tbsp. olive oil
- 2 tbsp. Parmesan cheese, shredded
- Salt and black pepper ground, to taste

Directions:

1. Add parmesan cheese, basil, pine nuts, salt, pepper, oil, lemon juice, and garlic to a food processor.
2. Blend this mixture well then transfer it to a large bowl.
3. Toss in shrimp and stir well to coat them well with the cheese mixture.
4. Allow the shrimp to marinate for 20 minutes.
5. Thread 2 to 3 shrimps over each wooden skewer.
6. Grill shrimp skewers in a preheated grill for 3 minutes per side.
7. Serve right away.

Nutrition:

Calories: 234, Fat: 11.9g, Fiber: 0.2g, Carbs: 2.7g, Protein: 28.5g

Red Shrimp Stew

Prep Time + Cook Time: 1 hour 10 minutes Servings: 3

Ingredients:

- Spicy sausage, sliced -½ lb.
- Celery stalk, chopped -1
- Garlic clove, minced -1

- Shrimp, peeled and deveined -½ lb.
- Green bell pepper, chopped -½
- Canned tomatoes, chopped -14 oz.
- Salt and black pepper- to taste

Directions:
1. Place a cooking pot over medium-high heat. Add sausage and sauté for 10 minutes.
2. Stir in garlic, celery, tomatoes, bell pepper, salt, and pepper.
3. Let this mixture simmer for 45 minutes on medium heat.
4. Gently toss in shrimp and cover the pot. Let the shrimp cook for 6 minutes until they are al dente.
5. Serve right away.

Nutrition:
Calories: 301, Fat: 4, Fiber: 7, Carbs: 12, Protein: 8

Roll in Salmon

Prep Time + Cook Time: 9 minutes Servings: 2

Ingredients:
- Nori sheets-3
- Canned salmon-5 ounces (dried and flaked)
- Red bell pepper-1 (cut into thin strips)
- Small avocado-1 small (pitted, peeled and cut into thin strips)
- Small cucumber-1 small (cut into thin strips)
- Spring onion-1 (chopped)
- Mayonnaise-1 tbsp.
- Coconut aminos-for serving

Directions:
1. Settle the nori sheets on a cutting board. Divide the salmon, bell pepper, avocado, cucumber, onion and mayonnaise.
2. Roll well and cut each roll in 2 pieces.
3. Serve with coconut aminos on the side.

Nutrition:
calories 200, fat 4, fiber 7, carbs 11, protein 6

Sage Shrimp Kebabs and Tomato Salad

Prep Time + Cook Time: 16 minutes Serves: 4

Ingredients:
- Chopped celery, 1 cup
- Grated lemon zest, 1 tsp.
- Chopped sage, 2 tbsps.
- Chopped chives, 2 tbsps.
- Salt
- Lemon juice, 1/3 cup
- Black pepper
- Peeled shrimp, 24
- Halved cherry tomatoes, 12
- Olive oil, 3 tbsps.

Directions:

1. Set a mixing bowl in position to whisk together the seasoning, lemon juice, sage, lemon zest, chives, and oil
2. Set aside 2 tbsps. of the mixture for later usage.
3. Put the remaining mixture into another bowl to combine with celery and the tomatoes
4. Preheat the grill over medium heat
5. Set the shrimp onto skewer then cook on the preheated grill for about three minutes each side.
6. Set on plates along with the reserved dressing and tomatoes mix as a side.

Nutrition:
Calories: 200, Fat: 3, Fiber: 4, Carbs: 5, Protein: 12

Salad Of Shrimp and Asparagus

Prep Time + Cook Time: 17 minutes Servings: 1

Ingredients:
- Shrimp-1 pound (peeled and deveined)
- Thyme-1 tsp. (dried)
- Garlic cloves-2 (minced)
- Basil-1 tsp. (dried)
- Salt and black pepper-A pinch
- Sweet paprika-2 tsps.
- Asparagus-2 bunches (trimmed and halved)
- Olive oil-1 tsp.
- Lettuce leaves-4 cups (torn)
- Basil-A handful of (torn)
- Red onion-1 small (chopped)
- Avocado-1 (peeled, pitted and cubed)
- Coconut cream-1/3 cup
- Lemon juice-1 tsp.
- Water-2 tbsp.

Directions:
1. Warm up oil in a pan.
2. Over medium heat.
3. Add shrimp, thyme, garlic, basil, salt, pepper, paprika and asparagus.
4. Toss and cook for 5 minutes.
5. Take a salad bowl.
6. Combine the shrimp and asparagus with the lettuce, basil, onion, avocado, coconut cream, lemon juice and water.
7. Toss well.
8. Serve for lunch.

Nutrition:
calories 251, fat 4, fiber 7, carbs 15, protein 7

Salmon Crust Fillet

Prep Time + Cook Time: 26 minutes Servings: 3

Ingredients:

- Garlic cloves-3 (peeled and minced)
- Salmon fillet-2 pounds
- Salt and ground black pepper to taste
- Parmesan cheese-1/2 cup (grated)
- Fresh parsley-1/4 cup (chopped)

Directions:

1. Keep the salmon on a lined baking sheet.
2. Season with salt, and pepper.
3. Cover with a parchment paper, place in an oven at 425°F.
4. Cook for 10 minutes.
5. Place the fish out of the oven.
6. Sprinkle Parmesan cheese, parsley, and garlic over fish.
7. Keep it in an oven again and cook for 5 minutes.
8. Distribute on plates and serve.

Nutrition:
Calories: 350, Fat: 17, Fiber: 1.5, Carbs: 0.2, Protein: 48.8

Salmon Fillets

Prep Time + Cook Time: 40 minutes Servings: 2

Ingredients:

- Salmon fillets-4
- Olive oil-1 tbsp.
- Salt and ground black pepper to taste
- Cumin-1 tsp.
- Sweet paprika-1 tsp.
- Chili powder-1/2 tsp.
- Onion powder-1 tsp.

For the salmon fillet serving salsa:

- Onion-1 (peeled and chopped)
- Avocado-1 (pitted, peeled, and chopped)
- Fresh cilantro-2 tbsps. (chopped)
- Limes-2 (juice)
- Salt and ground black pepper to taste

Directions:

1. Pick a bowl to mix salt, pepper, chili powder, onion powder, paprika, and cumin.
2. Marinate the salmon with this mixture, drizzle the oil, rub.
3. Bake on preheated grill pan for 4 minutes on each side.
4. Mix avocado with onion, salt, pepper, cilantro, lime juice in a bowl and stir.
5. Place the salmon on plates.
6. Layer on top of each fillet with avocado salsa.

Nutrition:
Calories: 379, Fat: 24.3, Fiber: 4, Carbs: 6.9, Protein: 35.8

Salmon Mix Salad

Prep Time + Cook Time: 1 hour 30 minutes Servings: 3

Ingredients:

- Salmon fillets-4 (boneless)
- Portobello mushroom caps-2 (sliced)
- Baby bok choy-4
- Sesame seeds-1 tbsp. (toasted)
- Green onion-1 (chopped)
- Olive oil-1 tbsp.
- Coconut aminos-1 tbsp.
- Sesame oil-1 tsp.
- Ginger-1 tsp. (grated)
- Lemon-1/2 (juiced)
- Salt and black pepper-A pinch

Directions:

1. Take a large mixing bowl.
2. Add the salmon with the olive oil, amines, sesame oil, ginger, salt, pepper and lemon juice.
3. Toss and cover. Keep in the fridge for 1 hour. Layer the salmon fillets on a lined baking sheet.
4. Add mushroom slices and bok choy.
5. Transfer in the oven and cook at 400 oF for 20 minutes.
6. Distribute everything between plates.
7. Sprinkle green onion and sesame seeds.
8. Top and serve for lunch.

Nutrition:

calories 261, fat 4, fiber 7, carbs 15, protein 7

Salmon with Mushroom Shrimp Filling

Prep Time + Cook Time: 40 minutes Servings: 2

Ingredients:

- ¼ cup mayonnaise
- 2 salmon fillets
- 2 cups spinach
- A drizzle of olive oil
- 6 mushrooms, diced
- ¼ cup macadamia nuts, toasted and roughly chopped
- 3 green onions, chopped
- Salt and black pepper ground, to taste
- A pinch of nutmeg
- 5 oz. tiger shrimp, peeled, deveined, and diced

Directions:

1. Pour oil in a pan, set over medium-high heat.
2. Toss in mushrooms, onions, pepper, and salt. Sauté this mixture for 4 minutes then add macadamia nuts.
3. Stir cook for 2 minutes and add spinach to the pan.
4. After cooking for 1 more minute add shrimp. Let them cook for 1 minute then remove the pan from the heat.
5. After 3-5 minutes, add nutmeg and mayonnaise to the shrimp and mix well.
6. Lengthwise carve an incision along one side of each salmon fillet.

7. Rub the fillet with salt and pepper from inside out. Stuff the incisions with shrimp and spinach mixture.
8. Place a large sized skillet over medium heat and heat oil in it.
9. Put the stuffed salmon in the hot oil with their skin side down.
10. Continue cooking for another minute then reduce the heat and cover the fish with a lid.
11. Continue cooking it for 8 minutes then transfer the pan to the broiler.
12. Broil it for 3 minutes then serve warm.

Nutrition:
Calories: 567, Fat: 34.6g, Fiber: 3.3g, Carbs: 13.9g, Protein: 53.9g

Sardine Cucumber Salad

Prep Time + Cook Time: 5 minutes Servings: 1

Ingredients:
- 1 tbsp. lemon juice
- ½ tbsp. mustard
- 5 oz. canned sardines in oil
- 1 small cucumber, diced
- Salt and black pepper ground, to taste

Directions:
1. Remove the sardines from its can and drain the excess liquid.
2. Place the fish in the medium-sized bowl and mash it using a fork,
3. Add cucumber, salt, pepper, lemon juice, and mustard.
4. Mix well and place the salad in the refrigerator for 30 minutes or more.
5. Enjoy fresh.

Nutrition:
Calories: 509, Fat: 32.5g, Fiber: 1.6g, Carbs: 11.3g, Protein: 42.1g

Sardines Tapenade Mix

Prep Time + Cook Time: 10 minutes Servings: 3

Ingredients:
- canned sardines - 14 ounces, drained and flaked
- capers - 1 tbsp.
- white vinegar - 1 tsp.
- garlic cloves - 3, minced
- celery sticks - 3, chopped
- A pinch of salt and black pepper
- Cucumber - ½, sliced

Directions:
1. Mix the sardines with the capers, vinegar, garlic, celery, cucumber, salt and pepper in a clean bowl.
2. Toss to ensure it is coated.
3. Then divide into different smaller bowls and serve.

Nutrition:
calories: 199, fat: 2, fiber: 4, carbs: 11, protein: 8

Sea Bass with Capers

Prep Time + Cook Time: 30 minutes Servings: 3

Ingredients:

- Lemon-1 (sliced)
- Sea bass-1 pound (fillet)
- Capers-2 tbsps.
- Fresh dill-2 tbsps.
- Salt and ground black pepper-to taste

Directions:

1. Place the sea bass fillet into a baking dish.
2. Do the seasoning with salt, and pepper, add capers, dill, and lemon slices on top.
3. Keep in an oven at 350°F.
4. Bake for 15 minutes.
5. Distribute on plates and serve.

Nutrition:

Calories: 150, Fat: 3.1, Fiber: 0.8, Carbs: 2.4, Protein: 27.4

Shrimp and Asparagus with Lime Flavor

Prep Time + Cook Time: 20 minutes Servings: 2

Ingredients:

- medium shrimp - 1 pound; peeled and deveined
- Lime juice: 1
- Asparagus - 1 pound; trimmed and chopped
- olive oil - 2 tsps.
- garlic cloves - 4, minced
- small yellow onion - 1, chopped
- small cilantro bunch - 1, chopped
- A pinch of salt and black pepper

Directions:

1. Put a pan containing oil over a medium-high heat source
2. Then add onion and garlic, stir gently and cook for about 5 minutes.
3. Add asparagus to the mixture and shrimp, stir gently.
4. Cook for close to 4 minutes, remove heat and sprinkle a pinch of salt and pepper.
5. Pour some lime juice and cilantro, and stir.
6. Divide between different plates and serve.

Nutrition:

calories: 215, fat: 2, fiber: 4, carbs: 8, protein: 22

Shrimp and Eggs Salad Mix

Prep Time + Cook Time: 35 minutes Servings: 4

Ingredients:

- green eggplants - 2 pounds
- big shrimp - ¼ pound, peeled and deveined
- eggs - 4, hard-boiled, peeled and cut into quarters
- shallots - 2, sliced
- lime juice - 3 tbsps.
- bird's eye chilies - 3, sliced
- Cilantro - 1 tbsp., chopped
- olive oil - 1 tbsp.

Directions:

1. Place the eggplants neatly on a lined baking dish, and transfer them to an oven, at 450 0F. Bake for about 20 minutes.
2. Remove the peels, cut into medium chunks and move the chunks into a bowl.
3. Add heat to a pan containing oil over medium heat, then add chilies and lime juice, and stir gently.
4. Cook the mixture for 1 minute.
5. Pour the shrimp into the mixture, cook them for 2 minutes on each side, and move to a clean bowl.
6. Then add some eggplant pieces, shallots, eggs, and cilantro.
7. Toss to ensure it is well coated and serve.

Nutrition:

calories: 200, fat: 5, fiber: 7, carbs: 10, protein: 12

Shrimp Mayo Side Salad

Prep Time + Cook Time: 25 minutes Servings: 4

Ingredients:

- 2 tbsp. lime juice
- 2 tbsp. mayonnaise
- 2 tbsp. olive oil
- 3 endives, leaves
- 1 lb. shrimp, peeled and deveined
- 1 tsp. lime zest
- Salt and black pepper ground, to taste
- 1 tbsp. lemon juice
- 3 tbsp. fresh parsley, roughly chopped
- 2 tsp. fresh mint, finely chopped
- 1 tbsp. fresh tarragon, chopped
- ½ cup sour cream

Directions:

1. Gently toss shrimps with olive oil, salt, and pepper in a bowl.
2. Spread these shrimps in a baking sheet lined with parchment paper.
3. Bake the shrimps for 10 minutes at 400 0F.
4. Transfer the baked shrimp to a bowl and toss them with lime juice.
5. Mix sour cream, with mayonnaise, lemon juice, lime zest, tarragon, mint, parsley, salt and pepper in another bowl.

6. Dice the cooked shrimp and add them to the mayo dressing.
7. Mix gently until well combined.
8. Spread the endive leaves in the serving plates.
9. Top the leaves with shrimp mixture.
10. Serve fresh.

Nutrition:
Calories: 332, Fat: 18g, Fiber: 8.1g, Carbs: 14.2g, Protein: 30.2g

Shrimp Mushroom Medley

Prep Time + Cook Time: 30 minutes Servings: 2

Ingredients:

- Mushrooms, chopped -4 oz.
- Shrimp, peeled and deveined -½ lb.
- Yellow onion, chopped-½
- Salt and black pepper-to taste
- Butternut squash, peeled and cubed -½
- Olive oil -1 tbsp
- Italian seasoning -1 tsp
- Red pepper flakes, crushed -½ tsp
- Ghee-2 tbsp
- Parmesan, grated-½ cup
- Garlic clove, minced-1
- Coconut cream -½ cup

Directions:

1. Place a pan with oil and ghee over medium-high heat.
2. Toss in onion and mushrooms, stir cook for 5 minutes.
3. Add Italian seasoning, pepper flakes, salt, pepper, and squash.
4. Stir cook this mixture for 6 minutes.
5. Add coconut cream, garlic, shrimp and Parmesan.
6. Stir well and cook well for 5 minutes.
7. Serve warm.

Nutrition:
Calories: 251, Fat: 6, Fiber: 2, Carbs: 9, Protein: 10

Shrimp, Calamari with Avocado Sauce

Prep Time + Cook Time: 35 minutes. Servings: 1

Ingredients:

- 1 egg
- 1 tbsp. coconut oil
- 1 tsp. tomato paste
- 8 oz. calamari, sliced into medium rings
- 1 tbsp. mayonnaise
- 1 tsp. lemon juice
- 3 tbsp. coconut flour
- 2 tbsp. avocado, cored and diced
- A splash of Worcestershire sauce
- 2 lemon slices
- Salt and black pepper ground, to taste
- 7 oz. shrimp, peeled and deveined

- ½ Tsp. turmeric

Directions:

1. Whisk egg with coconut oil in a medium-sized bowl.
2. Dip the calamari rings and shrimp in the egg mixture and coat them well.
3. Combine flour with turmeric, pepper, and salt in another shallow bowl.
4. Place the shrimps and calamari rings in the dry flour mixture.
5. Coat them well and shake off the excess flour.
6. Place the coated shrimp and calamari rings in a greased baking sheet
7. Bake the seafood for 10 minutes at 400 ºF in a preheated oven.
8. Remove the baking sheet from the oven and flip all the shrimp and rings.
9. Continue baking them for another 10 minutes.
10. Meanwhile, mash the avocado flesh in a glass bowl.
11. Stir in mayonnaise, tomato paste, lemon juice, salt, pepper and Worcestershire sauce. Mix well.
12. Divide the baked shrimp and calamari in the serving plates.
13. Serve them with avocado sauce and lemon slices.

Nutrition:

Calories: 2022, Fat: 86.1g, Fiber: 9.2g, Carbs: 129.6g, Protein: 163.8g

Simple Baked Catfish with Salad

Prep Time + Cook Time: 30 minutes Servings: 4

Ingredients:

- Parsley - 2 tbsps., chopped
- Basil - ½ tsp., dried
- Thyme - ½ tsp., dried
- Oregano - ½ tsp., dried
- sweet paprika - 1 tsp.
- A pinch of salt and black pepper
- medium catfish fillets - 4, boneless
- Lemon juice - 4
- garlic powder - ¼ tsp.
- ghee - 2 tbsps., melted

Directions:

1. Pour some melted ghee on a baking dish to act as grease and place the fish fillets neatly in the dish.
2. Then add parsley, basil, thyme, oregano, paprika, salt, pepper, lemon juice, and the garlic powder.
3. Toss gently to make sure it is properly coated, then move into an oven and bake at 350 ºF for about 20 minutes.
4. Divide the fish into different plates
5. Serve with side salad.

Nutrition:

calories: 212, fat: 2, fiber: 3, carbs: 13, protein: 7

Simple Sardines and Cucumber Mix

Prep Time + Cook Time: 10 minutes Servings: 2

Ingredients:

- canned sardines in oil - 10 ounces, cubed
- lemon juice - 2 tbsps.
- small cucumber - 2, chopped
- mustard - 1 tbsp.
- Salt and black pepper to the taste

Directions:

1. Mix the sardines with a pinch of salt, pepper, cucumber, lemon juice and mustard in a clean bowl.
2. Then stir gently and serve.

Nutrition:

calories: 190, fat: 10, fiber: 4, carbs: 10, protein: 10

Smoked Salmon with Eggs Salad

Prep Time + Cook Time: 6 minutes Servings: 4

Ingredients:

- Eggs - 8, hard-boiled, peeled and mashed with a fork
- smoked salmon - 8 ounces, cubed
- Salt and black pepper to the taste
- yellow onion - 1, chopped
- avocado mayonnaise - ¾ cup

Directions:

1. Pour eggs with mayo, salmon, salt, pepper, and onion in a clean bowl and mix together.
2. Toss to make sure it is well coated.
3. Then divide into different small cups and serve.

Nutrition:

calories: 202, fat: 8, fiber: 3, carbs: 9, protein: 7

Spicy Salmon Fillets with Salad

Prep Time + Cook Time: 20 minutes Servings: 4

Ingredients:

- salmon fillets - 4, boneless and skin-on
- chili pepper - 2 tbsps., chopped
- Juice lemon: 1
- olive oil - 2 tbsps.
- A pinch of salt and black pepper

Directions:

1. Place a pan containing oil over medium-high heat source, and add chili pepper. Stir gently and cook between 1-2 minutes.
2. Add the salmon, salt and pepper, cook each side for about 3 minutes.
3. Divide into different plates, then drizzle the lemon juice all over
4. Serve with salad on the side.
5. Enjoy your meal!

Nutrition:

calories: 231, fat: 8, fiber: 8, carbs: 12, protein: 4

Tangy Pepper Filled Oysters

Prep Time + Cook Time: 5 minutes Servings: 4

Ingredients:

- ¼ cup olive oil
- 1 Serrano chili pepper, chopped
- 12 oysters, shucked
- Juice from 1 lime
- ½ tsp. fresh ginger, shredded
- Juice of 2 lemons
- ¼ tsp. garlic, minced
- Zest from 2 limes
- ¼ cup scallions, chopped
- 1 cup tomato juice
- Salt, to taste
- ¼ cup fresh cilantro, chopped

Directions:

1. Arrange all the oysters in a baking tray and with their shell side downward.
2. Mix garlic, scallions, salt, olive oil, tomato juice, serrano chili, lime juice and zest, lemon juice and zest, ginger and cilantro in a medium bowl.
3. Top each oyster with a scoop of this mixture.
4. Serve fresh.

Nutrition:
Calories: 179, Fat: 14.6g, Fiber: 0.5g, Carbs: 6.4g, Protein: 7.1g

Tomatoes Stuffed With Tuna & Cheese

Prep Time + Cook Time: 11 minutes Servings: 2

Ingredients:

- Tomato-1 (top cut off and insides scooped)
- Balsamic vinegar-2 tsps.
- Canned tuna-5 ounces (drained)
- Mozzarella-1 tbsp. (chopped)
- Green onion-1 tbsp. (chopped)
- Basil-1 tbsp. (chopped)

Directions:

1. Take a bowl.
2. Mix the tune with the vinegar, mozzarella, onion and basil and stir well.
3. Stuff the tomato with this mix.
4. Serve for lunch.
5. Enjoy!

Nutrition:
calories 188, fat 4, fiber 1, carbs 7, protein 7

Tuna Salad Mix

Prep Time + Cook Time: 14 minutes Servings: 4

Ingredients:

- yellow onion - 1, chopped
- cilantro - ½ cup, chopped
- olive oil - 1/3 cup and 2 tbsps.
- jalapeno pepper - 1, chopped
- basil - 2 tbsps., chopped
- white vinegar - 3 tbsps.
- garlic cloves - 3, minced
- red pepper flakes - 1 tsp.

- thyme - 1 tsp., chopped
- A pinch of salt and black pepper
- sushi tuna - 1 pound, cubed
- arugula - 6 ounces

Directions:

1. Add heat to a pan containing about 2 tbsps. of oil over medium-high heat. Then add tuna and season with salt and black pepper.
2. Cook this for 2 minutes on each side, before moving to a salad bowl.
3. Add arugula to the mixture and toss well to make sure it is coated.
4. Mix onion with the cilantro, the rest of the oil, jalapeno, basil, vinegar, garlic, pepper flakes, thyme, salt and pepper and whisk in a clean bowl.
5. Add this to your salad, then toss.
6. Now you can serve.
7. Enjoy your meal!

Nutrition:

calories: 140, fat: 1, fiber: 1, carbs: 2, protein: 6

Tuna with Arugula Sauce

Prep Time + Cook Time: 15 minutes Servings: 4

Ingredients:

- 3 tbsp. balsamic vinegar
- 1 tsp. red pepper flakes
- 1 jalapeño pepper, roughly chopped
- ½ cup fresh cilantro, roughly chopped
- 1 onion, peeled and diced
- ⅓ cup, and 2 tbsp. olive oil
- 2 tbsp. fresh parsley, roughly chopped
- 2 tbsp. fresh basil, roughly chopped
- 1 lb. sushi tuna steak
- 2 avocados, pitted, peeled, and sliced
- Salt and black pepper ground, to taste
- A pinch of cayenne pepper
- 1 tsp. fresh thyme, finely chopped
- 6 oz. baby arugula
- 3 garlic cloves, peeled and minced

Directions:

1. Add 1/3 cup oil to a large bowl along with onion, jalapeno, vinegar, basil, cilantro, parsley, garlic, thyme, pepper flakes, salt, cayenne, and black pepper.
2. Mix all of those ingredients well and set their mixture aside.
3. Now pour the remaining oil into a flat pan and let it heat over medium heat.
4. Add tuna and sear it for 2 minutes per side.
5. Season the tuna with salt and pepper during cooking.
6. Once done, transfer the seared tuna to the cutting board and slice it.
7. Toss arugula with half of the prepared chimichurri mixture in a bowl.
8. Divide this arugula into the serving plates.
9. Top this mixture with tuna slices.
10. Garnish with a drizzle of remaining chimichurri mixture and avocado slices.

Nutrition:

Calories: 564, Fat: 37.6g, Fiber: 8.2g, Carbs: 13.8g, Protein: 48.6g

Chapter 6 Ketogenic Poultry Recipes

A pot filled Roasted Chicken

Prep Time + Cook Time: 50 minutes Servings: 12

Ingredients:

- Guar gum - 2 tsps.
- Garlic powder - ½ tsp.
- A whole chicken
- onion powder - ½ tsp.
- Coconut oil - 2 tbsps.
- Italian seasoning - 1 tsp.
- Chicken stock - 1½ cups
- Seasoning: Salt and ground black pepper

Directions:

1. Polish the chicken with half of the coconut oil, garlic powder, salt, pepper, Italian seasoning, and onion powder. Pour the rest of the oil into an Instant Pot, add chicken to the pot.
2. With stock been added, cover Instant Pot, cook on Poultry mode for 40 minutes.
3. Chicken should be transferred to a platter and set aside.
4. The instant pot should be set on Sauté mode, then add guar gum, mix thoroughly, and cook until it thickens.
5. Pour sauce over chicken and serve.

Nutrition:

Calories: 463, Fat: 31.8, Fiber: 0, Carbs: 0.4, Protein: 44.1

Almond Butter Chicken Stew

Prep Time + Cook Time: 50 minutes Serves: 4

Ingredients:

- Minced garlic clove, 1
- Black pepper
- Chopped yellow onion, ½
- Chicken stock, 1 cup
- Chopped collard greens, 1 cup
- Salt
- Chopped chicken breast, 8 oz.
- Grated ginger, 2 tbsps.
- Soft almond butter, ½ cup

Directions:

1. Set the pot on fire then stir in chicken, garlic, and onion to boil for 20 minutes over medium heat
2. Meanwhile, set another bowl in a clean working surface to mix almond butter with one tbsp. soup then mix in the pot.
3. Stir in the collard green, ginger, and seasonings to cook for five more minutes
4. Set on serving bowls and enjoy.

Nutrition:

Calories: 209, Fat: 5, Fiber: 5, Carbs: 8, Protein: 11

Artichokes and Chicken Breast Mix

Prep Time + Cook Time: 40 minutes Serves: 6

Ingredients:

- White vinegar, ¼ cup
- Chopped canned tomatoes, 28 oz.
- Veggie stock, 1½ cup
- Chopped kalamata olives, ½ cup
- Canned artichoke hearts, 28 oz.
- Chopped yellow onion, 1
- Chopped parsley, ¼ cup
- Dried basil, 2 tsps.
- Salt
- De-boned skinless chicken breasts, 2 lbs.
- Black pepper

Directions:

1. Set the baking dish in place then put on the chicken breast.
2. Add the artichokes, vinegar, pepper, tomatoes, salt, parsley, basil, and olives.
3. Set the oven for 30 minutes at 400ºF, allow to bake
4. Once the timer is up, set on plates to serve.

Nutrition:

Calories: 280, Fat: 5, Fiber: 4, Carbs: 6, Protein: 15

Arugula Chicken Bowls

Prep Time + Cook Time: 1 hour 30 minutes Serves: 4

Ingredients:

- Chopped cilantro, 1 tbsp.
- Minced garlic, 2 tsps.
- Coconut aminos, ¾ cup
- Olive oil, 1 tbsp.
- White vinegar, 2 tbsps.
- Salt
- Chopped onion, ½
- Black pepper
- Cubed chicken breasts, 2
- Arugula, 2 cup
- Orange juice, 2 tbsps.

Directions:

1. Set the pan on fire with oil to cook the onion for 3 minutes over medium heat.
2. Stir in orange juice, pepper, garlic, coconut aminos, vinegar, and salt.
3. Allow to simmer for five minutes then set in the blender to process until smooth.
4. Meanwhile, set a mixing bowl in place to coat the chicken with orange marinade then let it rest for one hour.
5. Set the pan on fire to fry the marinated chicken for six minutes on both sides over medium-high heat.
6. Divide into serving bowls.
7. Top with arugula and cilantro

Nutrition:

Calories: 500, Fat: 6, Fiber: 2, Carbs: 10, Protein: 7

Bacon, Chicken and Broccoli mix

Prep Time + Cook Time: 22 minutes Serves: 4

Ingredients:

- Cooked and crumbled bacon slices, 2
- Chopped broccoli florets, 12 oz.
- Vinegar, 2 tbsps.
- Olive oil, 5 tbsps.
- Salt
- Stripped medium chicken breasts, 3
- Black pepper
- Chopped chives, 1 tbsp.

Directions:

1. Set the mixing bowl in place to combine the seasonings, 4 tbsps. oil, broccoli, and vinegar and reserve

2. Set up the pan on fire with the remaining oil to fry the seasoned chicken for 6 minutes each sides over medium-high heat.
3. Set on plates,
4. Mix with the broccoli mix then serve with chopped chives and crumbled bacon on top.

Nutrition:

Calories: 200, Fat: 15, Fiber: 3, Carbs: 10, Protein: 16

Baked Turkey Delight

Cooking time: 55 minutes Servings: 8

Ingredients:

- Turkey meat (cooked and shredded): 3 cups
- Cream cheese: ½ cup
- Parmesan cheese (grated): ½ cup
- Zucchini (cut with a spiralizer): 4 cups
- Egg (whisked): 1
- Cabbage (shredded): 3 cups
- Poultry seasoning: 1 tsp.
- Cheddar cheese (grated): 2 cup
- Seasoning: salt and ground black pepper
- Turkey stock: ½ cup
- Garlic powder: ¼ tsp.

Directions:

1. Heat a pan with broth over medium heat.

2. Add the egg, cream, Parmesan cheese, cheddar cheese, salt, pepper, poultry herbs, and garlic powder, stir and bring to a boil gently.
3. Add turkey meat, cabbage, stir and remove heat.
4. Put the zucchini noodles in a casserole dish, add some salt and pepper, add the turkey mixture and divide it up.
5. Cover with aluminum foil, place in an oven at 400 ° F and bake for 35 minutes. Allow to cool before serving.

Nutrition:

Calories: 290, Carbs: 4.6, Fat: 18.5, Fiber: 1.3, Protein: 26.4

Balsamic-Plum Chicken Mix

Prep Time + Cook Time: 2 hours 10 minutes Serves: 6

Ingredients:

- Balsamic vinegar, 1tbsp.
- Salt
- Plum, 5 oz.
- Chopped red onion, 1
- Olive oil, 1 tbsp.
- Whole chicken, 1
- Chopped ginger pieces, 1
- Minced garlic cloves, 4
- Black pepper
- Coconut aminos, 6 tbsps.

Directions:

1. Prepare the roasting pan.
2. Season the chicken with pepper and salt topped with some oil, onion, ginger, aminos, plums, and vinegar.
3. Set the oven for 2 hours at 380ºF, allow to bake.
4. Once fully baked, set on serving plates.

Nutrition:
Calories: 350, Fat: 8, Fiber: 4, Carbs: 12, Protein: 17

Cauliflower Turkey Soup

Prep Time + Cook Time: 55 minutes Servings: 4

Ingredients:

- Shallots, chopped -4
- Turkey, ground -1 lb.
- Salt and black pepper - to taste
- Red bell pepper, chopped -1
- Chicken stock -5 cups
- Cauliflower florets, chopped -1 and ½ cups
- Olive oil -2 tbsp.
- Canned tomatoes, chopped -15 ounces

Directions:

1. Add oil to a cooking pot and preheat it over medium-high heat.
2. Toss in shallots, bell pepper, and cauliflower, saute for 10 minutes.
3. Stir in turkey, pepper, salt, tomatoes, and stock.
4. Cook this mixture for 30 minutes, after bringing it to a boil.
5. Serve warm.

Nutrition:
Calories: 250, Fat: 1, Fiber: 4, Carbs: 13, Protein: 15

Cheese Rich Turkey Bowls

Prep Time + Cook Time: 35 minutes Servings: 4

Ingredients:

- Turkey stock -1 cup
- Turkey meat, cooked and shredded -1 cup
- Salt and black pepper - to taste
- Thyme, chopped -1 tsp.
- Kale, torn -½ cup
- Butternut squash, peeled and cubed -½ cup

- Cheddar cheese, shredded -½ cup
- Paprika -¼ tsp.
- Garlic powder -¼ tsp.

Directions:
1. Warm stock in a pot over medium heat.
2. Add turkey meat and squash, cook it for 10 minutes.
3. Stir in kale, garlic powder, salt, pepper, thyme, cheddar cheese, and paprika.
4. Let it cook for 10 minutes.
5. Serve right away.

Nutrition:
Calories: 320, Fat: 23, Fiber: 8, Carbs: 6, Protein: 16

Cheesy Chicken and Kale Casserole

Prep Time + Cook Time: 40 minutes Serves: 8

Ingredients:
- Tomato passata, 1 cup
- Chopped cilantro, ½ cup
- Chopped jalapeno peppers, 2
- Chopped kale leaves, 10
- Chopped green onions, ½ cup
- Chili powder, 2 tsps.
- Cumin, 2 tsps.
- Shredded mozzarella cheese, 3 cup
- Garlic powder, 1 tbsp.
- Chopped canned tomatoes, 14 oz.
- Cooked and shredded chicken breast, 3 cup
- Cooking spray

Directions:
1. Spray a baking sheet with cooking spray.
2. Se the mixing bowl in a clean working surface to combine the chicken breast with kale, jalapenos, chili powder, mozzarella, cumin, tomato passata, cilantro, green onions, and garlic powder.
3. Set the oven for 30 minutes at 350°F, allow to bake.
4. Seton plates to serve

Nutrition:
Calories: 305, Fat: 12, Fiber: 6, Carbs: 12, Protein: 26

Chicken Chilies Soup

Prep Time + Cook Time: 40 minutes Servings: 2

Ingredients:
- Chicken breast, boneless and skinless and cubed-1
- Chicken stock -1.5 cups
- Canned tomatoes, chopped-8 oz.
- Canned green chilies, chopped-2 oz.
- Salt and black pepper- to taste
- Garlic clove, minced-1
- White onion, chopped -½ cup
- Oregano, dried -½ tsp
- Cilantro, chopped -½ tbsp

Directions:

1. Pour the stock into the cooking pot and warm up on medium heat on a simmer.
2. Add tomatoes, chicken, salt, pepper, onion, garlic, and oregano.
3. Stir gently and cover this mixture. Let it simmer for 30 minutes.
4. Add cilantro and mix gently.
5. Serve warm.

Nutrition:
Calories: 261, Fat: 7, Fiber: 7, Carbs: 13, Protein: 13

Chicken Fajitas With Paprika

Prep Time + Cook Time: 25 minutes Servings: 4

Ingredients:

- Garlic powder: 1 tsp.
- Chicken breasts (skinless, boneless, and cut into strips): 2 pounds
- Lime juice: 2 tbsps.
- Chili powder: 1 tsp.
- Coconut oil: 2 tbsps.
- Onion, peeled and sliced: 1
- Cumin: 2 tsps.
- Seasoning: Salt and ground black pepper
- Coriander: 1 tsp.
- Sweet paprika: 1 tsp.
- Avocado (pitted, peeled, and sliced): 1
- Red bell pepper, seeded and sliced: 1
- Fresh cilantro (chopped): 1 tbsp.
- Green bell pepper (seeded and sliced): 1
- Limes (cut into wedges): 2

Directions:

1. Mix the lime juice in a bowl with chili powder, cumin, salt, pepper, garlic powder, pepper, coriander, and stir.
2. Add chicken pieces and toss them well.
3. Heat a pan with half of the oil over medium heat, add chicken, cook on each side for 3 minutes and place in a bowl.
4. Heat the pan with the remaining oil over medium heat, add onions and paprika, stir and cook for 6 minutes.
5. Put the chicken back into the pan, add salt and pepper, stir and spread on plates.
6. Cover with avocado, lime wedges, coriander and serve.

Nutrition:
Calories: 643, Fiber: 6.2, Carbs: 17.2, Fat: 34, Protein: 68.1

Chicken Gumbo Recipe

Prep Time + Cook Time: 7 hours 10 minutes Servings: 5

Ingredients:

- Creole seasoning - 6 tbsps.
- Peeled and chopped onion- 1
- Dried oregano - 2 tbsps.
- Dried thyme - 3 tbsps.
- Canned diced tomatoes - 28 ounces
- 2 chopped and seeded bell peppers
- Garlic powder - 2 tbsps.
- 3 Cubed chicken breasts,
- Sliced sausages: 1
- Chili powder - 1 tbsps.
- Cayenne powder - 1 tsp.
- Dry mustard - 2 tbsps.
- Ground black pepper and Salt to taste

Directions:

1. With a low-pressure cooker, mix chicken with sausages, salt, pepper, bell peppers, oregano, onion, thyme, garlic powder, dry mustard, tomatoes, cayenne, chili, and Creole seasoning.
2. Cover the lid of the cooker and boil for 7 hours.
3. Unmount the lid again, shake the gumbo and split into cups. Serve it hot.

Nutrition:

Calories: 445, Fat: 20.7, Fiber: 3.8, Carbs: 13, Protein: 50.9

Chicken in Creamy Sauce Recipe

Prep Time + Cook Time: 1 hour and 10 minutes Servings: 4

Ingredients:

- Ground black pepper and Salt to taste
- Whipping cream - 1 cup
- Coconut oil - 1 tbsp.
- 8 chicken thighs
- Peeled and minced Garlic cloves– 4 pcs
- An onion, peeled and chopped
- Chardonnay - 2 cups
- 4 chopped bacon strips
- Cremini mushroom (Halved) - 10 ounces
- Chopped Fresh parsley - ½ cup

Directions:

1. With moderate temperature, heat a pan with oil, add bacon, mix, cook until crisp, transfer to paper towel while the heat is removed.
2. With medium temperature heat a pan with bacon fat, add chicken pieces, add salt and pepper, cover until brown on all sides, and place on a paper towel.
3. Heat the frying pan with moderate

temperature, add the onion, mix and cook for 6 minutes.

4. Add the garlic, mix and boil the mixture for one minute and place it next to pieces of bacon.

5. Put the frying pan back on the stove, reheat to medium temperature. Add the mushrooms and mix for 5 minutes and also add the chicken,

bacon, garlic, and onion to the pan.

6. Add wine, mix, cook, heat and simmer for 40 minutes.

7. Add cream and parsley, stir and cook for 10 minutes. Divide into plates and serve.

Nutrition:

Calories: 1044, Fat: 45.8, Fiber: 1.3, Carbs: 9.6, Protein: 125.4

Chicken Italian Style Servings

Prep Time + Cook Time: 26 minutes Servings: 3

Ingredients:

- Basil-2 tsps. (dried)
- Marjoram-2 tsps. (dried)
- Salt and black pepper-A pinch
- Thyme-2 tsps. (dried)
- Rosemary-2 tsps. (dried)
- Sweet paprika-1 tsp.
- Chicken breasts-2 pounds (skinless, boneless and cubed)
- Tomatoes-1 cup (cubed)
- Red onion-1 (chopped)
- Broccoli florets-1-1/2 cups
- Olive oil-2 tbsps.
- Garlic-2 tsps. (minced)
- Zucchini-1 (chopped)
- Cauliflower rice-4 cups (cooked)

Directions:

1. In a mixing bowl.
2. Add the chicken with basil, marjoram, salt, pepper, thyme, rosemary, paprika, tomatoes, onion, broccoli, olive oil, garlic and zucchini.
3. Toss and spread this mix on a lined baking sheet.
4. Transfer in the oven.
5. Cook at 425 0F for 20 minutes.
6. Divide the cauliflower rice between plates.
7. Add the chicken mix on top and serve.

Nutrition:

calories 251, fat 6, fiber 8, carbs 16, protein 7

Chicken Masala Curry

Prep Time + Cook Time: 1 hour 30 minutes Servings: 2

Ingredients:

- Chicken breast, skinless, boneless and chopped-1
- Lemon juice -½ tbsp

- Garam masala-½ tbsp
- Ginger, grated -1/8 tsp
- Salt and black pepper- to taste

Passata sauce:

- Garam masala -2 tsp
- Garlic cloves, minced -2
- Canned tomato passata -7.5 oz.
- Sweet paprika -¼ tsp
- Turmeric powder -¼ tsp

Directions:

1. Toss chicken with lemon juice, ginger, salt, pepper and 1 tbsp garam masala in a large bowl.
2. Cover the seasoned chicken and refrigerate for 1hour
3. Place a cooking pot on medium high heat.
4. Toss in the marinated chicken along with its marinade.
5. Stir cook this chicken for 10 minutes.
6. Add all the sauce ingredients to the chicken and mix well.
7. Cover this chicken mixture and let it simmer for 20 minutes.
8. Serve fresh.
9. Devour.

Nutrition:

Calories: 252, Fat: 4, Fiber: 7, Carbs: 9, Protein: 11

Chicken Mushroom Sautee

Prep Time + Cook Time: 40 minutes Servings: 2

Ingredients:

- Chicken thighs-2
- Mushrooms, sliced-1 cup
- Ghee -2 tbsp
- Salt and black pepper - to taste
- Onion powder-¼ tsp
- Garlic powder -¼ tsp
- Water -¼ cup
- Mustard -½ tsp
- Parsley, chopped- ½ tbsp

Directions:

1. Add half of the ghee to a pan and place it over medium-high heat.
2. Place the chicken thighs in the pan and season them with salt, pepper, onion powder, and garlic powder.
3. Sauté for 3 minutes for each side then transfer them to a suitable bowl.
4. Heat the remaining ghee in the same pan over medium-high heat.
5. Toss in mushrooms, water, and mustard.
6. Stir cook for 5 minutes then return the chicken to pan.
7. Cover this mixture and continue cooking for 15 minutes.
8. Garnish with parsley.
9. Serve fresh.

Nutrition:

Calories: 273, Fat: 32, Fiber: 6, Carbs: 12, Protein: 26

Chicken Soup, Chinese Style

Prep Time + Cook Time: 30 minutes Serves: 4

Ingredients:

- Salt
- Coconut aminos, 2 tbsps.
- Black pepper
- Olive oil, 2 tbsps.
- Garlic cloves, 2
- Chopped head bok choy, 1
- Chopped chili pepper, 1
- Cubed boneless chicken thighs, 3
- Chopped cilantro, ½ cup
- Five spice powder, 1 ½ tbsps.
- Chicken stock, 3 cup

Directions:

1. Set a mixing bowl in place to combine the five-spice powder with salt to rub on the chicken.
2. Set the pot with oil on fire to cook chili pepper and garlic to cook for 3 minutes over medium heat
3. Stir in the bok choy, chicken stock, and aminos o cook for 12 minutes.
4. Set on serving bowls then enjoy topped with chopped cilantro.

Nutrition:

Calories: 227, Fat: 4, Fiber: 5, Carbs: 10, Protein: 9

Chicken Soup, Indian Style

Prep Time + Cook Time: 2 hours 10 minutes Serves: 5

Ingredients:

- Chopped cilantro, 2 tbsps.
- Veggie stock, 3 ½ quarts
- Celery ribs, 4
- Minced garlic clove, 1
- Parsley springs, 6
- Salt
- Divided whole chicken, 1
- Black pepper
- Olive oil, ¼ cup
- Chopped tomatoes, 2
- Black peppercorns, 1 tsp.
- Grated ginger, 2 tbsps.
- Chopped yellow onion, 1
- Tomato paste, 1 tbsp.
- Coconut milk, 1 cup

Directions:

1. Set the pot on fire then add the chicken with onion and stock to simmer over medium heat
2. Stir in the parsley sprigs, peppercorns, and garlic
3. Bring to simmer for 1 hour 30 minutes while covered
4. In the meantime, set the pan on fire with some oil to cook ginger, tomatoes, curry powder, and tomatoes to cook for 7 minutes on medium-high heat
5. Mix in the coconut milk to cook for 30 minutes.
6. Give the soup a gentle stir, then serve topped with chopped cilantro.

Nutrition:

Calories: 219, Fat: 9, Fiber: 5, Carbs: 10, Protein: 9

Chicken Stroganoff

Prep Time + Cook Time: 4 hours and 10 minutes Servings: 4

Ingredients:

- Chicken stock - 1 cup
- 4 zucchini, cut with a spiralizer
- coconut milk - 1 cup
- fresh parsley, chopped - 2 tbsps.
- Ground black pepper and Salt to taste
- An onion, peeled and chopped
- Dried thyme - 1½ tsps.
- Celery seeds, ground - ¼ tsp.
- 2 peeled and minced garlic cloves,
- Chopped mushrooms - 8 ounces
- Chicken breasts, cut into medium-sized pieces - 1 pound

Directions:

1. Set a slow cooker and place the chicken. Add salt, pepper, onion, garlic, mushrooms, coconut milk, celery seeds, sauces, half parsley, and thyme.
2. For 4 hours, stir, cover and cook on high heat. Add the rest of the parsley, if necessary, and stir.
3. With moderate temperature, heat a little water, add a little salt, leave until boiling, add Zucchini pasta, and cook for 1 minute then drain it.
4. Divide the dish, add chicken mixture and serve.

Nutrition:

Calories: 413, Fat: 23.4, Fiber: 4.7, Carbs: 15.1, Protein: 38.9

Chicken Thighs with Mushrooms and Cheese

Prep Time + Cook Time: 55 minutes Servings: 4

Ingredients:

- 2 peeled and minced garlic cloves,
- Butter - 3 tbsps.
- Grated Gruyere cheese - 2 tbsps.
- Sliced Mushrooms, - 8 ounces
- Ground black pepper and Salt to taste
- 6 chicken thighs

Directions:

1. With moderate temperature, heat a frying pan then add 1 tbsp. of butter, add the chicken fillets, add salt and pepper, cook on each side for 3 minutes and place it in a baking dish.
2. Reheat the pan again with the same temperature, add the rest of the butter, garlic, mix and cook for 1 minute.
3. Add the mushrooms and mix well. Add salt and pepper, mix and cook for 10 minutes.
4. Mix over chicken with a spoon, sprinkle with cheese, place in an oven for 30minutes at 350°F.
5. Broil everything for 2 minutes in the oven. Divide them into dishes and serve them.

Nutrition:

Calories: 729, Fat: 34.2, Fiber: 0.6, Carbs: 2.4, Protein: 98

Chicken with Green Onion Sauce Recipe

Prep Time + Cook Time: 37 minutes Servings: 4

Ingredients:

- 1 peeled and chopped green onion
- Sour cream - 8 ounces
- Butter - 2 tbsps.
- 4 Halves Skinless and boneless chicken breast
- Seasoning: Salt and ground black pepper

Directions:

1. With medium-high meat, heat a pan with butter, put chicken pieces, season with salt and pepper, cover with a lid, lessen the heat, and cook slowly (bring to simmer) for 10 minutes.
2. Uncover the pan, turn over chicken pieces, cover and cook for 10 minutes.
3. Supplement with green onions, mix well and cook for another 2 minutes.
4. Put off the heat from the oven, put more salt and pepper if needed, put sour cream, stir well, cover pan, and put to one side for 5 minutes.
5. Stir thoroughly again, divide between plates then serve.

Nutrition:
Calories: 659, Fat: 36.6, Fiber: 0.1, Carbs: 2.7, Protein: 75.8

Chicken with Mustard Sauce

Prep Time + Cook Time: 40 minutes Servings: 3

Ingredients:

- Sweet paprika: ¼ tsp.
- Chicken stock: 1½ cups
- Seasoning: Salt and ground black pepper
- Onion (chopped): 1 cup
- Olive oil: 1 tbsp.
- Dijon mustard: ⅓ cup
- Chicken breasts (skinless and boneless): 3
- Bacon strips (chopped): 8

Directions:

1. Mix paprika with mustard, salt, and pepper in a bowl and stir well. Distribute on chicken fillets and massage.
2. Heat a pan over medium heat, add bacon, stir, cook until brown, and place on a plate.
3. Heat the same pan with oil over medium heat, add chicken fillets, cook on each side for 2 minutes and place on a plate.
4. Heat the pan again over medium heat, add the stock, stir and simmer.
5. Add bacon and onions, salt and pepper and stir.
6. Put the chicken back into the pan, stir gently and simmer for 20 minutes over medium heat, turning the meat in half.
7. Place the chicken on the plate, sprinkle with the sauce and serve.

Nutrition:
Calories: 793, Fat: 36.9, Carbs: 6.5, Fiber: 1.8, Protein: 103.6

Chicken with Olive Tapenade and Garlic

Prep Time + Cook Time: 20 minutes Servings: 2

Ingredients:

- Chicken breast (cut into 4 pieces): 1
- Coconut oil: 2 tbsps.
- Garlic (peeled and crushed): 3 cloves
- Olive tapenade: ½ cup

For the tapenade:

- Fresh parsley (chopped): ¼ cup
- Black olives (pitted): 1 cup
- Seasoning: Salt and ground black pepper
- Lemon juice: 1 tbsp.
- Olive oil: 2 tbsps.

Directions:

1. Mix olives with salt, pepper, 2 tbsps. olive oil, lemon juice and parsley in a food processor, mix well and put in a bowl.
2. Heat a skillet with coconut oil over medium heat, add the garlic, stir and cook for 2 minutes.
3. Add the chicken pieces and cook on each side for 4 minutes.
4. Place the chicken on the plate and cover with olive tapenade.

Nutrition:

Calories: 727, Fat: 61.6, Carbs: 7.5, Fiber: 2.5, Protein: 37.7

Chicken with Sour Cream Sauce

Prep Time + Cook Time: 50 minutes Servings: 4

Ingredients:

- Ground black pepper and Salt to taste
- Sour cream - ¼ cup
- 4 chicken thighs
- Sweet paprika - 2 tbsps.
- Onion powder - 1 tsp.

Directions:

1. In a bowl, mix the sweet pepper (paprika) with salt, pepper and onion powder.
2. Prepare the chicken pieces with the pepper mixture, place on a baking sheet with lid and turn the oven on for 40 minutes at temperature of400°F, and divide the chicken on a plate and set it aside.
3. Add sour cream to the juice dish. Mix the sauce well and spill over the chickens.

Nutrition:

Calories: 526, Fat: 22.4, Fiber: 1.3, Carbs: 2.5, Protein: 74.9

Chipotle Spiced Chicken

Prep Time + Cook Time: 55 minutes Serves: 4

Ingredients:

For the sauce:

- Chopped jalapeno pepper, 1
- Chopped dried chipotle chilies, 3
- Garlic cloves, 4
- Chopped cilantro, ½ cup
- Chopped canned tomatoes, 28oz.
- Hot water, 1 cup
- Olive oil, 2 tbsps.
- Salt
- Chopped yellow onion, 1
- Black pepper

For the chicken:

- Sliced avocados, 2
- Cooked and shredded chicken meat, 2 cup

Directions:

1. Set a mixing bowl in position to combine dried chipotle peppers with hot water then reserve for 20 minutes.
2. Drain and keep the water for later usage.
3. Move the peppers to the blender, reserved water, canned tomatoes, jalapeno, garlic, seasonings, onion, cilantro, and oil to process until smooth
4. Pour the mixture to a pan then allow to boil for 20 minutes over medium heat
5. Set the sauce into 6 ramekins divide the chicken and avocado to serve

Nutrition:

Calories: 190,Fat: 5, Fiber: 5, Carbs: 8, Protein: 12

Chunky Chicken Cheese Soup

Prep Time + Cook Time: 40 minutes Servings: 6

Ingredients:

- Chicken tights, skinless, boneless and cubed-1 ½ lb.
- Chunky salsa- 15 oz.
- Chicken stock -15 oz.
- Monterrey jack cheese, shredded -8 oz.

Directions:

1. Fill the pot with stock and place chicken in it.
2. Let this stock simmer over medium heat.
3. Stir in salsa and cover it. Cook for 30 minutes on a simmer.
4. Add cheese and mix well.
5. Serve warm.

Nutrition:

Calories: 300, Fat: 6, Fiber: 3, Carbs: 9, Protein: 18

Cranberry Turkey Salad

Prep Time + Cook Time: 15 minutes   Servings: 4

Ingredients:

- Romaine lettuce leaves, torn-4 cups
- Turkey breast, cooked and cubed -2 cups
- Red apple, cored and chopped -1
- Almonds, chopped -3 tbsp.
- Cranberries -¼ cup

Directions:

1. Take a salad bowl and toss in the turkey, lettuce, cranberries, almonds, and apples.
2. Mix well using a spatula.
3. Serve fresh and chilled.

Nutrition:

Calories: 200, Fat: 7, Fiber: 1, Carbs: 13, Protein: 7

Creamy Italian Chicken Soup

Prep Time + Cook Time: 35 minutes Servings: 3

Ingredients:

- Butternut squash, peeled and cubed-2/3 lb.
- Chicken meat, cooked and shredded -½ cup
- Green onions, chopped -¼ cup
- Ghee, melted-1 ½ tbsp
- Chicken stock-15 oz.
- Celery, chopped -¼ cup
- Garlic clove, minced -½
- Italian seasoning-¼ tsp
- 7.5 oz. Canned tomatoes, chopped
- Salt and black pepper - to taste
- Red pepper flakes, dried-½ pinch
- Coconut cream -2/3 cup

Directions:

1. Add ghee in a pot and preheat it over medium-high heat.
2. Stir in onions and celery, sauté for 5 minutes.
3. Toss in squash, garlic, chicken, tomatoes, Italian seasoning, salt, pepper, nutmeg, pepper flakes, and stock.
4. Let this squash mixture simmer on medium heat for 15 minutes.
5. Use a hand blender to puree this soup.
6. Stir in coconut cream and cook for 5 minutes.
7. Dish out and serve warm.
8. Enjoy.

Nutrition:

Calories: 282, Fat: 9, Fiber: 7, Carbs: 10, Protein: 7

Creamy Turkey Spinach Medley

Prep Time + Cook Time: 45 minutes Servings: 4

Ingredients:

- Turkey meat, minced-18 ounces
- Spinach-3 ounces
- Canned tomatoes, chopped-20 ounces
- Olive oil -2 tbsp.
- Coconut cream -2 tbsp.
- Garlic cloves, minced -2
- Yellow onions, sliced -2
- Ginger, grated -2 tbsp.
- Turmeric powder -1 tbsp.
- Chili powder -2 tbsp.
- Salt and black pepper - to taste

Directions:

1. Add oil in a pan and preheat it over medium heat.
2. Stir in onion and saute for 5 minutes.
3. Toss in the garlic, ginger, salt, pepper, tomatoes, chili powder, and turmericup
4. Stir cook for a minute then add coconut cream.
5. Cook this mixture for 10 minutes then puree this mixture using a hand-held blender.
6. Add spinach and turkey meat. Cook it on a simmer for 15 minutes.
7. Serve warm.

Nutrition:
Calories: 240, Fat: 4, Fiber: 3, Carbs: 9, Protein: 12

Duck Breast Salad

Prep Time + Cook Time: 25 minutes Servings: 4

Ingredients:

- Shallot (peeled and chopped): 1
- Olive oil: ¼ cup
- Swerve: 1 tbsp.
- Red vinegar: ¼ cup
- Raspberries: ¾ cup
- Water: ¼ cup
- Seasoning: Salt and ground black pepper
- Dijon mustard: 1 tbsp.

For the salad:

- Goats cheese (crumbled): 4 ounces
- Baby spinach: 10 ounces
- Duck breasts (medium & boneless): 2
- Pecans (halves): ½ cup
- Salt and ground black pepper
- Raspberries: ½ pint

Directions:

1. Mix in a blender with shallot, vinegar, water, oil, ¾ cup raspberries, mustard, salt, pepper and mix well.
2. Sift in a bowl and set aside.
3. Cut the duck breast, season with salt, pepper and place the skin side in a pan, which is heated over medium heat.
4. Cook for 8 minutes, turn over and cook for 5 minutes.
5. Spread the spinach on a plate, sprinkle with goat cheese, pecan halves and a ½ pint of raspberries.
6. Cut off duck breast and add raspberries.
7. Add the raspberry vinaigrette and serve.

Nutrition:
Calories: 628, Fat: 52, Fiber: 7.2, Carbs: 15.1, Protein: 32

Duck Breast with Vegetables

Prep Time + Cook Time: 20 minutes Servings: 2

Ingredients:

- Zucchini (sliced): 2
- Duck breasts (skin on and sliced thin): 2
- Green onion bunch (chopped): 1
- Coconut oil: 1 tbsp.
- Daikon (chopped): 1
- Seasoning: Salt and ground black pepper
- Green bell peppers (seeded and chopped): 2

Directions:

1. Heat a pan with oil over medium heat, add spring onions, stir and cook for 2 minutes.
2. Add zucchini, daikon, pepper, salt, pepper, stir and cook for 10 minutes.
3. Heat another pan over medium heat, add duck slices, cook on each side for 3 minutes and place in the pan.
4. Cook for 3 minutes, spread over the plates and serve.

Nutrition:
Calories: 558, Fiber: 5.2, Fat: 20.3, Carbs: 19.3, Protein: 75.2

Easy Chicken Stir–fry

Prep Time + Cook Time: 22 minutes Servings: 2

Ingredients:

- Broccoli florets- 2 cups
- Water - ½ cup
- Stevia- 1 tbsp.
- Tamari sauce -¼ cup
- Garlic powder- ½ tsp.
- Sesame oil -1 tbsp.
- Red pepper flakes - 1 tsp.
- onion powder - 1 tsp.
- Two skinless and boneless chicken thighs (cut into thin strips)
- Xanthan gum - ½ tsp.
- Chopped scallions - ½ cup
- Grated fresh ginger - 1 tbsp.

Directions:

1. With a medium-high temperature, heat a pan with oil, add ginger and chicken, mix well and cook for 3 minutes.
2. Put water, onion powder, tamari sauce, garlic powder, pepper flakes, xanthan gum, stevia, mix carefully, and cook for another 5 minutes.
3. Put scallions and broccoli, mix well, cook for another 2 minutes, and divide into plates then Serve hot.

Nutrition:
Calories: 392, Fat: 19.1, Fiber: 3.6, Carbs: 11.3, Protein: 43.9

Flavorsome Turkey Chili

Prep Time + Cook Time: 1 hour and 35 minutes Servings: 6

Ingredients:

- Olive oil -3 tsp.
- Green bell pepper, chopped -1
- Turkey meat, ground -1 lb.
- Garlic, minced -1 tbsp.
- Yellow onion, chopped -1
- Ancho chilies, ground -1 tsp.
- Chili powder -1 tbsp.
- Canned green chilies and juice, chopped-8 ounces
- Tomato paste -8 ounces
- Canned tomatoes, chopped -15 ounces
- Beef stock -2 cups
- Salt and black pepper - to taste

Directions:

1. Add 2 tsp. of oil to a pan and preheat it over medium heat.
2. Stir in turkey and saute until it is brown then transfer to a pot.
3. Add remaining oil to the pan and preheat it over medium heat.
4. Toss in green bell pepper, onion, garlic, ancho chilies, chili powder, pepper, and salt. Saute for 6 minutes.
5. Add this mixture to the turkey meat along with tomato sauce, green chilies, and chopped tomatoes.
6. Stir well then cover this pot. Cook this mixture for 1 hour on medium-low heat.
7. Serve right away.

Nutrition:

Calories: 250, Fat: 8, Fiber: 4, Carbs: 11, Protein: 20

Fried Chicken

Prep Time + Cook Time: 44 hours Servings: 4

Ingredients:

- Crushed pork rinds - 4 ounces
- Jarred pickle juice - 16 ounces
- Whisked egg- 2
- Coconut oil - 2 cups
- 3 chicken breasts, cut into strips

Directions:

1. Mix the chicken breast pieces in a bowl with pickle juice, mix rigorously, cover and place in the refrigerator for a day.
2. In two separate bowls, Place eggs in a bowl and pork rinds in the other.
3. Put the chicken pieces in the egg and then into the pork skin and coat well.
4. With moderate temperature, heat a pan with oil, add chicken pieces, grill on all side for 3 minutes, put on a paper towel, drain grease then serve.

Nutrition:

Calories: 1488, Fat: 134.8, Fiber: 0, Carbs: 2.4, Protein: 73.8

Garlic Chicken Meatloaf

Prep Time + Cook Time: 50 minutes Servings: 8

Ingredients:

- Ground chicken- 2 pound
- Chopped fresh parsley- 2 tbsps.
- Minced garlic - 1 tsp.
- Dried basil -1 tsp.
- Onion powder -2 tsps.
- Italian seasoning- 2 tsps.
- Tomato sauce -1 cup
- Dried rosemary - ½ tsp.
- Peeled and minced garlic cloves-Four
- Seasoning: Salt and ground black pepper

For the filling:

- Grated Parmesan cheese - 1 cup
- Mozzarella cheese (shredded)- 1 cup
- Chopped fresh parsley - 2 tbsps.
- 1 Peeled and minced garlic clove
- Ricotta cheese - ½ cup
- Chopped fresh chives - 2 tsps.

Directions:

1. Mix chicken with half of 4 garlic cloves, tomato paste, garlic, basil, rosemary, salt and pepper, onion powder, Italian seasoning, 2 tbsps. parsley in a container(bowl), and stir properly.
2. In a separate container, add together ricotta cheese with half of the mozzarella cheese, half of Parmesan cheese, chives, 1 garlic clove, salt, pepper, 2 tbsps. of parsley, and mix thoroughly.
3. Add half of the chicken, then mix into a loaf pan and spread evenly, also add cheese filling and spread evenly. Top with rest of meat and spread again.
4. Place meatloaf in oven for 20 minutes at a temperature 400°F.
5. Remove the meatloaf out of the oven, then spread rest of tomato paste, garlic, basil, rosemary and rest of the cheese evenly, heat for 20 minutes.
6. Remove the meatloaf and allow to cool, slice then divide between plates, and serve.

Nutrition:

Calories: 334, Fat: 15.6, Fiber: 0.5, Carbs: 3.7, Protein: 43.9

Grilled Wings with Green Sauce

Prep Time + Cook Time: 45 minutes Servings: 3

Ingredients:

- Chicken wings -9
- Turmeric powder -½ tbsp
- Ginger, grated-½ tbsp
- Coriander, ground-½ tbsp
- Sweet paprika-½ tbsp
- Salt and black pepper -to taste
- Olive oil-1 tbsp

Green sauce:

- Juice of ¼ lime
- Mint leaves-½ cup
- Ginger, grated -½ -inch
- Cilantro-¼ cup

- Olive oil-½ tbsp
- Water -½ tbsp
- Salt and black pepper -to taste

Directions:

1. Toss 1 tbsp ginger, paprika, turmeric, pepper, salt, coriander and 2 tbsp oil in a suitable bowl.
2. Add the chicken wings to the bowl and mix well to season.
3. Cover these wings and refrigerate for 20 minutes to marinate.
4. Preheat a grill over high heat and grease it grilling grates.
5. Place the wings in the grill and cook for 25 minutes while flipping them after 5 minutes.
6. Meanwhile blend cilantro, mint, lime juice, 1 tbsp oil, salt, pepper, water, and 1-inch ginger in a processor until smooth.
7. Serve the grilled chicken wings with mint sauce.
8. Enjoy fresh.

Nutrition:

Calories: 260, Fat: 5, Fiber: 7, Carbs: 15, Protein: 11

Hot Wings (Buffalo Sauce Style)

Prep Time + Cook Time: 34 minutes Servings: 1

Ingredients:

- Chicken wings-6 (cut in halves)
- Garlic powder-A pinch
- Hot sauce-1/2 cup
- Sweet paprika-1/2 tsp.
- Ghee-2 tbsps.
- Cayenne pepper-A pinch
- Salt and black pepper-To taste

Directions:

1. Pick a mixing bowl.
2. Coat the chicken pieces with half of the hot sauce, salt and pepper.
3. Shake well.
4. Settle the chicken pieces on a lined baking dish.
5. Shift in preheated broiler and broil 8 minutes.
6. Turn the sides of the chicken pieces.
7. Leave to broil for further 8 minutes.
8. Warm up a pan with the ghee and put it over medium heat.
9. Combine rest of the hot sauce, salt, pepper, cayenne and paprika.
10. Toss and cook for a couple of minutes.
11. Slide the broiled chicken pieces to a bowl.
12. Stir ghee and hot sauce mix.
13. Drizzle over the pieces.
14. Again, toss well to coat well.
15. Serve them right away!

Nutrition :

Calories:- 500; Fat : 45; Fiber : 12; Carbs : 1; Protein : 45

Leek and Chicken Mix

Prep Time + Cook Time: 1 hour 40 minutes Serves: 4

Ingredients:

- Lemon juice, ½ cup
- Salt
- Olive oil, 3 tbsps.
- Black pepper
- Tomato passata, 1` cup
- Sliced leek, 1
- Whole chicken, 1
- Sliced carrot, 1
- Veggie stock, 1 c
- Chopped yellow onion, 2 cup

Directions:

1. Prepare the baking tray with some greasing.
2. Set the chicken on the baking tray.
3. Season with pepper and salt then top with carrots, leek, tomato passata, onion, veggie stock, and lemon juice
4. Ensure they coat evenly
5. Set the oven for 1 hour 3 minutes, allow to bake
6. Once fully baked, carve the chicken and divide the vegetables on plates to serve.
7. Enjoy topped with cooking juices

Nutrition:

Calories: 219, Fat: 3, Fiber: 5, Carbs: 6, Protein: 20

Lemon Chicken and Fennel Salad

Prep Time + Cook Time: 10 minutes Serves: 4

Ingredients:

- Walnut oil, 2 tbsps.
- Chopped fennel, 1½ cup
- Black pepper.
- Chopped fennel fronds, 2 tbsps.
- Lemon juice, 2 tbsps.
- Toasted and chopped walnuts, ¼ cup
- Mayonnaise, ¼ cup
- Cooked, chopped and de-boned chicken breasts, 3.
- Salt.
- Cayenne pepper

Directions:

1. Set a mixing bowl in place to combine walnuts and chicken
2. Combine mayo with the seasonings, walnut oil, fennel fronds, lemon juice, garlic, and cayenne in another bowl.
3. Spread the mixture over chicken and fennel mix to coat evenly
4. Refrigerate until service time.

Nutritional :

calories: 200, fiber: 1, fat: 10, carbs: 3, protein: 7

Lettuce Wrapped Turkey

Prep Time + Cook Time: 17 minutes Serves: 6

Ingredients:

- Tomato passata, ½ cup
- Olive oil, 1 tbsp.
- Salt
- Romaine lettuce head, 1
- Black pepper
- Sweet paprika, ½ tsp.
- Ground turkey meat, 1 lb.
- Chopped yellow onion, ¾ cup
- Chili powder, 1 tbsp.
- Ground cumin, 1 tsp.
- Chicken stock, ½ cup
- Minced garlic cloves, 2

Directions:

1. Set the pan on fire to fry the onion for 2 minutes over medium-high heat
2. Stir in pepper, turkey, and salt to cook for 5 minutes
3. Mix in the stock, paprika, chili powder, tomato sauce, and cumin to simmer for 5 minutes
4. Wrap the turkey into lettuce leaves to serve.

Nutrition:

Calories: 205, Fat: 5, Fiber: 1, Carbs: 9, Protein: 10

Luscious Chicken thigh Stew

Prep Time + Cook Time: 50 minutes Servings: 3

Ingredients:

- Chicken thighs -3
- Olive oil -½ tsp
- Salt and black pepper -to taste
- Yellow onion, chopped -½
- Celery stalk, chopped -½
- Parsley, chopped -½ tbsp
- Chicken stock -1 ¼ cups
- Canned tomatoes, chopped-7.5 oz.

Directions:

1. Add oil to a pot and place it over medium-high heat.
2. Place chicken in the pot and season it with salt and pepper.
3. Sear it for 4 minutes per side.
4. Add onion and celery, sauté for 4 minutes.
5. Stir in tomatoes and stock. Let it simmer for 25 minutes.
6. Transfer the cooked chicken thighs to a cutting board.
7. Remove the thighs bones and shred the meat using a fork.
8. Return these shreds to the pot and mix well.
9. Garnish with parsley.
10. Enjoy fresh.

Nutrition:

Calories: 272, Fat: 4, Fiber: 4, Carbs: 7, Protein: 14

Mango Habanero Chicken

Prep Time + Cook Time: 30 minutes Serves: 2

Ingredients:

For the sauce:

- Mango juice, ¾ cup
- Coconut aminos, ½ tbsp.
- Minced garlic, 1 tsp.
- Coconut oil, 2 ½ tsps.
- Minced ginger, 1 ½ tsps.
- Minced habanero pepper, ½ tsp.

For the chicken:

- Tapioca flour, 3 tbsps.
- Chicken breast, 8 oz.
- Salt
- Coconut oil, 1 tbsp.
- Black pepper

Directions:

1. Set the pan on fire with 2½ tsp. of coconut oil to fry the ginger, habanero, and garlic for one minute over medium-high heat

2. Stir in the juice and coconut aminos to cook for 10 minutes then remove from heat.

3. Set another bowl in place to combine the coconut flour with seasonings and chicken to coat evenly

4. Set the pan on heat with 2 tbsps. of coconut oil to cook the coated chicken for five minutes over medium heat the set move to the pan with the sauce.

5. Allow the mixture to cook for 10 minutes

6. Serve and enjoy.

Nutrition:

Calories: 260, Fat: 32, Fiber: 6, Carbs: 13, Protein: 35

Mayonnaise Chicken Salad

Prep Time + Cook Time: 10 minutes Serves: 4

Ingredients:

- Mayonnaise, ¼ cup
- Halved cherry tomatoes, 10.
- Salt
- Garlic pesto, 2 tbsps.
- Cooked and crumbled bacon slices, 6.
- Cooked and cubed chicken meat, 1lb.
- Pitted and cubed avocado, 1.
- Black pepper.

Directions:

1. Combine chicken with avocado, bacon, salt, tomatoes, and pepper in a mixing bowl.

2. Mix in garlic pesto and mayo to coat evenly.

3. Serve and enjoy.

Nutrition :

calories: 357, fat: 23, fiber: 5, carbs: 3, protein: 26

Mexican Cheesy Casserole

Prep Time + Cook Time: 49 minutes Servings: 7

Ingredients:

- Chicken thighs-1 pound (skinless, boneless and chopped)
- Red enchilada sauce-1 cup
- Chipotle peppers-2 (chopped)
- Jalapenos-2 (chopped)
- Olive oil-1 tbsp.
- Heavy cream-1/4 cup
- Pepper jack cheese-1 cup (shredded)
- Cream cheese-4 ounces
- Cooking spray-As required
- Cilantro-2 tbsps. (chopped)
- Tortillas-2
- White onion-1 (small and chopped)
- Salt and black pepper-To taste

Directions:

1. Heat up a pan with the oil over medium heat.
2. Add the chipotle and jalapeno peppers. Toss and cook for a few seconds.
3. Add onion and stir. Cook for 5 minutes.
4. Combine the cream cheese and heavy cream. Shake well until the cheese melts.
5. Add the chicken, salt, pepper and enchilada sauce. Mix well and take off the heat.
6. Grease baking dish with cooking spray.
7. Fix in the tortillas on the bottom. Spread chicken mix all over.
8. Sprinkle shredded cheese.
9. Cover with tin foil. Place in the oven at 350 ºF.
10. Prepare for 15 minutes. Remove the tin foil.
11. Bake for 15 minutes more.
12. Sprinkle cilantro on top.

Nutrition:
Calories:- 240; Fat : 12; Fiber : 5; Carbs : 5; Protein : 20

Minced Chicken Burgers

Prep Time + Cook Time: 20 minutes Serves: 6

Ingredients:

- Sweet paprika, 1 tsp.
- Medium egg, 1
- Minced garlic clove, 1
- Salt
- Chopped yellow onion, 1
- Black pepper
- Minced chicken breast, 2 lbs.
- Olive oil, 3 tbsps.

Directions:

1. Set the mixing bowl in place to combine the chicken meat with paprika, egg, pepper, garlic, salt, and onion.
2. Stir gently then mold 6 burgers from the mixture.
3. Set the pan on fire to cook the burgers for 5 minutes each side
4. Serve warm and enjoy

Nutrition:
Calories: 189, Fat: 3, Fiber: 3, Carbs: 9, Protein: 8

Olive Braised Chicken

Prep Time + Cook Time: 35 minutes Serves: 6

Ingredients:

- Chopped green bell peppers, 2
- Chopped celery, ½ cup
- Lemon juice, 1 tbsp.
- Salt
- Chopped chicken, 2 lbs.
- Chopped garlic, ½ tsp.
- Olive oil, 2 tbsps.
- Veggie stock, 1 cup
- Black pepper
- Chopped plum tomatoes, 4
- Chopped red onion, 1
- Tomato sauce, 1 cup
- Halved olives, ¼ cup
- Chopped coriander, 1 bunch

Directions:

1. Set a medium mixing bowl in a clean working surface.
2. Combine the chicken pieces with celery, onion, pepper, garlic, salt, and lemon juice. Allow to rest for 15 minutes while covered
3. Set the pot on fire over medium heat with some oil to fry the chicken and vegetable ix for 15minutes
4. Mix in the stock, tomato sauce, bell pepper, tomatoes, and olives to cook for 7 minutes while covered
5. Gently stir in the chopped coriander and serve.
6. Enjoy

Nutrition:
Calories: 230, Fat: 3, Fiber: 5, Carbs: 6, Protein: 19

Oregano Chicken Breasts

Prep Time + Cook Time: 40 minutes Serves: 6

Ingredients:

- Olive oil, 2 tbsps.
- Stripped De-boned, skinless chicken breasts, 3
- Minced garlic, 1 tbsp.
- Whisked eggs, 2
- Dried oregano, 1 tsp.
- Salt
- Ground almonds, 1¼ cup
- Black pepper

Directions:

1. Set a mixing bowl in place to combine almonds with oregano, pepper, garlic, and salt.
2. Coat the chicken strips in the almond mixture
3. Set the pan on fire with the oil to fry the chicken strips for 10 minutes each side over medium-high heat.
4. Set on plates to serve and enjoy.

Nutrition:
Calories: 183, Fat: 8, Fiber: 1, Carbs: 8, Protein: 7

Pan-Fried Sour Chicken Thighs

Prep Time + Cook Time: 50 minutes Serves: 6

Ingredients:

- Chopped green onions, 1 bunch
- Chicken thighs, 4 lbs.
- Soy sauce, 1 cup

Directions:

1. Set the pan on fire to brown the chicken thighs for four minutes evenly over medium-high heat
2. Mix in the soy sauce and onions to coat well then cook for 30 minutes
3. Set on serving plates and enjoy.

Nutrition:

Calories: 200, Fat: 4, Fiber: 2, Carbs: 12, Protein: 10

Pan-seared Duck Breast Recipe

Prep Time + Cook Time: 30 minutes Servings: 1

Ingredients:

- Medium duck breast (skin scored): 1
- Heavy cream: 1 tbsp.
- Swerve: 1 tbsp.
- Fresh sage: ¼ tsp.
- Orange zest: ½ tsp.
- Butter: 2 tbsps.
- Seasoning: Salt and ground black pepper
- Baby spinach: 1 cup

Directions:

1. Heat a frying pan with butter over medium heat. Once it has melted, add it and mix until the butter is brown.
2. Add orange peel and sage, stir and cook for 2 minutes. Add the heavy cream and stir again.
3. Heat another skillet over medium heat, add the duck breast, skin, cook for 4 minutes, turn and cook for another 3 minutes.
4. Pour the orange sauce over the duck breast, mix and cook for a few minutes.
5. Add the spinach to the pan with the sauce, mix and cook for 1 minute.
6. Remove the duck from the heat, cut the duck breast and place on a plate.
7. Sprinkle orange sauce and serve with spinach separately.

Nutrition:

Calories: 1088, Fat: 54.3, Carbs: 6.6, Fiber: 0.7, Protein: 142.2

Parmesan Chicken Cal zone

Prep Time + Cook Time: 1 hour 10 minutes Servings: 12

Ingredients:

- keto marinara sauce- ½ cup
- Onion powder - 1 tsp.
- Garlic powder - 1 tsp.
- Seasoning: Salt and ground black pepper
- Two eggs
- Grated Parmesan cheese - ½ cup
- Skinless and boneless chicken breasts and each sliced in half - 1 pound
- Italian seasoning - 1 tsp.
- Flaxseed (ground) - ¼ cup
- Provolone cheese - 8 ounces

For pizza crust:

- Four eggs
- Shredded mozzarella - 6 oz.

Directions:

1. Add the Italian seasoning with onion powder, salt, pepper, flaxseed, garlic powder, and Parmesan cheese in a container(bowl), and mix well.
2. Mix and whisk together eggs with a pinch of salt and pepper, in another container.
3. Prepare the chicken pieces, and dip in eggs, and then in seasoning mixture, arrange all pieces on a lined baking sheet, and bake in the oven for 30 minutes at a temperature of 350°F.
4. For pizza crust: Break eggs in a container (bowl), add cheese, mix thoroughly and spread the mixture on a baking sheet lined with parchment paper. Bake for 3 minutes at a temperature of 350°F.
5. Place pizza crust on a lined baking sheet and spread half of the provolone cheese on half.
6. Remove the chicken out of the oven, cut it into pieces, and sprinkle over provolone cheese.
7. The marinara sauce and the rest of the cheese should be added, then cover with another half of the dough and shape calzone.
8. Place in an oven, while all edges are sealed, and heat for 20 minutes at a temperature of at 350°F.
9. Let cal zone cool down before slicing and serving.

Nutrition:
Calories: 247, Fat: 14.9, Fiber: 0.7, Carbs: 2.4, Protein: 25.2

Passata Chicken Soup

Prep Time + Cook Time:4 hours 10 minutes Servings: 6

Ingredients:

- Chicken stock- 15 ounces
- Skinless and boneless chicken tights (cubed)- 1½ pounds
- Tomato passata- 15 ounces
- Monterey jack- 8 ounces

Directions:

1. Add chicken with stock, tomato passata, cheese in a pot and set on a slow cooker, mix properly, cover with a lid, and cook for 4 hours.
2. Remove the lid, mix the soup then divide into bowls, and serve.

Nutrition:
Calories: 397, Fat: 27.7, Fiber: 0, Carbs: 4.2, Protein: 34.4

Pecan–Crusted Chicken

Prep Time + Cook Time: 30 minutes Servings: 4

Ingredients:

- 4 chicken breasts
- Coconut oil - 3 tbsps.
- Ground black pepper and Salt to taste
- 1 whisked egg
- Chopped Pecans- 1½ cups

Directions:

1. In two separate bowl, add pecans in a bowl and whisked egg in the other.
2. Season the chicken with salt and ground black pepper to taste, dip it in egg and then in pecans.
3. With medium temperature heat a pan with oil, add chicken, fry until its brown on both sides.
4. Place the chicken pieces on a baking tray in the oven and cook for 10 minutes at 350 ° F. Serve and serve on plates.

Nutrition:

Calories: 930, Fat: 65.2, Fiber: 5.3, Carbs: 7.1, Protein: 80.6

Pepperoni Chicken Bake

Prep Time + Cook Time: 65 minutes Servings: 6

Ingredients:

- Coconut oil - 1 tbsp.
- sliced mozzarella cheese - 6 ounces
- Garlic powder - 1 tsp.
- Salt and ground black pepper, to taste
- Medium chicken breasts, skinless and boneless - 4
- Tomato passata - 14 ounces
- Dried oregano - 1 tsp.
- Pepperoni, sliced - 2 ounces

Directions:

1. Put the tomato paste in a pot, Preset the oven to medium temperature, boil for 3 minutes and then put off the heat.
2. Season the chicken with salt, pepper, garlic powder and oregano in a bowl.
3. Preset the oven to a moderate temperature, then heat a pan with coconut oil, add chicken pieces, cook for two minutes on both sides then transfer it onto a baking pan.
4. Put the mozzarella cheese slices on top, sprinkle with sauce with the pepperoni slices and place in the oven at 400° F and bake for 30 minutes. Separate plates and serve.

Nutrition:

Calories: 491, Fat: 24.4, Fiber: 0.2, Carbs: 4.7, Protein: 60.3

Salsa Chicken with Veggies spray

Prep Time + Cook Time: 1 hour and 25 minutes Servings: 6

Ingredients:

- Chicken breasts (skinless & boneless): 6
- Vegetable cooking spray
- Seasoning: Salt and ground black pepper
- Cheddar cheese (shredded): 1 cup
- For keto salsa:
- Chili peppers: 2
- Roasted tomatoes (medium): 8
- Whole limes juiced: 1
- Salt: 1 tbsp.
- Garlic: 4 cloves

Directions:

1. Spray a casserole dish with cooking oil, put chicken fillets on top and season with salt and pepper.
2. Combine all salsa ingredients in a blender, pulsing well.
3. Cover chicken fillets with salsa. Place in a 425°F oven and bake for 1 hour.
4. Spread cheese and bake for 15 minutes.
5. Divide into plates and serve.

Nutrition:

Calories: 788, Fiber: 0.7, Carbs: 18, Fat: 39.3, Protein: 89.5

Savory Chicken Recipe

Prep Time + Cook Time:1 hour 10 minutes Servings: 4

Ingredients:

- Ground black pepper and Salt to taste
- Bacon slices, chopped: 5
- ¼ cup onion, peeled and chopped
- Mayonnaise - ½ cup
- Cheddar cheese, grated - 1 cup
- Jalapeños, chopped - ¼ cup
- 6 chicken breasts, skinless and boneless
- Parmesan cheese, grated - ½ cup
- Cream cheese - 8 ounces

For the topping:

- Melted butter - 4 tbsps
- Parmesan cheese - ½ cup
- Pork skins, crushed - 2 ounces

Directions:

1. Put the chicken fillets in a casserole dish, season with salt and pepper, place in an oven for and bake for 40 minutes at a temperature of 425 °F.
2. With moderate temperature heat a pan and add the bacon, stir and boil until crisp, pour it on a plate.
3. Heat the pan again, with moderate temperature, add the onion, stir and cook for 4 minutes.
4. Put off the heat, add bacon, jalapeño, cream cheese,

mayonnaise, cheddar cheese, and ½ cup Parmesan cheese, mix well and sprinkle over the chicken.

5. Mix the pork with the butter and a quarter cup of Parmesan and stir in a bowl.

6. Pour over the chicken, put it in the oven and bake for 15 minutes. Serve hot.

Nutrition:
Calories: 1452, Fat: 95.2, Fiber: 0.2, Carbs: 11.2, Protein: 133.4

Seared Cheesy Meatballs

Prep Time + Cook Time: 21 minutes Servings: 6
Ingredients:
- Egg -1
- Salt and black pepper - to taste
- Almond flour -¼ cup
- Turkey meat, ground -1 lb.
- Garlic powder-½ tsp.
- Sun-dried tomatoes, chopped -2 tbsp.
- Mozzarella cheese, shredded -½ cup
- Olive oil -2 tbsp.
- Oregano, chopped -2 tbsp.

Directions:
1. Thoroughly mix turkey with egg, garlic powder, salt, pepper, mozzarella, oregano, flour and sun-dried tomatoes in a bowl.

2. Make medium sized meatballs out of this mixture.

3. Place a skillet with cooking oil over medium-high heat.

4. Sear these meatballs for 3 minutes per side.

5. Serve warm with fresh salad.

Nutrition:
Calories: 140, Fat: 6, Fiber: 3, Carbs: 8, Protein: 14

Simple Chicken Salad

Prep Time + Cook Time: 10 minutes Serves: 3
Ingredients:
- Dill relish, ½ tbsps.
- Chopped celery rib, 1.
- Roasted and chopped chicken breast, 5 oz.
- Mustard, 1 tsp.
- Chopped parsley, 2 tbsps.
- Hard-boiled and chopped egg, 1.
- Chopped green onion, 1.
- Mayonnaise, 1/3 cup
- Black pepper.
- Salt.
- Granulated garlic

Directions:
1. Combine onion, parsley, and celery in a blender to process until done then reserve on a bowl.

2. Again, place the chicken in the blender to process until done then combine with the veggies.

3. Stir in the seasoning and egg pieces.

4. Mix in mayo, mustard, granulated garlic, and dill relish to coat evenly.
5. Serve right away and enjoy.

Nutritional :

calories: 283, fat: 23, fiber: 5, protein: 12, carbs: 3

Skillet Chicken and Mushrooms Recipe

Prep Time + Cook Time: 40 minutes Servings: 4

Ingredients:
- Butter: ¼ cup
- Chicken thighs: 4
- Mushrooms (sliced): 2 cups
- Water: ½ cup
- Seasoning: Salt and ground black pepper
- Garlic powder: ½ tsp.
- Onion powder: ½ tsp.
- Fresh tarragon (chopped): 1 tbsp.
- Dijon mustard: 1 tsp.

Directions:
1. Heat a pan with half of the butter over medium heat, add chicken legs, season with salt, pepper, garlic powder, and onion powder, cook on each side for 3 minutes and place in a bowl.
2. Heat the same pan with the remaining butter over medium heat, add the mushrooms, stir and cook for 5 minutes.
3. Supply mustard and water and stir well. Put back the chicken pieces inside the pan, stir, cover and cook for 15 minutes.
4. Add tarragon, stir, cook for 5 minutes, divide between plates and dish.

Nutrition:

Calories: 664, Fiber: 0.4, Fat: 33.3, Carbs: 1.2, Protein: 85.7

Spiced Turkey Mix

Prep Time + Cook Time: 1 hour 20 minutes Serves: 2

Ingredients:
- Spinach, 6 cup
- Minced garlic cloves, 2
- Cubed avocados, 2
- Salt
- Melted ghee, 2 tbsps.
- Black pepper
- Ground turkey meat, ½ lb.
- Cayenne pepper, ¼ tsp.
- Garlic powder, 1 tsp.
- Hot sauce, 2 tbsps.
- Chopped yellow onion, ½

Directions:
1. Set the pan on fire to fry the garlic and onion for six minutes over medium-high heat
2. Mix in the hot sauce, turkey meat, pepper, garlic powder, salt, and

cayenne pepper to cook for 10 minutes

3. Stir in the spinach and avocado to cook for one minute.

4. Set on serving plates and enjoy.

Nutrition:

Calories: 270, Fat: 12, Fiber: 3, Carbs: 12, Protein: 18

Spinach Artichoke Chicken

Prep Time + Cook Time: 60 minutes Servings: 4

Ingredients:

- Onion powder- 1 tbsp.
- Garlic powder - 1 tbsp.
- Seasoning: Salt and ground black pepper
- Four chicken breasts
- Chopped Canned artichoke hearts- 10 ounces
- Spinach- 10 ounces
- Grated Parmesan cheese - ½ cup
- Shredded Mozzarella cheese- 4 ounces
- Cream cheese- 4 ounces

Directions:

1. Arrange chicken breasts on a lined baking sheet, season with pepper and salt.

2. Place in an oven and set the temperature to 400°F and bake for 30 minutes.

3. Add artichokes with onion, spinach, cream cheese, Parmesan cheese, garlic, salt, pepper in a bowl then stir until its even.

4. Remove the chicken from the oven, cut each Chicken piece in the middle, divide artichokes mixture, sprinkle with mozzarella cheese, bake in an oven for 15 minutes at a temperature of 400°F. Serve hot.

Nutrition:

Calories: 573, Fat: 30.6, Fiber: 5.4, Carbs: 12.5, Protein: 63.5

Stuffed Chicken Breast Recipe

Prep Time + Cook Time: 25 minutes Servings: 3

Ingredients:

- Garlic (peeled and minced): 1 clove
- Chicken breasts: 3
- Seasoning: Salt and ground black pepper
- Spinach (cooked & chopped): 8 ounces
- Feta cheese (crumbled): 3 ounces
- Cream cheese (softened): 4 ounces
- Coconut oil: 1 tbsp.

Directions:

1. Mix feta cheese in a bowl with cream cheese, spinach, salt, pepper, garlic and stir well.

2. Place chicken fillets on a work surface, cut into a bag, fill with a spinach mixture and season with salt and

pepper.

3. Heat a pan of oil over medium heat, add stuffed chicken, cook on each side for 5 minutes and place in the oven at 450 ° F.

4. Bake for 10 minutes, divide between plates and serve.

Nutrition:

Calories: 912, Carbs: 5.2, Fat: 49.3, Fiber: 1.7, Protein: 107.7

Turkey and Cranberry Salad Recipe

Prep Time + Cook Time: 10 minutes Servings: 4

Ingredients:

- Cranberry puree: ½ cup
- Turkey breast (cooked and cubed): 2 cups
- Cranberries: ¼ cup
- Walnuts (chopped): 3 tbsps
- Lemon juice: 1 cup
- Lemon (peeled & cut into small segments): 1
- Romaine lettuce leaves (torn): 4 cups
- Kiwis (peeled and sliced): 3 slices

Directions:

1. Mix salad in a salad bowl with turkey, lemon segments, apple pieces, cranberries, walnuts and discard the coat.

2. In another bowl, mix cranberry puree with lemon juice and stir.

3. Sprinkle the turkey salad over it, throw it in the mantle and serve it with the kiwis.

Nutrition:

Calories: 347, Fat: 15.4, Carbs: 12.3, Fiber: 3.6, Protein: 40.1

Turkey Chili Recipe

Prep Time + Cook Time: 30 minutes Servings: 8

Ingredients:

- Fresh cilantro (chopped):1 tbsp.
- Chicken stock: 6 cups
- Seasoning: Salt and ground black pepper
- Squash (chopped): 2 cups
- Canned chipotle peppers (chopped): 1 tbsp.
- Turkey meat (cooked and shredded): 4 cups
- Cumin: 2 tsps
- Garlic powder: ½ tsp.
- Salsa verde: ½ cup
- Coriander: 1 tsp.
- Sour cream: ¼ cup

Directions:

1. Heat a pan with broth over medium heat. Add the pumpkin, stir and cook for 10 minutes.

2. Add turkey, chipotles, garlic powder, salsa verde, cumin, coriander, salt, pepper, stir and cook for 10 minutes.

3. Add sour cream, stir, remove heat and divide into bowls.
4. Sprinkle with a little chopped coriander and serve.

Nutrition:
Calories: 153, Fat: 5.6, Fiber: 0.5, Carbs: 2.9, Protein: 21.9

Turkey Pie

Prep Time + Cook Time: 50 minutes Servings: 6
Ingredients:
- meat (cooked and shredded) - 1 cup turkey
- butternut squash, peeled and chopped - ½ cup
- cheddar cheese, shredded - ½ cup
- fresh thyme, chopped - 1 tsp.
- turkey stock - 2 cups
- paprika - ¼ tsp.
- Garlic powder - ¼ tsp.
- Xanthan gum - ¼ tsp.
- Vegetable oil cooking spray
- kale, chopped - ½ cup
- Salt and ground black pepper, to taste

For the crust:
- Butter - ¼ cup
- Xanthan gum - ¼ tsp.
- almond flour - 2 cups
- A pinch of salt
- 1 egg
- cheddar cheese - ¼ cup

Directions:
1. Heat a pan with broth over medium heat. Add the pumpkin and turkey, stir and cook for 10 minutes.
2. Add garlic powder, kale, thyme, pepper, salt, pepper, ½ cup cheddar cheese and stir well. In a bowl, add ¼ tsp of xanthan gum with a ½ cup of broth from the pan, mix everything and put everything in the pan.
3. Leave the fire and set aside. Mix the flour with a ¼ tsp. of xanthan gum and a pinch of salt in a bowl and stir.
4. Add butter, egg and ¼ cup cheddar cheese and stir until a dough crust is formed. Form a ball and place it in the fridge.
5. Spray a casserole dish with cooking spray and spread the cake filling on the floor.
6. Transfer the dough to a work surface, roll it in a circle and fill it with the top.
7. Press the edges together well and seal the edges, place them at 350 ° F in an oven and bake 35 minutes.
8. Allow the cake to cool and serve.

Nutrition:
Calories: 241, Fiber: 1.3, Fat: 18.9, Carbs: 4.9, Protein: 14

Turkey Soup

Prep Time + Cook Time: 40 minutes Servings: 4

Ingredients:

- Onion (peeled and chopped): 1
- Butter 1 tbsp.
- Turkey stock: 6 cups
- Celery (chopped): 3 stalks
- Turkey (cooked & shredded): 3 cups
- Fresh parsley (chopped): ¼ cup
- Seasoning: Salt and ground black pepper
- Baked spaghetti squash (chopped): 3 cups

Directions:

1. Heat a pan with butter over medium heat, add celery and onion, stir and cook for 5 minutes.
2. Add parsley, broth, turkey, salt and pepper, stir and cook for 20 minutes.
3. Add spaghetti squash, stir and cook for 10 minutes. Divide into bowls and serve.

Nutrition:

Calories: 272, Carbs: 13.7, Fat: 8.5, Fiber: 2.5, Protein: 33.6

Turkey Squash Curry

Prep Time + Cook Time: 35 minutes Servings: 6

Ingredients:

- Turkey meat, cooked and shredded-4 cups
- Squash, chopped -2 cups
- Chicken stock -1 cup
- Salt and black pepper - to taste
- Garlic, minced -1 tsp.
- Sugar-free salsa verde -½ cup
- Coriander, ground -1 tsp.
- Cumin, ground -2 tsp.
- Tomato, chopped -¼ cup
- Parsley, chopped-1 tbsp.

Directions:

1. Add stock to a pan and heat it up over medium heat.
2. Stir in squash and let it cook for 10 minutes.
3. Add cumin, garlic, salsa, turkey, coriander, tomato, salt, pepper and cilantro.
4. Cook this mixture for 10 minutes with occasional stirring.
5. Enjoy fresh and warm.

Nutrition:

Calories: 254, Fat: 5, Fiber: 3, Carbs: 9, Protein: 27

Turkey Stuffed Chive Rolls

Prep Time + Cook Time: 15 minutes Servings: 4

Ingredients:

- Chives, 2 of them sliced -6
- Peach, cut into 8 wedges -1
- Turkey breast, cooked and cut into 8 pieces -3 ounces

Directions:

1. Spread the 2 turkey slices and place 2 peaches wedges and chopped chives over them.
2. Roll these turkey slices and then wrap them in the chive leaf.
3. Tie a knot and place them aside.
4. Repeat the same steps using the remaining material.
5. Serve with fresh salad.

Nutrition:

Calories: 180, Fat: 2, Fiber: 5, Carbs: 9, Protein: 17

Turkey Tarragon Bake

Prep Time + Cook Time:1 hour 15 minutes Servings: 6

Ingredients:

- Onion, chopped -¼ cup
- Turkey meat, ground -1 lb.
- Eggplant, chopped -1
- Garlic, minced -1 tbsp.
- Tomato paste -8 ounces
- Canned tomatoes, chopped -15 ounces
- Salt and black pepper - to taste
- Chili powder -¼ tsp.
- Cumin, ground -¼ tsp.
- Cooking spray
- Tarragon, dried -½ tsp.

Directions:

1. Place a nonstick skillet over medium heat and add turkey, onion, and garlic
2. Saute until turkey turns brown then transfer this to a bowl.
3. Add tomatoes, eggplant, salt, black pepper, cumin, chili powder, tomato paste and tarragon to the same pan.
4. Stir cook this mixture for 4 minutes then transfer this to a greased baking dish.
5. Spread the sauteed turkey over this layer then bake it for 1 hour at 350 0F.
6. Slice and serve.

Nutrition:

Calories: 278, Fat: 3, Fiber: 7, Carbs: 9, Protein: 18

Turkey Zucchini Lasagna

Prep Time + Cook Time: 60 minutes Servings: 8

Ingredients:

- Zucchinis, cubed -4 cups
- Egg whisked -1
- Cabbage, shredded -3 cups
- Turkey meat, cooked and shredded -3 cups
- Veggie stock -½ cup
- Cream cheese -½ cup
- Cheddar cheese, grated -2 cup
- Salt and black pepper - to taste
- Garlic powder -¼ tsp.

Directions:

1. Heat stock in a pan over medium-low heat.
2. Add cream cheese, salt, pepper, cheddar cheese, and garlic powder to the pan.
3. Let it simmer then add cabbage and turkey meat. Remove it from the heat.
4. Spread the zucchinis in a baking dish and top this layer with turkey mixture.
5. Cover this dish with the aluminum foil then bakes it for 35 minutes at 400 0F in a preheated oven.

Nutrition:

Calories: 240, Fat: 11, Fiber: 4, Carbs: 13, Protein: 25

Chapter 7 Ketogenic Meat Recipes

Almond Glazed Beef Meatloaf

Prep Time + Cook Time: 1 hour and 20 minutes Servings: 6

Ingredients:

- Chopped fresh parsley- 2 tbsps.
- Almond flour - ½ cup
- Grated Parmesan cheese- ⅓ cup
- 3 eggs
- White mushrooms (chopped)- 1 cup
- Ground beef - 3 pounds
- 2 Peeled and minced garlic cloves
- Chopped Onion - ½ cup
- Balsamic vinegar- 1 tsp.
- Red bell pepper (seeded and chopped)- ¼ cup
- Seasoning: Salt and ground black pepper

For the glaze:

- Tomato passata -2 tbsps.
- Balsamic vinegar - 2 cups
- Swerve - 1 tbsp.

Directions:

1. Mix beef with salt, pepper, mushrooms, garlic, onion, bell pepper, parsley, almond flour, Parmesan cheese, 1 tsp. vinegar, salt, pepper, eggs in a bowl, and mix well.
2. Prepare for baking by Placing into a loaf pan and bake for 30minutes in an oven at 375°F.
3. With medium temperature, heat a small pan over medium heat, put tomato passata, swerve, and 2 cups vinegar, mix well and cook for 20 minutes.
4. Remove the meatloaf from the oven, spread the glaze on meatloaf.
5. Place in oven at the same temperature and bake for 20 minutes.
6. Allow the meatloaf cool, slice, and serve it.

Nutrition:

Calories: 606, Fat: 26.4, Fiber: 2, Carbs: 8.3, Protein: 79.8

Avocado-Beef Zucchini Cups

Prep Time + Cook Time: 45 minutes Servings: 4

Ingredients:

- Coconut oil - 1 tbsp.
- Smoked paprika - 1 tsp.
- 3 zucchini, sliced in half lengthwise, and insides scooped out
- Chopped fresh cilantro- ¼ cup
- Shredded cheddar cheese- ½ cup
- Tomato paste - 1½ cups
- Avocado (chopped for serving)
- Green onions (chopped for serving)
- Tomatoes (cored and chopped for serving)

- 2 Peeled and minced garlic cloves
- Cumin - 1 tsp.
- Ground beef - 1 pound
- Chopped onion- ½ cup
- Seasoning: Salt and ground black pepper

Directions:
1. With medium-high heat, heat the oil in a pan, put onions, mix well, and cook for 2 minutes.
2. Put beef, mix well, and ensure it brown on both sides for a couple of minutes.
3. Supplement with paprika, salt, pepper, cumin, and garlic, mix well and cook for 2 minutes.

4. In a baking pan place zucchini halves into the pan, stuff each with the beef, pour enchilada sauce on top and drizzle with cheddar cheese.
5. Cover and heat in the oven for 20 minutes at a temperature of 350°F.
6. Disclose the pan, drizzle with the cilantro, and heat in the oven for 5 minutes.
7. Also drizzle with the following ingredients avocado, green onions, and tomatoes on top.
8. Divide between plates and serve.

Nutrition:
Calories: 622, Fat: 17.1, Fiber: 16.7, Carbs: 74.6, Protein: 55.4

Awesome Pilaf

Prep Time + Cook Time: 45 minutes Servings: 5

Ingredients:
- Lamb-1 pound (ground)
- Goat cheese-4 ounces (crumbled)
- Egg-1
- Cauliflower florets-12 ounces
- Garlic cloves-2 (minced)
- Coconut oil-2 tbsps.
- Mint-1 bunch (chopped)
- Lemon zest-1 tbsp.
- Fennel seed-1 tsp.
- Paprika-1 tsp.
- Garlic powder-1 tsp.
- Yellow onion-1 (small and chopped)
- Salt and black pepper-To taste

Directions:
1. Add the cauliflower florets in your food processor.
2. Put the salt and pulse well.

3. Take a pan and grease with some of the coconut oil.
4. Heat up over medium heat.
5. Combine the cauliflower rice.
6. Prepare for 8 minutes.
7. Do season with salt and pepper to the taste.
8. Take off from the heat and keep it warm.
9. Pick a-mixing bowl.
10. Marinate the lamb with salt, pepper, egg, paprika, and garlic powder and fennel seed.
11. Coat and then stir very well.
12. Shape them into 12 meatballs.
13. Arrange them on a plate for now.
14. Warm up a pan with the coconut oil over medium heat.

15. Put in the onion.
16. Toss and cook them for 6 minutes.
17. Add garlic and stir to cook for a minute.
18. Place the meatballs and cook them well from all sides.
19. And take off from the heat.
20. Divide cauliflower rice between plates.
21. Add meatballs and onion mix on top.
22. Sprinkle mint, lemon zest and goat cheese at the end.
23. Serve.

Nutrition Values:
Calories:- 470; Fat : 43; Fiber : 5; Carbs : 4; Protein : 26

Bacon Burger

Prep Time + Cook Time: 40 minutes Serves: 4

Ingredients:
For the sauce:
- Water, 1 cup
- Almond butter, 1 cup
- Minced garlic cloves, 4.
- Coconut aminos, 6 tbsps.
- Swerve, 1 tsp.
- Chopped chili peppers, 4.
- Rice vinegar, 1 tbsp.

For the burgers:
- Pepper jack cheese slices, 4.
- Lettuce leaves, 8.
- Black pepper.
- Bacon slices, 8.
- Ground beef, 1½ lbs.
- Sliced red onion, 1.
- Salt.

Directions:
1. Set the pan on fire to melt the almond butter over medium heat
2. Sir in water then allow to simmer
3. Mix in the coconut aminos stirring gently
4. Set the blender in place to combine garlic, chili peppers, vinegar, and swerve to blend until done.
5. Combine the mixture with almond butter
6. Remove from heat then reserve.
7. Set a mixing bowl in place to combine the seasoning and beef then mold into 4 patties then set them on a pan.
8. Preheat the broiler then broil the patties for seven minutes each side.
9. Arrange the cheese slices on burger then set in the broiler to broil for 4 minutes
10. Heat a pan with oil to fry the bacon slices over medium heat
11. Set 2 lettuce leaves on a platter, add 1 burger on top followed by 1 onion slice and then topped with 1 and some almond butter sauce
12. Do the same with the remaining lettuce leaves, burgers, onion, bacon and sauce

Nutrition:
calories: 700, fiber: 10, protein: 40, fat: 56, carbs: 7

Baked beef with mushroom bowls

Prep Time + Cook Time: 3 hours 10 minutes Serves: 7

Ingredients:

- Cubed beef chuck roast- 2 Ib.
- Beef stock- 1 cup
- Water- 1 cup
- Almond flour- 3 tbsp.
- Chopped celery stalks- 2
- Mushrooms: sliced- ½ Ib.
- Canned diced tomatoes- 15 oz.
- Chopped butternut squash- 10 oz.
- Dry mustard- ½ tsp.
- Chopped fresh thyme- 1 tbsp.
- Salt and black pepper

Directions:

1. Put an ovenproof pot on medium heat and add the beef cubes
2. to brown for some minutes.
3. Mix in the thyme, tomatoes, mustard, squash, onions, stock, celery, pepper, salt and pepper.
4. Mix water with flour in a bowl until it blends in well.
5. Pour flour mix into the pot and bake for 3 hours at 350°F.
6. Mix every 30 minutes.
7. Serve into bowls.

Nutrition:

Calories- 547, carbs- 12.4, protein- 37.6, fiber- 3.2, fats- 38.5

Baked beef with mushrooms and celery

Prep Time + Cook Time: 3 hours 10 minutes Serves: 7

Ingredients:

- Beef chuck roast: cubed- 2 Ib.
- Chopped celery ribs- 2
- Chopped canned tomatoes- 15 oz.
- Sliced mushrooms- ½ Ib.
- Mustard powder- ½ tsp.
- Chopped yellow onions- 2
- Chopped thyme- 1 tbsp.
- Almond flour- 3 tbsp.
- Water- 1 cup
- Beef stock- 1 cup
- Chopped carrots: 4
- Salt and pepper

Directions

1. Brown beef cubes in an oven proof pot on all sides and add mushrooms, carrots, tomatoes, onions, celery, mustard, salt , stock, thyme, and pepper and mix.
2. Mix water and flour in a bowl and pour into the pot.
3. Mix everything and bake for 3 hours at 325°F.
4. Serve.

Nutrition:

Calories 275, carbs 7, protein 28, fiber 18, fat 13

Baked lamb chops with cranberry tomato sauce

Prep Time + Cook Time: 2 hours 30 minutes Serves: 4

Ingredients:

- Chopped shallot- 1
- Olive oil
- Half lemon: juiced
- Beef stock- 2 cups
- Garlic powder- 1 tsp.
- White wine- 1 cup
- Lamb chops- 8
- Crushed mint- 2 tsp.
- Bay leaf- 1
- Salt and black pepper
- Chopped parsley

Sauce

- Cranberries- 2 cups
- Dried mint- 1 tsp.
- Chopped rosemary- ½ tsp.
- Half lemon: juiced
- Grated ginger- 1 tsp.
- Water- 1 cup
- Harissa paste- 1 tsp.
- Swerve- ½ cup

Instructions

1. Rub the lamb with a mixture of garlic powder, mint, pepper and salt and let it coat the lamb well.
2. Drizzle olive oil in an heated pan over medium-high and brown the lamb chops on all sides. Remove and set aside.
3. Return the pan and add the shallots, let it cook for 1 minute and then pour in the wine and the bay leaf. Let it cook for 4 minutes.
4. Add the lemon juice, parsley and the beef stock and let it cook for 5 minutes.
5. Add the lamb chops to the pan and cook for 10 minutes.
6. Cover the pan and bake in the oven for 2 hours at 350°F.
7. Sauce: pour the cranberries in a pan over medium high and add the remaining sauce ingredients to it. Let it cook on low heat for 15 minutes.
8. Serve lamb chops drizzled with cranberry sauce.

Nutrition:

Calories 450, carbs 6, protein 26, fiber 2, fat 34

Baked lamb with fennel and figs

Prep Time + Cook Time: 50 minutes Serves: 4

Ingredients:

- Lamb racks- 12 oz.
- Apple cider vinegar- ⅛ cup
- Swerve- 1 tbsp.
- Olive oil- 2 tbsp.
- Figs: halved- 4
- Sliced fennel bulbs- 2
- Salt and black pepper

Instructions

1. Combine swerve, vinegar, figs and fennel in a bowl and flip to coat and put in a baking dish.

2. Sprinkle with salt and pepper and bake for 15 minutes at 400°F.
3. Season lamb with pepper and salt and put on a pan over medium-high for some minutes.
4. Put the lamb in the dish with figs and fennel and bake for 20 minutes.

Nutrition:
Calories 230, carbs 5, protein 10, fiber 3, fat 3

Baked Parmesan veal with tomatoes sauce

Prep Time + Cook Time: 1 hour 20 minutes Serves: 6

Ingredients:
- Veal cutlets- 8
- Tomato sauce- 5 cups
- Butter- 2 tbsp.
- Melted coconut oil- 2 tbsp.
- Grated parmesan cheese- ⅔ cup
- A pinch of garlic salt
- Provolone cheese slices- 8
- Vegetable oil cooking spray
- Italian seasoning- 1 tsp.
- Salt and black pepper

Directions:
1. Sprinkle garlic salt, pepper and salt on veal cutlets.
2. Dissolve bitter on a pan and add some oil. Sear veal until brown on all sides.
3. Spray the baking tray and spread half of the tomato sauce on it.
4. Lay veal cutlets on the sauce and season with Italian seasoning.
5. Spread the remaining sauce over the veal and cover with a foil.
6. Let bake for 40 minutes at 350°F.
7. Remove the foil and spread the provolone cheese over it and bake for another 15 minutes.
8. Serve warm.

Nutrition:
Calories- 620, carbs- 12.3, protein- 58.7, fiber- 3.1, fat- 37.6

Baked pork sausage and mushrooms

Prep Time + Cook Time: 1 hour 10 minutes Serves: 6

Ingredients:
- Swerve- 1 tbsp.
- Sliced pork sausage: 2 Ib.
- Portobello mushrooms: sliced- 2 Ib.
- Red bell peppers: seeded and chopped- 3
- Sweet onions: chopped- 2
- A drizzle of olive oil.

Directions:
1. Mix sliced sausage with pepper, salt, bell peppers, swerve, onions, mushrooms and oil together in a baking dish.
2. Place in an oven to bake for 1 hour at 300° F.
3. Serve hot.

Nutrition:
Calories- 585, carbs- 11.8, protein- 34.2, fiber- 1.6, fats- 43.1

Baked veal and green beans

Prep Time + Cook Time: 50 minutes Serves: 4

Ingredients:

- Chopped canned tomatoes- 15 oz.
- Steamed green beans
- Veal leg steaks- 4 medium sized
- Chopped parsley- 2 tbsp.
- Sliced bocconcini- 1 oz.
- Chopped red onion- 1
- Chopped sage-2 tsp.
- Minced garlic- 2 cloves
- Drizzle of avocado oil
- Salt and black pepper

Directions:

1. Sear veal on a pan with oil over medium-high for 2 minutes on both sides and place on a baking dish.

2. Put the onions on the pan over medium-high and cook for 4 minutes.
3. Mix in the garlic and the sage and cook for 1 minute.
4. Add in the tomatoes, mix and cook for 10 minutes.
5. Pour sauce mix over veal and add the parsley and bocconcini to bake in the oven for 20 minutes at 350°F.
6. Serve with steamed beans on the side.

Nutrition:

Calories 276, carbs 5, protein 36, fiber 4, fat 6

Beef Cabbage Casserole

Prep Time + Cook Time: 1 hour and 45 minutes Servings: 4

Ingredients:

- Cabbage head, shredded -½
- Yellow onion, chopped -1
- Garlic cloves, minced -3
- Beef, ground -1 ½ lbs.
- Tomatoes, crushed -1 ½ cups
- Cauliflower rice -2 cups
- A drizzle of olive oil
- Salt and black pepper - to taste
- Red pepper, crushed -½ tsp.
- Parsley, chopped -½ cup

Directions:

1. Take a baking dish and grease it with cooking oil.

2. Spread the cabbage shred in the dish, in an even layer.
3. Add onion beef, garlic, tomatoes, crushed pepper, salt, and pepper.
4. Cover the baking dish and bake it for 1hr. 30 minutes at 375 0F.
5. Garnish with parsley.
6. Serve warm.

Nutrition:

Calories: 301, Fat: 6, Fiber: 8, Carbs: 12, Protein: 28

Beef Keto Stew

Prep Time + Cook Time: 3 hours 49 minutes Servings: 5

Ingredients:

- Beef shanks-5 pounds
- Tomatoes-8 (chopped)
- Carrots-3 (chopped)
- Garlic cloves-8 (minced)
- Onions-2 (chopped)
- Chicken stock-1 quart
- Parsley-2 tsps. (dried)
- Basil-2 tsps. (dried)
- Garlic powder-2 tsps.
- Water-2 cups
- Apple cider vinegar-2 tbsps.
- Bay leaves-3
- Red pepper-3 tsps. (crushed)
- Tomato sauce-1/4 cup
- Onion powder-2 tsps.
- Cayenne pepper-A pinch
- Salt and black pepper-To taste

Directions:

1. Warm up a pot over medium heat.
2. Put the garlic, carrots and onions.
3. Mix and brown for a few minutes.
4. Heat a pan over medium heat again. Put the beef shank.
5. Let this brown for a few minutes on each side and take off heat.
6. Add stock over carrots, the water and the vinegar and stir.
7. Combine tomatoes, tomato sauce, salt, pepper, cayenne pepper, crushed pepper, bay leaves, basil, parsley, onion powder and garlic powder.
8. Then stir everything.
9. Toss the beef shanks and cover the pot.
10. Bring it to a simmer and cook for 3 hours.
11. Waste the bay leaves.
12. Divide into bowls and serve.

Nutrition :

Calories:- 500; Fat : 22; Fiber : 4; Carbs : 6; Protein : 56

Beef Patties with coconut flour

Prep Time + Cook Time: 45 minutes Servings: 6

Ingredients:

- Canned onion soup -10 ounces
- Ketchup- ¼ cup
- Worcestershire sauce - 3 tsps.
- Dry mustard - ½ tsp.
- 1 egg
- Ground beef -1½ pounds
- Coconut flour-1 tbsp.
- Cauliflower rice -½ cup
- water -¼ cup
- Seasoning: Salt and ground black pepper

Directions:

1. Mix ⅓ cup of onion soup with beef, salt, pepper, egg, cauliflower rice in a bowl and stir well.

2. With medium-high temperature, heat a pan, shape 6 patties from beef mixture, place into the pan, and brown on both sides.

3. Carefully mix the rest of soup with coconut flour, water, dry mustard, Worcestershire sauce, ketchup in a bowl and stir well.

4. Pour over the beef patties, cover pan, and cook for 20 minutes stirring from occasionally. Divide among plates and serve.

Nutrition:
Calories: 846, Fat: 28.2, Fiber: 1.4, Carbs: 10.1, Protein: 130.3

Braised veal and capers

Prep Time + Cook Time: 25 minutes Serves: 2

Ingredients:
- Veal scallops- 8 oz.
- White wine- ¼ cup
- Ghee- 2 tbsp.
- Chicken stock- ¼ cup
- Capers- 1½ tbsp.
- Minced garlic- 1 clove
- Salt and black pepper

Directions
1. Dissolve half of the ghee on a pan over medium-high and sear the veal seasoned with pepper and salt on both sides for 2 minutes and set aside.

2. Put the garlic in the pan and fry for 1 minute.

3. Pour in the wine and simmer for 2 minutes then add the veal, remaining ghee, capers, stock, salt and pepper.

4. Mix and close the lid. Cook on medium-low until veal is soft.

5. Serve.

Nutrition:
Calories 204, carbs 5, protein 10, fiber 1, fat 12

Brisket and Beef Burgers

Prep Time + Cook Time: 35 minutes Serves: 8

Ingredients:
- Mayonnaise, 2 tbsps.
- Ground beef, 1 lb.
- Salt.
- Minced garlic, 1 tbsp.
- Ground brisket, 1 lb.
- Butter slices, 8.
- Italian seasoning, 1 tbsp.
- Ghee, 1 tbsp.
- Olive oil, 2 tbsps.
- Chopped yellow onion, 1.
- Black pepper.
- Water, 1 tbsp.

Directions:
1. Using a medium bowl, stir in pepper, mayo, beef, Italian seasoning, brisket,

salt and garlic Ensure they are mixed well

2. Form 8 patties and let each have a pocket.
3. Take a butter slice and fill into each burger. Seal them.
4. Set a pan over medium high heat. Add olive oil and heat. Stir in onions and let cook until done for about 2 minutes.
5. Stir in the water and set them to one side of the pan. Add in the burgers and cook for 10 minutes while heat is set to medium-low.
6. You then flip them to the other side, place in the ghee and continue cooking for another 10 minutes.
7. Set your buns ready and divide the burgers amongst them. Top with caramelized onions and serve.

Nutrition :
calories: 180, fiber: 1, fat: 8, carbs: 4, protein: 20

Cheesy ham and cauliflower soup bowls

Prep Time + Cook Time: 4 hours 10 minutes Serves: 6
Ingredients:

- Cauliflower florets- 16 oz.
- Chopped ham- 3 cups
- Chicken stock- 14 oz.
- Grated cheddar cheese- 8 oz.
- Garlic cloves: minced- 4
- Heavy cream- ½ cup
- Onion powder- ½ tsp.
- Garlic powder- ½ tsp.
- Salt and ground black pepper

Directions:

1. Add stock, cheese, ham, onion and garlic powder, cauliflower, heavy cream, garlic, salt and pepper to a crock pot.
2. Mix and cook for 4 hours on high pressure.
3. Serve into bowls.

Nutrition:
Calories- 306, carbs- 8.4, protein- 22.6, fiber- 2.8, fats- 20.4

Cheesy sausage with tomatoes

Prep Time + Cook Time: 40 minutes Serves: 4
Ingredients:

- Sugar-free pork sausage: chopped- 2 Ib.
- Orange bell peppers: chopped- 3
- Yellow bell peppers: chopped- 3
- Thinly sliced sun-dried tomatoes- 4
- Melted coconut oil- 2 oz.
- Grated gouda cheese- ½ Ib.
- Onion: sliced- 1
- A pinch of red pepper flakes
- Parsley: sliced thin- ½ cup
- Salt and black pepper

Directions:

1. Put a pot on medium heat and add

the sausage slices to brown for 3 minutes on each side. Remove and keep aside.
2. On medium heat, add in bell peppers, tomatoes, and onion. Mix and cook for 5 minutes.
3. Add in red pepper flakes, pepper and salt and cook for 1 minute.
4. Place the sliced sausages on a baking dish and add the bell pepper mix over it. Sprinkle parsley and gouda cheese over it and bake for 15 minutes at 350°F.
5. Serve hot.

Nutrition:
Calories- 1176, carbs- 7.7, protein- 61.2, fiber 3.7, fats- 94.7

Cheesy veal and beans

Prep Time + Cook Time: 50 minutes Serves: 4
Ingredients:
- Medium veal leg steaks- 4
- Green beans: steamed
- Canned diced tomatoes- 15 oz.
- Sliced semi-soft cheese- 1 oz.
- Chopped fresh sage- 2 tsp.
- Chopped fresh parsley- 2 tsp.
- Onion: chopped- 1
- Garlic cloves: minced- 2
- Drizzle of avocado oil.
- Salt and pepper

Directions:
1. Put a pot on medium heat and add the veal to brown for 2 minutes on both sides, remove and set aside.
2. Add onions an brown for 4 minutes.
3. Mix in garlic and safe for 1 minute and then add the tomatoes and boil for 10 minutes.
4. Place the veal on a baking dish and pour tomatoes over it.
5. Spread cheese and parsley over the tomatoes and bake I am oven for 20 minutes on 350°F.
6. Serve.

Nutrition:
Calories- 759, carbs- 37.6, protein- 44, fiber- 17.1, fats 54.1

Cheesy veal dish

Prep Time + Cook Time: 1 hour 20 minutes Serves: 6
Ingredients:
- Melted coconut oil- 2 tbsp.
- Cooking spray,
- Salt and pepper
- Italian seasoning- 1 tsp.
- Garlic salt
- Tomato sauce- 5 cups
- Ghee- 2 tbsp.
- Grated Parmesan - ⅔ cup
- Provolone cheese slices- 8
- Veal cutlets- 8

Instructions

1. Sprinkle salt and pepper on veal and brown on all sides in a pan with melted ghee over medium-high.
2. Spray a baking dish and spread half of the tomato sauce on the bottom.
3. Put the veal and sprinkle the Italian seasoning over it then pour the rest of the sauce.
4. Bake covered for 40 minutes at 350°F.
5. Open and spread the cheese over it an spread parmesan over it.
6. Bake for 15 minutes and serve.

Nutrition:
Calories 362, carbs 6, protein 26, fiber 2, fat 21

Coconut Smoked Beef Mix

Prep Time + Cook Time: 6 hours 10 minutes Serves: 6

Ingredients:
- Stevia, 2 tbsps.
- Stripped beef, 2½ lbs.
- Liquid smoke, 2 tbsps.
- A drizzle of olive oil
- Apple cider vinegar, ¼ cup
- Grated ginger, 1 tbsp.
- Coconut aminos, ½ cup
- Black pepper

Directions:
1. Set the mixing bowl in place to combine the liquid smoke, vinegar, black pepper, stevia, beef strips, and aminos then refrigerate for 6 hours while covered
2. Set the pan on fire with oil to fry the beef strips for 10 minutes over medium-high heat.
3. Set on plates and serve.

Nutrition:
Calories: 280, Fat: 11, Fiber: 3, Carbs: 7, Protein: 16

Creamy lamb sauce

Prep Time + Cook Time: 30 minutes Serves: 4

Ingredients:
- Lemon juice- 2 tsp.
- Chopped shallots- 1 tbsp.
- Heavy cream- ⅔ cup
- Beef stock- ½ cup
- Ghee- 2 tbsp.
- Mustard- 1 tbsp.
- Erythritol- 1 tsp.
- Gluten-free Worcestershire sauce- 2 tsp.
- Chopped fresh rosemary- 1 tbsp.
- Lamb chops- 1½ Ib.
- Olive oil- 2 tbsp.
- Thyme sprig
- Rosemary sprig
- Black pepper

- Salt

Directions

1. Combine garlic, salt, rosemary, salt, pepper and 1 tbsp. of oil together in bowl.
2. Add in the lamb chops and let the spices coat it then set aside.
3. Pour the remaining oil on the pan over medium-high and arrange the lamb chops in it.
4. Reduce the heat to medium and let it cook for 14 minutes on both sides. Remove and set aside.
5. Add the shallots to the pan on medium heat and cook for 3 minutes.
6. Pour in the stock and let it cook for 1 minute then add the sprigs, erythritol, mustard, Worcestershire sauce and heavy cream. Let it cook for 8 minutes.
7. Mix in the lemon juice, ghee, pepper and salt and remove the sprigs.
8. Remove and serve lamb chops drizzled with sauce.

Nutrition:

Calories 435, carbs 5, protein 32, fiber 4, fat 30

Creamy veal with mushrooms and squash

Prep Time + Cook Time: 2 hours 20 minutes Serves: 12

Ingredients:

- Cubed veal- 3 Ib.
- Heavy cream- ½ cup
- Egg yolks- 3
- Water- 1 cup
- Dried oregano- 2 tsp.
- Avocado oil: 2 tbsp.
- Masala wine- 1½ cups
- Chopped butternut squash- 4 oz.
- Canned tomato paste- 10 oz.
- Chopped mushrooms- 7 oz.
- Garlic clove: minced- 1
- Chopped onion- 1
- Salt
- Black pepper

Directions:

1. Put a pot on medium heat and add the cubed veal to brown for some minutes.
2. Mix in the onion and garlic to cook for 2-3 minutes.
3. Pour in water and wine and add the pepper, salt, mushrooms, squash, oregano and tomato paste.
4. Mix and lose the lid.
5. Let it cook for 1 hour 45 minutes on low heat.
6. Whisk egg yolks and cream in a bowl and pour it into the pot and mix.
7. Let it cook for 15 minutes and season with salt and pepper.
8. Serve.

Nutrition:

Calories- 284, carbs- 8.9, protein- 24.3, fiber- 1.7, fat- 9.6

Crusty Pork Cheese Pie

Prep Time + Cook Time: 60 minutes Servings: 6

Ingredients:

Pie crust:

- Flax meal -¼ cup
- Cracklings -2 cups
- Eggs -2
- Almond flour -1 cup

Filling for Pie:

- Eggs -4
- Pork loin, chopped -12 oz.
- Ghee, melted -2 tbsp
- Chives, chopped -¼ cup
- Cheddar cheese, grated -1 cup
- Coconut cream -½ cup
- Red onion, chopped -1
- Salt and black pepper -to taste
- Garlic cloves, minced -2

Directions:

1. Add crackling, flour, 2 eggs and flax meal to a food processor.
2. Blend this mixture to form a smooth dough then transfer it to a pie plate.
3. Spread it evenly then bake this crust for 15 minutes at 350 0F.
4. Meanwhile, add ghee to a skillet and place it over medium-high heat.
5. Add onion and garlic to sauté for 5 minutes.
6. Place pork loin and bacon in the skillet and sear the meat for 6 minutes until brown then remove it from the heat.
7. Whisk 4 eggs with cheese, salt, pepper, cream and chives in a bowl.
8. Spread the pork filling in the baked crust and pour the egg mixture over it.
9. Bake this pie for 25 minutes at 350 0F.
10. Slice and serve.
11. Devour.

Nutrition:

Calories: 405, Fat: 14, Fiber: 3, Carbs: 13, Protein: 33

Dijon Beef Fillets and Coconut Sauce

Prep Time + Cook Time: 40minutes Serves: 4

Ingredients:

- Beef fillets, 4
- Minced garlic cloves, 2
- Dijon mustard, ¼ cup
- Beef stock, ¼ cup
- Chopped shallot, 1
- Coconut cream, 1¼ cup
- Chopped parsley, 2 tbsps.
- Salt
- Sliced mushrooms, 12
- Black pepper
- Olive oil, 2 tbsps.

Directions:

1. Set the pan on fire with oil to fry the garlic and shallots for 3 minutes over medium-high heat
2. Stir in the mushroom and stock to cook for 10 minutes
3. Mix in the mustard, pepper, coconut cream, salt, and parsley to cook for 5 minutes then remove from heat.
4. Season the fillets with pepper and salt.
5. Set another pan on fire to cook the seasoned beef fillets for 4 minutes each side.
6. Set on plates to serve topped with Dijon and coconut sauce.

Nutrition:
Calories: 300, Fat: 12, Fiber: 1, Carbs: 9, Protein: 23

Garlic and Lemon Pork

Prep Time + Cook Time: 40 minutes Servings: 4

Ingredients:

- A pinch of lemon pepper
- Chopped fresh parsley- 2 tbsps.
- Chopped mushrooms- 8 ounces
- 1 Sliced lemon
- Butter - 3 tbsps.
- 4 pork steaks (bone–in)
- Chicken stock - 1 cup
- Coconut oil - 3 tbsps.
- 6 Peeled and minced garlic cloves
- Seasoning: Salt and ground black pepper

Directions:

1. With medium-high temperature, heat the 2 tbsps. butter and 2 tbsps. oil in a pan, add pork steaks, season with salt and pepper, cook until its brown on both sides, and transfer to a plate.
2. Put the pan on the oven while the temperature is set to medium, add the remaining butter, oil, and half of the stock. Mix properly, and cook for a minute.
3. Mushrooms and garlic should be added, stir carefully, and cook for 4 minutes. Also add lemon slices and the rest of the stock, salt, pepper, and lemon pepper, stir well and cook everything for another 5 minutes.
4. Take back pork steaks to the pan and cook slowly for 10 minutes. Divide steaks and sauce between plates and serve.

Nutrition:
Calories: 665, Fat: 49.2, Fiber: 1.1, Carbs: 5, Protein: 47.6

Garlic Beef Chili

Prep Time + Cook Time:8 hours 10 minutes Servings: 4

Ingredients:

- Coconut aminos - 2 tbsps.
- A pinch of cayenne pepper
- Cumin - 2 tbsps.
- Onion powder - 1 tsp.

- Garlic powder - 1 tsp.
- 1 peeled and chopped onion
- Ground beef - 2½ pounds
- Canned tomatoes and green chilies (chopped)- 15 ounces
- Tomato paste - 6 ounces
- Chili powder - 4 tbsps.
- 1 bay leaf
- Dried oregano - 1 tsp.
- Pickled jalapeños (chopped) - ½ cup
- Garlic, minced -4 tbsps.
- 3 Chopped celery stalks
- Seasoning: Salt and ground black pepper

Directions:

1. With medium-high temperature, heat a pan, add half of onion, beef, half of the garlic, salt, and pepper, stir, and cook until meat browns on all sides.
2. Place to a slow cooker, add rest of the onion and garlic, plus jalapeños, celery, tomatoes, chilies, tomato paste, canned tomatoes, coconut aminos, chili powder, salt, pepper, cumin, garlic powder, onion powder, oregano, and bay leaf, stir, cover, and cook on low for 8 hours.
3. Divide into separate bowls and serve.

Nutrition:
Calories: 626, Fat: 19.3, Fiber: 4, Carbs: 19.7, Protein: 89.7

Garlic Beef Meatball Casserole

Prep Time + Cook Time: 1 hours Servings: 8
Ingredients:

- Garlic powder-½ tsp.
- Tomato paste - 2 cups
- Minced garlic - 2 tsps.
- Dried basil - 2 tsps.
- Dried rosemary - 1 tsp.
- Shredded mozzarella cheese- 1½ cups
- Almond flour- ⅓ cup
- 2 eggs
- Chopped Beef sausage -1 pound
- Ground beef- 1 pound
- Dried oregano- ¼ tsp.
- Ricotta cheese - 1 cup
- Grated Parmesan cheese- ¼ cup
- Onion powder - ¼ tsp.
- Dried parsley - 1 tbsp.
- Red pepper flakes - ¼ tsp.
- Seasoning: Salt and ground black pepper

Directions:

1. Combine and mix sausage with beef, salt, pepper, almond flour, parsley, pepper flakes, onion powder, garlic powder, oregano, Parmesan cheese, eggs in a bowl and stir well.
2. Arrange shape meatballs on a lined baking sheet, bake for 15 minutes then place in an oven for 15 minutes at 375°F.
3. Remove meatballs out of oven, place into a baking dish, and cover with half of the tomato paste, garlic, basil, and rosemary.
4. Put ricotta cheese all over and then pour rest of the tomato mixture.
5. Mozzarella cheese should be sprinkled all over, place the dish in the oven for 30 minutes at 375°F.
6. Cool casserole before cutting and serving.

Nutrition:
Calories: 531, Fat: 33.6, Fiber: 3, Carbs: 17.5, Protein: 40.9

Garlicy sausage and tomatoes stew

Prep Time + Cook Time: 30 minutes Serves: 9

Ingredients:

- Sliced smoked sausage- 1 Ib.
- Gluten-free hot sauce- 1 tbsp.
- Chopped canned tomatoes- 28 oz.
- Garlic cloves- 6
- Chopped green onions- 8
- Beef stock- 1 cup
- Avocado oil- ¼ cup
- Chopped parsley- 1 cup
- Chopped green bell pepper- 1
- Coconut aminos- 2 tbsp.
- Chopped yellow onions- 2
- Tomato sauce- 8 oz.
- Chopped okra- 16 oz.
- Salt and pepper

Instructions

1. Pour oil on a pan over medium-high and fry sausages for 2 minutes.
2. Add the green onions, bell pepper, onions, salt, pepper, and parsley and cook for 2 minutes.
3. Pour in the stock, coconut aminos, tomatoes, garlic, hot sauce and okra and simmer for 15 minutes.
4. Season with pepper and salt.

Nutrition:

Calories 274, carbs 7, protein 10, fiber 4, fat 20

Greek Beef Mix

Prep Time + Cook Time: 40 minutes   Serves: 4

Ingredients:

- Olive oil, 4 tbsps.
- Broccoli head, 1
- Chopped red onion, 1
- Halved cherry tomatoes, 8
- Thyme springs, 4
- Minced garlic cloves, 4
- Salt
- Sweet paprika, ½ tbsp.
- Sirloin steaks, 4
- Black pepper

Directions:

1. Set a mixing bowl in place to whisk together paprika, garlic, pepper, and salt.
2. Set the broccoli, tomatoes, and onions on a well-lined baking tray
3. Set the oven for 10 minutes at 425ºF, allow to bake.
4. Season the steak with pepper and salt
5. Set the pan on fire cook the seasoned steaks for 2 minutes each side then add to the baking sheet.
6. Drizzle the garlic mix and oil to coat evenly then top with thyme and bake in the oven for 15 minutes more
7. Set on plates and serve.
8. Enjoy

Nutrition:

Calories: 290, Fat: 14, Fiber: 2, Carbs: 9, Protein: 29

Grilled Cajun Beef and Apricots Sauce

Prep Time + Cook Time: 32 minutes Serves: 2

Ingredients:

- Coconut aminos, ¼ cup
- Olive oil, ¼ cup
- Lemon juice, 1/3 cup
- Cajun seasoning, 2 tbsps.
- Chopped apricots, 2 tbsps.
- Medium beef steaks, 2

Directions:

1. Set a mixing bowl in a working surface to combine lemon juice, ½ of the Cajun seasoning, apricots, and aminos.
2. Pour the mixture into a pan then simmer for 10 minutes over medium-high heat.
3. Set an immersion blender in place then process the mixture until done.
4. Rub the steaks with the remaining seasoning and apricot sauce.
5. Set on the preheated grill to cook for 6minutes each side over medium-high heat.
6. Set on plates to serve topped with the remaining sauce.
7. Enjoy.

Nutrition:

Calories: 280, Fat: 6, Fiber: 8, Carbs: 9, Protein: 22

Grilled Ginger Lamb Chops

Prep Time + Cook Time: 20 minutes Serves: 6

Ingredients:

- Coconut aminos, 3 tbsps.
- Minced garlic cloves, 3
- Salt
- Black pepper
- Grated ginger, 2 tbsps.
- Lamb chops, 8
- Olive oil, 4 tbsps.
- Chopped parsley, 1 tbsp.

Directions:

1. Set a mixing bowl in place to whisk together parsley, oil, ginger, aminos, and garlic
2. Set the lamb chops on a preheated grill to cook for five minutes for 5 minutes each side over medium-high heat.
3. Serve basted with the ginger mix

Nutrition: Calories: 270, Fat: 11, Fiber: 3, Carbs: 8, Protein: 20

Grilled lamb chops

Prep Time + Cook Time: 35 minutes Serves: 4

Ingredients:

- Lamb chops- 1½ Ib.
- Pieces of orange peel- 2
- Minced garlic- 2 cloves
- Halved red oranges- 3
- Chopped rosemary- 2 tbsp.
- Ghee- 1 tsp.

- Drizzle of olive oil
- Chopped lavender- 1 tbsp.
- Salt and pepper

Directions

1. Mix the salt, pepper, lavender, garlic, rosemary, and orange peel together and coat the lamb chops with the spice mix and let it marinate for some hours.
2. Rub ghee on grill pan and heat under medium high.
3. Grill lamb chops on one side for 3 minutes, turn and squeeze one orange half over it and cook for another 3 minutes.
4. Turn over again and squeeze another half over it and cook for 2 minutes.
5. Remove lamb chops and set aside
6. Grill remaining orange halves for 6 minutes flipping after 3 minutes.
7. Serve lamb chops drizzled with olive oil and orange halves.

Nutrition:

Calories 250, carbs 5, protein 8, fiber 1, fat 5

Ground Beef Casserole with keto mayonnaise

Prep Time + Cook Time: 45 minutes Servings: 6

Ingredients:

- keto mayonnaise - ½ cup
- sesame seeds (toasted) - 2 tbsps.
- 20 dill pickle slices
- Onion flakes - 2 tsps.
- Gluten-free Worcestershire sauce-1 tbsp.
- Ground beef -2 pounds
- Shredded mozzarella cheese-1 cup
- Shredded cheddar cheese-2 cups
- 1 romaine lettuce head (torn)
- 2 Peeled and minced garlic cloves
- Seasoning: Salt and ground black pepper

Directions:

1. With medium temperature, heat a pan, put the following ingredients in a pan, beef, onion flakes, Worcestershire sauce, salt, pepper, and garlic, stir and cook for 5 minutes.
2. Place mixture into a baking dish, put 1 cup of cheddar cheese, mozzarella cheese, and half of the mayonnaise. Mix properly and spread evenly.
3. Arrange pickle slices on top, drizzle remaining cheddar and sesame seeds, place in an oven and bake for 20 minutes at 350°F. Then turn oven to broil and broil casserole for 5 minutes.
4. Divide lettuce between plates put beef casserole and the remaining mayonnaise on top.

Nutrition:

Calories: 577, Fat: 36.1, Fiber: 1, Carbs: 4.8, Protein: 57.6

Ground Beef Goulash

Prep Time + Cook Time: 30 minutes Servings: 5

Ingredients:

- Canned diced tomatoes-14 ounces
- Garlic powder -¼ tsp.
- Tomato paste -1 tbsp.
- Ground beef -1½ pounds
- Cauliflower florets -2 cups
- Water-14 ounces
- Bell pepper (seeded and chopped)-2 ounces
- Peeled and chopped onion- ¼ cup
- Seasoning: Salt and ground black pepper

Directions:

1. With medium temperature, heat a pan, put beef, stir, and ensure its brown on all sides for 5 minutes.
2. Put onion and bell pepper, mix thoroughly and cook for 4 minutes.
3. Put tomatoes, cauliflower, water, stir well, cook slowly (bring to simmer), cover pan, and cook for another 5 minutes.
4. Put garlic powder, tomato paste, salt, and pepper bring to the commotion by stirring properly.
5. Putt off the heat and divide into separate bowls then serve.

Nutrition:

Calories: 972, Fat: 31.4, Fiber: 2.9, Carbs: 10.1, Protein: 153.6

Healthy Beef Pot Roast Recipes

Prep Time + Cook Time: 1 hour and 25 minutes Servings: 4

Ingredients:

- Onion powder - 1 ounce
- Beef roast - 3½ pounds
- Sliced mushrooms - 4 ounces
- Beef stock- 12 ounces
- Olive oil - ½ cup

Directions:

1. Combine and stir stock with onion powder, olive oil in a bowl.
2. In a pan, put beef roast put mushrooms, stock mixture, cover with aluminum foil, bake in an oven for 1 hour and 15 minutes, while the temperature is set to 300°F.
3. Cool roast, slice, then serve.

Nutrition:

Calories: 990, Fat: 50.3, Fiber: 0.7, Carbs: 6.7, Protein: 123

Healthy Beef with Tzatziki Recipe

Prep Time + Cook Time: 25 minutes Servings: 6

Ingredients:

- Chopped fresh mint- ¼ cup
- Almond milk -¼ cup
- Ground beef -17 ounces
- 1 peeled and grated onion
- 5 oz cauliflower rice
- 1 cucumber (sliced thin)

- Baby spinach- 1 cup
- Lemon juice -1½ tbsps.
- 7 ounces jarred tzatziki
- 1 egg (whisked)
- Chopped fresh parsley-¼ cup
- 2 Peeled and minced garlic cloves
- Dried oregano -2½ tsps.
- Olive oil- ¼ cup
- Cherry tomatoes (cut in half) - 7 ounces
- Seasoning: Salt and ground black pepper

Directions:
1. In a clean bowl, put cauliflower rice, add milk, and for 3 minutes put to one side.
2. Drain, then put beef, egg, salt, pepper,

oregano, mint, parsley, garlic, onion, and mix well.
3. From mixture, Shape balls and place on a clean working surface.
4. With medium-high temperature, heat a pan, put meatballs, cook for 8 minutes, and flip from time to time, and transfer them to a tray.
5. Mix spinach with cucumber and tomato in a salad bowl.
6. Put meatballs, remaining oil, and some salt, pepper and lemon juice.
7. Put tzatziki, toss to coat, and serve.

Nutrition:
Calories: 322, Fat: 18.6, Fiber: 1.7, Carbs: 9.9, Protein: 29.2

Healthy Italian Pork Chops Recipes

Prep Time + Cook Time: 50 minutes Servings: 4

Ingredients:
- Chopped fresh oregano- 1 tbsp.
- Tomato paste- 1 tbsp.
- Tomato juice- ¼ cup
- 4 pork chops
- 2 Peeled and minced garlic cloves
- Canola oil - 1 tbsp.
- Canned diced tomatoes -15 ounces
- Seasoning: Salt and ground black pepper

Directions:
1. With medium-high temperature, heat the oil in a pan with oil, put pork chops, and season with salt and pepper, cook for 3 minutes, flip to other side and cook for another 3 minutes, transfer to a plate.

2. Put garlic in the pan while it on medium temperature, mix well, and cook for 10 seconds.
3. Add the following ingredients, tomato juice, tomatoes, tomato paste, mix well and bring to a boil and reduce heat to medium-low.
4. Put pork chops, mix well, cover the pan, cook slowly for 30 minutes. Place pork chops to plates
5. Add oregano to the pan, mix well, and cook for 2 minutes. Pour over the pork and serve.

Nutrition:
Calories: 318, Fat: 23.8, Fiber: 2, Carbs: 6.8, Protein: 19.4

Healthy Lemon Pork Chops

Prep Time + Cook Time: 25 minutes Servings: 4

Ingredients:

- Water- 1 tbsp.
- butter - 1 tbsp.
- Chopped fresh chives- 1 tbsp.
- Dijon mustard - 1 tsp.
- Worcestershire sauce- 1 tbsp.
- 4 medium pork loin chops
- lemon pepper - 1 tsp.
- lemon juice- 1 tsp.
- Seasoning: Salt and ground black pepper

Directions:

1. Mix and whisk water with Worcestershire sauce, mustard, and lemon juice in a bowl.

2. With medium temperature, heat butter in a pan, add pork chops, season with salt, pepper, and lemon pepper, cook for 6 minutes, flip, and cook for another 6 minutes.

3. Place pork chops into a dish and keep it warm.

4. Reheat the pan again, put mustard sauce, and cook slowly. Pour over pork, drizzle with chives, and serve it.

Nutrition:

Calories: 847, Fat: 66.3, Fiber: 0.1, Carbs: 0.9, Protein: 57.4

Healthy Thai Beef Recipes

Prep Time + Cook Time: 20 minutes Servings: 6

Ingredients:

- Peanut butter - 4 tbsps.
- Lemon pepper -1½ tsps.
- Beefsteak (cut into strips) -1 pound
- 1 green bell pepper (seeded and chopped)
- 3 green onions (chopped)
- Beef stock -1 cup
- Garlic powder - ¼ tsp.
- Onion powder -¼ tsp.
- Coconut aminos - 1 tbsp.
- Seasoning: Salt and ground black pepper

Directions:

1. Combine and mix peanut butter with stock, aminos, lemon pepper in a bowl, mix well and put to one side.

2. With medium-high temperature, heat a pan, put beef, season with salt, pepper, onion, garlic powder, and cook for 7 minutes.

3. Put green pepper, then bring to commotion, and cook for 3 minutes.

4. Put green onions and peanut sauce, mix well and cook for 1 minute.

5. Divide between plates, and serve.

Nutrition:

Calories: 222, Fat: 10.3, Fiber: 1.6, Carbs: 5.9, Protein: 26.6

Herb Beef and zucchini soup bowls

Prep Time + Cook Time: 30 minutes Serves: 5

Ingredients:

- Ground beef- 1 Ib.
- Dried oregano- 1 tbsp.
- Minced garlic- 2 cloves
- Dried sage- 1 tbsp.
- Zucchini: cut with a spiralizer: 2
- Dried rosemary- 1 tbsp.
- Dried basil- 1 tbsp.
- Chopped canned tomatoes
- Dried marjoram- 1 tbsp.
- Chopped yellow onion- 1
- Salt and black pepper

Directions

1. Brown onions and garlic on a pan over medium heat.
2. Mix in the beef and cook for 6 minutes.
3. Mix in the tomatoes, rosemary, sage, oregano, marjoram, basil, salt and pepper and simmer for 15 minutes.
4. Serve herb soup on noodles and beef.

Nutrition:

Calories 320, carbs 12, protein 40, fiber 4, fat 13

Hot and spicy beef stew with olives

Prep Time + Cook Time:- 6 hours 10 minutes Serves: 8

Ingredients:

- Cubed beef roast- 2 Ib.
- Chopped habanero pepper- 1
- Chopped jalapenos- 4
- Chopped onions- 2
- Garlic cloves: minced- 6
- Avocado oil- 2 tbsp.
- Green bell peppers: seeded and chopped- 2
- Cumin- 1 ½ tsp.
- Chopped fresh cilantro- 2 tbsp.
- Bouillon granules- 4 tsp.
- Water- ½ cup
- Dried oregano- 1 tsp.
- Black olives: pitted and chopped- ½ cup

Directions:

1. Put an ovenproof pot on medium heat and add the beef cubes to brown for some minutes and move it to the crock pot.
2. Add the jalapeños, habanero, green bell peppers, water, granules, onions, tomatoes, cilantro, garlic, cumin, oregano, salt and pepper to the pot and mix well.
3. Seal the crock pot and let it cook for 6 hours on low pressure.
4. Mix in the olives.
5. Serve into bowls.

Nutrition:

Calories- 267, carbs- 9.7, protein- 36, fiber- 2.5, fat- 9

Italian Style Beef Casserole

Prep Time + Cook Time: 2 hours 10 minutes   Serves: 6

Ingredients:

- Tomato paste, 2 tbsps.
- Sliced eggplants, 3
- Chopped tomatoes, 2 cup
- Tomato passata, 4 cup
- Chopped basil, ¼ cup
- Ground beef, 1 lb.
- Minced garlic cloves, 2
- Chopped parsley, 1 tbsp.
- Olive oil, 2 tbsps.
- Salt
- Chopped red bell pepper, 1
- Black pepper
- Chopped yellow onion, 1

Directions:

1. Set the pan on fire with oil to fry the garlic and onion for 2 minutes over medium-high heat
2. Stir in the beef to brown for 5 minutes
3. Gently stir in the tomatoes, bell pepper, parsley, basil, tomato paste, black pepper, tomato passata, and salt. Remove from heat.
4. Arrange the eggplant slices and beef mix to form layers in a baking dish.
5. Set the oven for 2 hours at 350ºF, allow to bake.
6. Set on plates and serve.
7. Enjoy.

Nutrition: Calories: 370, Fat: 10, Fiber: 5, Carbs: 7, Protein: 28

Juicy Pork Chops with Stock Chicken

Prep Time + Cook Time: 55 minutes Servings: 4

Ingredients:

- 2 Peeled and chopped onions
- 6 bacon slices (chopped)
- 4 pork chops
- Chicken stock- ½ cup
- Seasoning: Salt and ground black pepper

Directions:

1. Heat a pan with medium temperature, put bacon, mix thoroughly, cook until crispy and transfer mixture to a bowl.
2. Place back the pan to medium heat, put onions, some salt, and pepper, mix well, cover then cook for 15 minutes, and pour into the same bowl with bacon.
3. Return to heat, increase to medium-high temperature, put pork chops, season with salt and pepper, brown for 3 minutes on one side, flip, reduce heat to medium, and cook for 7 minutes.
4. The next on the list is to add the stock, mix well, and cook for another 2 minutes.

5. Bacon and onions are returned to the pan, mix well, cook for 1 minute.
6. Divide between plates, and serve.

Nutrition:
Calories: 433, Fat: 31.9, Fiber: 1.2, Carbs: 5.6, Protein: 29.2

Lamb and vegetables

Prep Time + Cook Time: 25 minutes Serves: 4

Ingredients:

- Lamb cutlets- 12
- Red wine vinegar- 1 tbsp.
- Olive oil- ¼ cup
- Sumac- 2 tbsp.
- Radishes: thinly sliced- 6
- Dried oregano- 2 tsp.
- Water- 2 tbsp.
- Mixed garlic- 2 cloves
- Ground cumin- 2 tsp.
- Paprika- 2 tsp.
- Sliced carrots- 4
- Black olives: pitted and sliced- 2 tbsp.
- Chopped parsley- ¼ cup
- Harissa- 2 tsp.
- Salt and black pepper

Directions

1. Mix lamb with garlic, oregano, paprika, half oil, salt, pepper, sumac, and water together in a bowl and coat the lamb well.
2. Boil carrots in water in a pot over medium-high for 2 minutes.
3. Drain and put in a salad bowl then add radishes and olives.
4. Mix the oil, harissa, cumin, parsley and vinegar together in a bowl and mix with the carrots. Season with salt and pepper.
5. Grill lamb on medium-high for 3 minutes on all sides.
6. Serve with carrots salad.

Nutrition:
Calories 245, carbs 4, protein 34, fiber 6, fat 32

Lamb Leg Curry

Prep Time + Cook Time: 3 hours and 40 minutes Servings: 2

Ingredients:

- Lamb leg -2 lbs.
- Salt and black pepper- to taste
- Thyme, dried -2/3 tsp
- Oregano, dried -½ tsp
- Tomato, chopped -1
- Yellow onion, chopped-½
- Garlic clove, minced -1
- Olive oil -½ tbsp
- Beef stock -1.5 cups

Directions:

1. Place lamb leg in a Dutch oven and add salt, pepper, oregano, thyme, tomatoes, garlic, onion, oil, and stock.
2. Cover the lamb leg mixture with a lid then place it in the oven for 3.5 hours at 370 0F.
3. Once done, remove the lamb leg from the cooked mixture.

4. Place it on the cutting board and slice it into pieces.
5. Serve warm with remaining curry on the top.
6. Devour!

Nutrition:
Calories: 363, Fat: 12, Fiber: 4, Carbs: 13, Protein: 15

Lamb pot pie

Prep Time + Cook Time: 1 hour 50 minutes Serves: 2

Ingredients:
- Lamb fillets: cut into medium pieces: 10 oz.
- Chopped carrots -2
- Ghee- 2 tbsp.
- Chopped rosemary- ½ tbsp.
- Half cauliflower: separated into florets
- Tomato puree: 1 tbsp.
- Half Celeriac: chopped
- Stevia- 1 tsp.
- Minced garlic- 2 cloves
- Mint sauce- 1 tbsp.
- Lamb stock- 1¼ cups
- Celery stick: chopped- 1
- Red onion: chopped: 1
- Olive oil- 1 tbsp.
- Chopped leek- 1
- Salt and black pepper

Directions

1. Pour oil in a pan over medium heat and fry celery, garlic and onion for 5 minutes.
2. Mix in the lamb pieces and cook for 3 minutes then add stevia, carrot, leek, mint sauce, rosemary, stock, and tomato puree. Close the lid and cook for 1 hour 30 minutes.
3. Pour some water in a pot over medium heat and add the celeriacup Simmer for 10 minutes and add the cauliflower florets.
4. Cook for 15 minutes and remove the liquid. Season with pepper, salt, and ghee.
5. Mash with a masher and serve with lamb and veggies over it.

Nutrition:
Calories 324, carbs 8, protein 20, fiber 5, fat 4

Lemon Cranberry Pork Roast

Prep Time + Cook Time:8 hours 10 minutes Servings: 4

Ingredients:
- Cranberries- ½ cup
- Pork loin - 1½ pounds
- A pinch of dry mustard
- ½ lemon sliced
- water - ¼ cup

- Ginger - ½ tsp.
- Erythritol- 2 tbsps.
- Coconut flour- 1 tbsp.
- 2 Peeled and minced garlic cloves
- Seasoning: Salt and ground black

pepper

Directions:

1. Mix and stir ginger with mustard, salt, pepper, and flour in a bowl.
2. Transfer meat to a slow cooker after roast was added and toss to coat.
3. Put erythritol, cranberries, garlic,

water, and lemon slices.
4. Cook on low for 8 hours while the slow cooker was covered.
5. Divide between plates and sprinkle pan juices on top, and serve.

Nutrition:
Calories: 1523, Fat: 86.9, Fiber: 0.9, Carbs: 7.7, Protein: 170.7

Mediterranean Pork Recipes

Prep Time + Cook Time: 45 minutes Servings: 4

Ingredients:

- 3 Peeled and minced garlic cloves
- 4 pork chops (bone–in)
- Dried rosemary -1 tsp.
- Seasoning: Salt and ground black pepper

Directions:

1. With salt and pepper season pork chops, and place in a roasting pan.
2. Put dried rosemary and garlic
3. Place in an oven while the oven is set

to a temperature of 425°F, heat for 10 minutes.
4. Lessen heat to 350°F and roast for 25 minutes.
5. Slice pork, divide between plates and sprinkle with pan juices all over.

Nutrition:
Calories: 259, Fat: 19.9, Fiber: 0.1, Carbs: 0.7, Protein: 18.1

Mexican Cilantro Beef Dish

Prep Time + Cook Time: 30 minutes Serves: 4

Ingredients:

- Cayenne pepper sauce.
- Water, ½ cup
- Black pepper.
- Ground beef meat, 2 lb.
- Chopped cilantro, ¼ cup
- Salt.
- Taco seasoning, ¼ cup
- Sour cream, 2 cup
- Minced garlic, 1 tsp.
- Chopped white onion, ¼ cup
- Sliced cherry tomatoes, 6.
- Pitted avocados, 2.
- Shredded lettuce leaves, 2 cup
- Lime juice, 1 tbsp.
- Shredded cheddar cheese, 2 cup

Directions:

1. Using a bowl, stir in salt, avocado, garlic, onion, cilantro, tomatoes, lime juice and pepper. Combine well and set in the refrigerator.

2. Set a pan over medium high heat. Stir in the beef and cook for 10 minutes until browned.
3. Stir in the water and taco seasoning. Reduce the heat to medium-low and cook for 10 more minutes.
4. Set the mixture into 4 plates in equal shares.
5. Add in cheddar cheese, sour cream, lettuce pieces and the avocado mixture.
6. Top up with a drizzling of cayenne pepper sauce and enjoy your lunch!

Nutrition:
calories: 340, fat: 30, protein: 32, fiber: 5, carbs: 3

Mint lamb

Prep Time + Cook Time: 8 hours 10 minutes Serves: 6
Ingredients:
- Lamb leg- 2 Ib.
- Thyme sprigs- 4
- Mint leaves- 6
- Pinch of dried rosemary
- Maple extract- 1 tbsp.
- Minced garlic- 1 tsp.
- Mustard- 2 tbsp.
- Olive oil- ¼ cup
- Salt and black pepper
- Salt and black pepper

Directions

1. Pour some oil in the slow cooker and add the lamb, maple extract, rosemary, garlic, salt and pepper. Close and cook for 7 hours on low.
2. Add in the thyme and mint and cook for 1 hour.
3. Leave to cool and slice.
4. Serve drizzled with juices.

Nutrition:
Calories 400, carbs 3, protein 26, fiber 1, fat 34

Mushroom Sauce with Meatballs

Prep Time + Cook Time: 35 minutes Servings: 6
Ingredients:
- Almond flour-¾ cup
- Chopped fresh parsley - 1 tbsp.
- Dried onion flakes - 1 tbsp.
- Garlic powder-½ tsp.
- Ground beef - 2 pounds
- Coconut aminos- 1 tbsp.
- Seasoning: Salt and ground black

pepper
- Beef stock - ¼ cup

For the sauce:
- Bacon fat -2 tbsps.
- Butter- 2 tbsps.
- Sour cream - ¼ cup
- Beef stock- ½ cup

- Chopped Onion- 1 cup
- Sliced mushrooms- 2 cups
- Coconut aminos- ½ tsp.
- Seasoning: Salt and ground black pepper

Directions:
1. Mix and stir beef with salt, pepper, garlic powder, 1 tbsp. coconut aminos, ¼ cup beef stock, almond flour, parsley, and onion flakes in a clean bowl,
2. Shape 6 patties, arrange them on a baking sheet, place in an oven and bake for 18 minutes at 375°F.
3. With medium temperature, heat heat butter in a pan, and also heat bacon fat over medium temperature, put mushrooms, mix well, and cook for 4 minutes.
4. Put onions, mix well and cook for 4 minutes, also put ½ tsp. coconut aminos, sour cream, and ½ cup beef stock, bring to the commotion by stirring well and cook slowly.
5. Put off heat, add salt and pepper, and stir well. Divide the beef patties into plates.
6. Serve with mushroom sauce on top.

Nutrition:
Calories: 452, Fat: 23.5, Fiber: 1.3, Carbs: 4.9, Protein: 53.2

Nutmeg Meatballs Curry

Prep Time + Cook Time: 40 minutes Servings: 3

Ingredients:
- Pork meat, ground- 2/3 lbs.
- Egg -½
- Parsley, chopped-1 tbsp
- Coconut flour-2 tbsp
- Garlic clove, minced-1
- Salt and black pepper - to taste
- Veggie stock -¼ cup
- Tomato passata-½ cup
- Nutmeg, ground -¼ tsp
- Sweet paprika -¼ tsp
- Olive oil-1 tbsp
- Carrot, chopped -1

Directions:
1. Thoroughly mix the meat with egg, parsley, salt, pepper, garlic, nutmeg, and paprika in a suitable bowl.
2. Mix well and make small meatballs out of this mixture.
3. Dredge these balls through dry flour or dust the balls with flour.
4. Place a pot with oil over medium-high heat.
5. Add dusted meatballs in the pot and sear them for 4 minutes per side.
6. Toss in tomato passata, carrots, and stock.
7. Cover this mixture and let it simmer for 20 minutes.
8. Serve right away.
9. Devour.

Nutrition:
Calories: 281, Fat: 8, Fiber: 6, Carbs: 10, Protein: 15

Pan seared sausage and kale

Prep Time + Cook Time: 35 minutes Serves: 4

Ingredients:

- Chopped kale- 5 Ib.
- Italian pork sausage: sliced- 1½ Ib.
- Minced garlic- 1 tsp.
- Water- 1 cup
- Onion: chopped- 1 cup
- Red bell pepper: seeded and chopped ½ cup
- Red chili pepper: chopped ½ cup
- Black pepper
- Salt

Directions:

1. Put a pan on medium heat and add the sausage to brown for 10 minutes.
2. Mix in onions and town for 3-4 minutes.
3. Add in the garlic and bell pepper and cook for 1 minute.
4. Mix in the chili, kale, water, pepper and salt and let cook for 10 minutes.
5. Serve

Nutrition:

Calories- 872, carbs- 63.1, protein- 50.4, fiber- 9.3, fats- 48.3

Pan-Fried Chorizo Mix

Prep Time + Cook Time: 35 minutes Serves: 4

Ingredients:

- Chopped tomato, 1
- Olive oil, 1 tbsp.
- Sugar-free chorizo sausages, 2
- Chopped zucchini, 1
- Chopped red bell pepper, 1
- Minced garlic cloves, 2
- Black pepper
- Chicken stock, 2 cup
- Chopped parsley, 2 tbsps.
- Lemon juice, 1 tbsp.
- Salt
- Chopped yellow onion, 1

Directions:

1. Set the pan on fire to fry the chorizo and onion for 3 minutes over medium-high heat.
2. Stir in the bell pepper, garlic, lemon juice, tomato, pepper, stock, and salt.
3. Allow to simmer for 10 minutes while covered
4. Mix in the zucchini and parsley to cook for 12 minutes.
5. Set in serving bowls and enjoy

Nutrition:

Calories: 280, Fat: 8, Fiber: 3, Carbs: 5, Protein: 17

Pork Rolls

Prep Time + Cook Time: 30 minutes Servings: 6

Ingredients:

- 3 Peeled and minced garlic cloves
- Italian seasoning - ½ tsp.
- 6 prosciutto slices
- Chopped fresh parsley - 2 tbsps.
- Thinly sliced pork cutlets- 1 pound
- Coconut oil - 1 tbsp.
- Chopped onion- ¼ cup
- Canned diced tomatoes - 15 ounces
- Chicken stock - ⅓ cup
- Grated Parmesan cheese - 2 tbsps.
- Ricotta cheese- ⅓ cup e
- Seasoning: Salt and ground black pepper

Directions:

1. Flatten pork pieces with a meat pounder.
2. Put prosciutto slices on top of each piece and then divide ricotta cheese, parsley, and Parmesan cheese.
3. Each piece of pork should be rolled and secure with a toothpick.
4. With medium-high temperature, heat the oil in a pan, add pork rolls, cook until brown on both sides, and transfer to a plate.
5. Heat the pan again over medium temperature, put onion and garlic, mix well. Cook for 5 minutes.
6. The stock should be added and cook for another 3 minutes.
7. Remove toothpicks from pork rolls and return into the pan.
8. Put tomatoes, Italian seasoning, salt, and pepper, bring to commotion by stirring, bring to a boil, reduce heat to medium-low, cover the pan with lid, and cook for 30 minutes.
9. Divide between plates and serve it.

Nutrition:
Calories: 256, Fat: 13.9, Fiber: 2.1, Carbs: 15.7, Protein: 17.2

Roasted Beef and pepperoncini

Prep Time + Cook Time: 2 hours 10minutes Serves: 4

Ingredients:

- Melted ghee, 2 tbsps.
- Veggie stock, 1 cup
- Coconut aminos, 1 tbsp.
- Beef chuck roast, 5 lbs.
- Pepperoncini, 10

Directions:

1. Prepare the baking tray with some greasing.
2. Set on the baking tray the meat, pepperoncini, stock, and aminos then cover.
3. Set the oven for 2 hours at 375°F, allow to bake.

4. Set the meat on a chopping board to slice and serve topped with the pepperoncini mix.

Nutrition:
Calories: 371, Fat: 11, Fiber: 8, Carbs: 13, Protein: 27

Rosemary lamb bowls

Prep Time + Cook Time: 3 hours 10 minutes Serves: 4

Ingredients:
- Chopped carrots: 2
- Rosemary sprigs
- Beef stock- 1 cup
- Cubed lamb- 2 Ib.
- Chopped tomato- 1
- Ghee- 2 tbsp.
- Chopped thyme- 1 tsp.
- Garlic cloves- 1
- Yellow onion: chopped- 1
- White wine- 1 cup
- Salt and black pepper

Instructions
1. Pour oil on the Dutch oven over medium-high and brown beef seasoned with salt and pepper on all sides and set aside.
2. Add in the onions to fry for 2 minutes.
3. Mix in the garlic, wine, rosemary, thyme, carrots, salt, pepper and tomatoes and cook for some minutes.
4. Mix in the lamb and turn down the heat to medium-low. Close and cook for 4 hours.
5. Season with salt and pepper and remove the sprigs.
6. Serve into bowls.

Nutrition:
Calories 700, carbs 10, protein 67, fiber 6, fat 43

Sauerkraut Soup and Beef

Prep Time + Cook Time: 1 hour and 30 minutes Servings: 8

Ingredients:
- Ground beef -1 pound
- Chopped fresh parsley- 3 tbsps.
- 1 onion (peeled and chopped)
- Dried sage - 1 tsp.
- Olive oil - 3 tsps.
- Beef stock -14 ounces
- Chicken stock -2 cups
- Canned tomatoes and juice -14 ounces
- Gluten-free Worcestershire sauce -1 tbsp.
- 4 bay leaves
- Garlic (minced) -1 tbsp.
- water - 2 cups
- Stevia - 1 tbsp.
- Chopped sauerkraut- 14 ounces
- Seasoning: Salt and ground black pepper

Directions:
1. With medium temperature, heat 1 tsp. oil in a pan, put beef, stir properly, and brown for 10 minutes.

2. Mix and stir chicken, beef stock, sauerkraut, stevia, canned tomatoes, Worcestershire sauce, parsley, sage, and bay leaves in a pot, cool slowly (brings to simmer) with medium heat.
3. Put beef into soup, mix well, and continue to cook slowly.
4. Pour the remaining oil in a pan and heat with medium temperature, Supplement with onions, mix well, and cook for 2more minutes.
5. Also, put garlic, stir, cook for 1 minute, and pour into the soup.
6. Lessen heat to soup, and cook slowly for 1 hour.
7. Put salt, pepper, water, mix carefully and cook for 15 minutes.
8. Divide between bowls and serve it.

Nutrition:
Calories: 152, Fat: 1.7, Fiber: 2.5, Carbs: 6, Protein: 19

Seared beef soup bowls

Prep Time + Cook Time: 4 hours 20 minutes Serves: 4
Ingredients:
- Cubed beef- 4 Ib.
- Thyme sprigs- 4
- Chopped pancetta- 8 oz.
- Chopped parsley
- Ghee- 2 tbsp.
- Lemon peel strips- 3
- Tomato paste- 2 tbsp.
- Olive oil- 2 tbsp.
- Cinnamon sticks- 2
- Minced garlic- 4 cloves
- Chopped brown onions- 2
- Red vinegar- 4 tbsp.
- Beef stock- 4 cups
- Salt and black pepper

Directions

1. Put pancetta, garlic, oil, and onion in a pan over medium-high and fry for 5 minutes.
2. Add the beef cubes to brown then mix in the salt, pepper, vinegar, cinnamon, lemon peel, tomato paste, ghee and thyme and cook for 3 minutes.
3. Put everything in a crock pot and cook for 4 hours on high.
4. Remove thyme, lemon peel and cinnamon and mix in the parsley.
5. Serve.

Nutrition:
Calories 250, carbs 7, protein 33, fiber 1, fat 6

Seared beef with peanut sauce

Prep Time + Cook Time: 20 minutes Serves: 6

Ingredients:

- Beef stock- 1 cup
- Green onions: chopped- 3
- Beef steak: cut into strips: 1 Ib.
- Green bell pepper: chopped- 1
- Lemon pepper- 1½ tsp.
- Coconut aminos- 1 tbsp.
- Peanut butter- 4 tbsp.
- Onion powder- ¼ tsp.
- Garlic powder- ¼ tsp.
- Salt and Pepper to taste

Directions

1. Combine lemon pepper, stock, peanut butter, stock and coconut aminos together in a bowl and set aside.

2. Sprinkle the beef with salt, onion powder, garlic powder and pepper and sear it on a pan over medium-high for 7 minutes.
3. Mix in the green pepper and let it cook for 3 minutes.
4. Add in the green onions and the peanut sauce and let it cook for 1 minute.
5. Serve.

Nutrition:

Calories 224, carbs 3, protein 19, fiber 1, fats 15

Seared veal and capers

Prep Time + Cook Time: 25 minutes Serves: 2

Ingredients:

- Veal scallops: 8 oz.
- Capers 1½ tbsp.
- Butter- 2 tbsp.
- Chicken Stock- ¼ cup
- Minced garlic clove- 1
- White wine- ¼ cup
- Salt and ground black pepper.

Directions:

1. Dissolve butter on a pan on medium-high.
2. Sprinkle salt and pepper on veal and brown each side for 1 minute. Set aside

3. On medium, add garlic to the pan and cook for 1 minute.
4. Pour in the wine and let it boil for 2 minutes.
5. Pour in stock, butter, capers, pepper and salt and then add the veal to the broth and mix well.
6. Close the pan and cook until veal is soft.

Nutrition:

Calories- 434, carbs- 10.6, protein- 57.9, fiber- 0.8, fat- 14.4

Shredded lamb topped with lemon dressing

Prep Time + Cook Time: 4 hours 10 minutes Serves: 4

Ingredients:

- Lamb shanks- 2
- Half lemon- zest
- Half lemon- juiced
- Olive oil- 4 tbsp.
- Peeled garlic head- 1
- Dried oregano- ½ tsp.
- Sat and black pepper

Directions

1. Combine lamb, pepper, garlic, and salt together in a slow cooker and cook on high for 4 hours.
2. Whisk zest, juice, oil, oregano, salt and pepper in a bowl.
3. Shred the lamb meat and remove the bone.
4. Serve topped with lemon dressing.

Nutrition:
Calories 160, carbs 5, protein 12, fiber 3, fat 7

Slow cook lamb chili

Prep Time + Cook Time: 4 hours 10 minutes Serves: 6

Ingredients:

- Cubed lamb meat- 1 Ib.
- Ground coriander- 2 tsp.
- Spinach: 1 Ib.
- Turmeric- 1 tsp.
- Cloves- 6
- Ga ram masala- 1 tsp.
- Chopped canned tomatoes- 14 oz.
- Minced garlic- 2 cloves
- Cumin powder- 2 tsp.
- Cardamom- 2 tsp.
- Red onion: chopped- 1

Directions

1. Put all your ingredients in the slow cooker and mix then cook on high for 4 hours.
2. Open and mix and serve into bowls.

Nutrition: Calories 160, carbs 7, protein 20, fiber 3, fat 6

Smokey Baked Pork

Prep Time + Cook Time:4 hours 15 minutes Servings: 2

Ingredients:

- Pork shoulder -1.5 lbs.
- Liquid smoke -½ tbsp
- Pink salt -1 ½ tbsp

Directions:

1.Place pork shoulder in a cooking pot and rub it with salt and smoke.

2.Transfer this pot to the oven and bake it for 4 hours at 350 °F.

3.Once cooked then slice the pork to serve. Enjoy with fresh salad.

Nutrition:
Calories: 382, Fat: 8, Fiber: 4, Carbs: 10, Protein: 17

Spicy Beef and Scallops Mix

Prep Time + Cook Time: 30 minutes Serve: 2

Ingredients:

- A drizzle of olive oil
- Chopped parsley, 2 tbsps.
- Minced garlic cloves, 4
- Beef steaks, 2
- Chopped shallot, 1
- Chopped basil, 2 tbsps.
- Grated lemon zest, 1 tsp.
- Melted ghee, ¼ cup
- Salt
- Sea scallops, 10
- Black pepper
- Lemon juice, 2 tbsps.
- Beef stock, ¼ cup

Directions:

1. Season the beef steaks with pepper and salt
2. Set the pan on fire with oil to fry the seasoned steaks for 5 minutes each side over medium-high heat.
3. Stir in the shallots to cook for 2 minutes
4. Mix in lemon juice, basil, lemon zest, stock, seasonings, and parsley to cook for 5 more minutes.
5. Set on plates to serve.
6. Enjoy.

Nutrition:

Calories: 290, Fat: 9, Fiber: 2, Carbs: 8, Protein: 20

Spicy Cinnamon Pork Chops

Prep Time + Cook Time: 4 hours and 25 minutes Servings: 4

Ingredients:

- 2 Peeled and minced garlic cloves
- Ground cinnamon -1 tsp.
- 2 tsps. cumin
- 4 pork rib chops
- Coconut oil (melted) -1 tbsp.
- Chili powder- 1 tbsp.
- chili powder - ½ tsp.
- lime juice - ¼ cup
- Seasoning: Salt and ground black pepper

Directions:

1. Mix and whisk lime juice with oil, garlic, cumin, cinnamon, chili powder, salt, pepper, chili powder, in a bowl.
2. Put pork chops, toss in order to coat, and put to one side in the refrigerator for 4 hours.
3. Place pork on a preheated grill pan over medium heat, cook for 7 minutes, flip, and cook for 7 minutes. Divide among plates and serve.

Nutrition:

Calories: 507, Fat: 32.7, Fiber: 0.1, Carbs: 1.4, Protein: 51.9

Spicy Mexican Luncheon

Prep Time + Cook Time:3 hours 10 minutes Servings: 8

Ingredients:

- Beef stew meat, cubed-2 lbs.
- Tomatoes, chopped -6
- Red onion, chopped -2
- Canned green chilies, chopped -10 oz.
- Chili powder -4 tsp
- Cumin powder -2 tsp
- Oregano, dried -2 tsp
- Veggie stock -4 cups
- Salt and black pepper- to taste

Directions:

1. Place a cooking pot over medium heat.
2. Toss in onion, chilies, tomatoes, cumin powder, chili powder, stock, oregano, salt and pepper.
3. Mix well and cook on a simmer for 30 minutes.
4. Add meat to the cooking mixture and cover it.
5. Cook for 2.5 hours on medium heat.
6. Dish out and serve warm.

Nutrition:
Calories: 338, Fat: 6, Fiber: 8, Carbs: 12, Protein: 15

Stewed Beef

Prep Time + Cook Time: 20 minutes Serves: 4

Ingredients:

- Chili powder, 2 tbsps.
- Cubed beef meat, 2 lbs.
- Hot sauce, 2 tbsps.
- Chopped red onion, 1
- Sliced zucchini, 1
- Juice of 1 lime
- Salt
- Chopped red bell peppers, 2
- Black pepper
- Olive oil, ¼ cup

Directions:

1. With your mixing bowl set, whisk together the hot sauce, lime juice, salt, oil, pepper, and chili powder
2. Set the beef, bell peppers, zucchini, and onion on the skewers.
3. Rub with the chili mix.
4. Set them on the preheated grill to cook for 5 minutes each side over medium-high heat.
5. Set on plates to serve.

Nutrition:
Calories: 270, Fat: 11, Fiber: 2, Carbs: 13, Protein: 19

Sweet Jamaican Pork

Prep Time + Cook Time: 55 minutes Servings: 12

Ingredients:

- Jamaican jerk spice mix - ¼ cup
- Pork shoulder - 4 pounds
- Coconut oil - 1 tbsp.
- Beef stock- ½ cup

Directions:

1. With Jamaican mixture, polish pork shoulder put it inside an Instant Pot.
2. The pot should be set to Sauté mode, add oil to the pot.
3. Put pork shoulder, ensure its brown on all sides.
4. Cover Instant Pot while stock is added, cook on Meat/Stew mode for 45 minutes.
5. Uncover, then transfer pork to a dish, shred, and serve.

Nutrition:

Calories: 452, Fat: 33.5, Fiber: 0, Carbs: 0, Protein: 35.3

Tasty Zucchini Noodles and Beef

Prep Time + Cook Time: 30 minutes Servings: 5

Ingredients:

- Dried oregano -1 tbsp.
- Ground beef -1 pound
- 1 onion (peeled and chopped)
- 2 garlic cloves (peeled and minced)
- Canned diced tomatoes -14 ounces
- Dried marjoram -1 tbsp.
- Dried rosemary - 1 tbsp.
- Dried sage - 1 tbsp.
- Dried basil - 1 tbsp.
- 2 Zucchini (cut with a spiralizer)
- Seasoning: Salt and ground black pepper

Directions:

1. With medium temperature, heat a pan, add garlic and onion, mix well, and ensure its brown on all sides for a couple of minutes.
2. Put beef, stir, and cook for 6 minutes.
3. Put the following ingredients tomatoes, salt, pepper, sage, rosemary, oregano, marjoram, basil, mix well and cook slowly for 15 minutes.
4. Divide zucchini noodles into separate bowls, top with beef mixture, and serve.

Nutrition:

Calories: 206, Fat: 6, Fiber: 2.3, Carbs: 8.2, Protein: 29.5

Tomato–stuffed Squash and Beef

Prep Time + Cook Time:1 hour 10 minutes Servings: 2

Ingredients:

- Dried thyme- ½ tsp.
- 3 Peeled and minced garlic cloves
- 1 Peeled and chopped onion
- 1 Portobello mushroom (sliced)
- Canned diced tomatoes - 28 ounces
- Dried oregano - 1 tsp.
- Ground beef - 1 pound
- 1 green bell pepper (seeded and chopped)
- Spaghetti squash, pricked with a fork - 1 pound
- Cayenne pepper - ¼ tsp.
- Seasoning: Salt and ground black pepper

Directions:

1. Arrange squash on a lined baking sheet, place in oven and bake for 40 minutes at 400°F.
2. Slice into half, put to one side to cool, take away seeds, and put aside.
3. With medium-high temperature, heat a pan, put meat, garlic, onion, mushroom, mix well and cook until meat brown on all sides.
4. Put the following ingredients, pepper, salt, oregano, thyme, cayenne, tomatoes, green pepper, stir, and cook for 10 minutes.
5. Stuff squash halves with beef mixture, place in an oven and bake for 10 minutes at 400°. Divide between 2 plates and serve.

Nutrition:

Calories: 616, Fat: 16.6, Fiber: 7.3, Carbs: 43.1, Protein:75.5

Turmeric Jamaican Beef Pies

Prep Time + Cook Time: 45 minutes Servings: 12

Ingredients:

- Turmeric -½ tsp.
- 3 peeled and minced garlic cloves
- Ground beef -½ pound
- Ground pork- ½ pound
- Stevia powder -¼ tsp.
- Butter -2 tbsps.
- Water -½ cup
- 1 small onion (peeled and chopped)
- 2 habanero peppers (chopped)
- Cumin- 2 tsps.
- Garlic powder - 1 tsp.
- Seasoning: Salt and ground black pepper

For the crust:

- Turmeric- 1 tsp.
- Stevia - ¼ tsp.
- water - 2 tbsps.
- Coconut flour - ½ cup
- Cream cheese -6 ounces

- A pinch of salt
- Baking powder -½ tsp.
- Flax meal -1½ cups
- Butter (melted) -4 tbsps.

Directions:

1. Blend onion with habaneros, garlic, and ½ cup water together in a blender.
2. With medium temperature, heat a pan, put pork and beef, mix well, and cook for 3 minutes.
3. Put onions mixture then stir, and cook for 2 minutes. Also supplement with the following ingredient, garlic, onion, curry powder, ½ tsp. turmeric, salt, pepper, stevia powder, and garlic powder, stir well, and cook for 3 minutes.
4. Also, put 2 tbsps. butter, mix until it melts, and put off heat. Combine and stir 1 tsp. turmeric, with ¼ tsp. stevia, baking powder, flax meal, and coconut flour in a bowl.
5. In another bowl, mix and stir 4 tbsps. butter with 2 tbsps. water and cream cheese.
6. Carefully combine the 2 mixtures, and mix until you obtain a dough, then shape 12 balls from this mixture, arrange them on a parchment paper, and roll each to form a circle.
7. Beef and pork should be divided.
8. Mix on one-half of the dough circles, cover with another half, seal edges, and arrange them all on a lined baking sheet.
9. Bake pies in the oven for 25 minutes at 350°F. Serve warm.

Nutrition:
Calories: 198, Fat: 13.6, Fiber: 2.6, Carbs: 5.7, Protein: 13

Vegetable Beef Stew

Prep Time + Cook Time: 2 hours and 40 minutes Servings: 2

Ingredients:

- Beef meat, cubed-½ lb.
- Yellow onion, chopped -½
- Tomato paste -3 oz.
- Garlic clove, minced -1
- Thyme, chopped -½ tbsp
- Carrot, chopped -1
- Celery stalks, chopped -1.5
- Parsley, chopped -1 tbsp
- White vinegar -1 tbsp
- Salt and black pepper- to taste

Directions:

1. Place a large cooking pot over medium heat.
2. Add beef, tomato paste, onion, garlic, carrots, thyme, parsley, celery, salt, pepper, and vinegar.
3. Mix well and let this beef mixture simmer for on medium heat.
4. Make sure to cover the pan and cook for 2.5 hours.
5. Dish out and serve warm.

Nutrition:
Calories: 360, Fat: 4, Fiber: 7, Carbs: 9, Protein: 15

Chapter 8Ketogenic Side Dish Recipes

Almond Cheddar Soufflés

Prep Time + Cook Time: 35 minutes Serves: 8

Ingredients:

- Dry mustard, 1 tsp.
- Heavy cream, ¾ cup
- Almond flour, ½ cup
- Large eggs, 6
- Black pepper
- Vegetable oil
- Tartar cream, ¼ tsp.
- Salt
- Cayenne pepper, ¼ tsp.
- Xanthan gum, ½ tsp.
- Shredded cheddar cheese, 2 cup
- Chopped fresh chives, ¼ cup
- Cooking spray

Directions:

1. Whisk together salt, cayenne, almond flour, xanthan gum, pepper, and mustard
2. Mix in eggs, tartar cream, cheese, chives, and cream as you whisk gently
3. Set the ramekins with cooking spray then pour in the mixture.
4. Set your oven for 25 minutes at 3500 F

Nutrition:

Calories: 211, Fat: 17.7, Fiber: 0.2, Carbs: 1.4, Protein: 11.8

Asian Salad with Cucumber

Prep Time + Cook Time: 50 minutes Servings: 4

Ingredients:

- A packet of Shiritaki noodles: 1
- Medium cucumber, sliced thin: 1
- Green onion, peeled and chopped: 1
- Salt: to taste
- Ground black pepper: to taste
- Red pepper flakes: ¼ tsp.
- Sesame seeds: 1 tsp.
- Balsamic vinegar: 1 tbsp.
- Coconut oil: 2 tbsps.
- Sesame oil: 1 tbsp.

Directions:

1. Prepare noodles by cooking them as per instruction on the packet, then drain and rinse well.
2. Place a medium skillet pan over medium-high heat, add oil and when hot, add noodles and cook for 5 minutes or until crispy, stirring frequently.
3. When done, transfer noodles to a plate lined with paper towels to absorb excess grease and then transfer into a bowl.
4. Add remaining ingredients, toss until well mixed and place the bowl in the refrigerator for 30 minutes or until chilled.
5. Serve straightaway.

Nutrition:

Calories: 110, Fat: 10.9, Fiber: 1.6, Carbs: 4.7, Protein: 0.9

Asian Style Braised Eggplant

Prep Time + Cook Time: 25 minutes Serves: 4

Ingredients:

- Minced garlic, 2 tsps.
- Coconut milk, ¼ cup Sliced onion, 1
- Vegetable oil, 2 tbsps.
- Chopped green onions, 4
- Vietnamese sauce, ½ cup
- Water, ½ cup
- Asian eggplant, 1
- Chili paste, 2 tsps.

For the Vietnamese sauce:

- Chicken stock, ½ cup
- Erythritol, 1 tsp.
- Fish sauce, 2 tbsps.

Directions:

1. Set your pan over medium heat then add stock
2. Mix in fish sauce and erythritol as you sir gently then reserve.
3. Stir fry the eggplant pieces over medium-high heat until browned evenly then set on a plate.
4. Again, sauté the onion and garlic on a pan until fragrant.
5. Add in the eggplant and cook for 2 more minutes
6. Pour in the water with chili paste, Vietnamese sauce, and coconut milk to cook for 5 minutes as you stir gently.
7. Top the green onions and cook for another minute.

Nutrition:

Calories: 125, Fat: 10.9, Fiber: 1.3, Carbs: 6.4, Protein: 1.7

Asparagus Deal

Prep Time + Cook Time: 23 minutes Servings: 5

Ingredients:

- Asparagus spears-40
- Ghee-1/4 cup
- Lemon juice-1 tbsp.
- Cayenne pepper-A pinch
- Egg yolks-2
- Salt and black pepper-To taste

Directions:

1. Take a bowl.
2. Beat the egg yolks very well.
3. Deliver this to a small pan over low heat.
4. Pour lemon juice and whisk well.
5. Combine ghee and whisk until it melts.
6. Add salt, pepper and cayenne pepper.
7. Whisk again well.
8. Meanwhile; heat up a pan over medium high heat.
9. Put in the asparagus spears and fry them for 5 minutes with tossing.
10. Divide asparagus on plates.
11. Drizzle the sauce you've made on top.
12. Serve.

Nutrition :

Calories:- 150; Fat : 13; Fiber : 6; Carbs : 2; Protein : 3

Avocado Fries with Almond Mix

Prep Time + Cook Time: 15 minutes Servings: 3

Ingredients:

- Avocados: 3; pitted, peeled, halved and sliced
- almond meal - 1½ cups
- A pinch of cayenne pepper
- sunflower oil - 1½ cups
- Salt and black pepper to the taste.

Directions:

1. Mix almond meal with salt, pepper and cayenne in a bowl and stir gently.
2. Whisk some eggs with a pinch of salt and pepper in another clean bowl.
3. Cover the avocado pieces in egg and then in almond meal mix.
4. Add heat to a pan which has oil on medium-high heat source; then add avocado fries and cook them until they show a golden coloration.
5. Move to paper towels, drain grease and divide into different plates
6. Serve as a side dish.

Nutrition :

Calories:- 450; Fat : 43; Fiber : 4; Carbs : 7; Protein : 17

Baked Brussels sprouts with ranch dressing

Prep Time + Cook Time: 40 minutes Serves: 4

Ingredients:

- Halved Brussels sprouts- 1 Ib.
- Minced garlic cloves- 3
- Keto ranch dressing- 2 tbsp.
- Hot paprika- ½ tsp.
- Parmesan: grated- 1 tbsp.
- Olive oil- 1 tbsp.
- Dried oregano- 1 tsp.
- Salt
- Black pepper

Directions:

1. Lay the Brussels sprouts on a baking sheet.
2. Sprinkle with salt, pepper, oregano, paprika, oil, and garlic
3. Mix well and put in the oven to bake for 30 minutes at 425°F.
4. Drizzle with ranch dressing and parmesan and mix well.

Nutrition:

Calories- 222, carbs- 12, protein- 8, fiber- 6, fats- 4

Baked Eggplant Salad with Oregano

Prep Time + Cook Time: 3 hours and 45 minutes Servings: 8

Ingredients:

- Eggplants: 6
- Minced garlic: ½ tsp.
- Salt: 1 tsp.
- Ground black pepper: 1 tsp.
- Stevia: 2 tbsps.
- Dried parsley: 1 tsp.

- Dried oregano: 1 tsp.
- Dried basil: ¼ tsp.
- Olive oil: 3 tbsps.
- Balsamic vinegar: 1 tbsp.

Directions:
1. Set oven to 350 0F and let preheat.
2. In the meantime, use a fork to prick eggplants and place on a baking sheet.
3. Then place this baking sheet into the oven and bake for 1 hour and 30 minutes.
4. When done, remove baking sheet from the oven, cool eggplants for 10 minutes and then peel them.
5. Chop eggplants into bite-size pieces and place into a bowl.
6. Season with salt and black pepper, add stevia, parsley, oregano, and basil and toss to coat.
7. Then place the salad into the refrigerator and chill for 2 hours.
8. Serve straightaway.

Nutrition:
Calories: 100, Fat: 4, Fiber: 9.7, Carbs: 16.3, Protein: 2.7

Baked green bean fries

Prep Time + Cook Time: 25 minutes Serves: 6

Ingredients:
- Green beans- 1½ Ib.
- Grated Parmesan- ½ cup
- Coconut flour- ½ cup
- Whisked eggs- 2
- Olive oil
- Black pepper and salt

Directions:
1. Mix salt, pepper, and Parmesan together in a bowl.
2. Dunk the beans in the flour and then in the eggs, then coat it with the Parmesan mix.
3. Lay the coated beans on a baking sheet drizzled with oil.
4. Bake in the oven for 15 minutes at 425°F.

Nutrition:
Calories 188, carbs 14, protein 5, fiber 6, fats 2

Baked Parmesan Egg plant and Tomatoes

Prep Time + Cook Time: 45 minutes Servings: 4

Ingredients:
- Medium tomato, sliced: 1
- Medium eggplant, sliced into thin rounds: 1
- Salt: to taste
- Ground black pepper: to taste
- Grated Parmesan cheese: ¼ cup
- Olive oil: 1 tbsp.

Directions:
1. Set oven to 400 0F and let preheat.

2. In the meantime, take a lined baking dish, line it with some eggplant slices in a single layer and drizzle with oil.
3. Sprinkle half of the cheese on top, then top with remaining eggplant slices in a single layer and then layer with tomato slices.
4. Season with salt and black pepper and sprinkle remaining cheese on tomato slices.
5. Place the baking dish into the oven and bake for 15 minutes or until cheese melts and the top is nicely golden brown.
6. Serve straightaway.

Nutrition:
Calories: 73, Fat: 4.5, Fiber: 4.5, Carbs: 7.2, Protein: 2.4

Balsamic Steak Salad

Prep Time + Cook Time: 30 minutes Serves: 4

Ingredients:
- Italian seasoning, 1 tsp.
- Balsamic vinegar, ¼ cup
- Thinly sliced steak, 1½ lb.
- Black pepper.
- Chopped lettuce head, 1.
- Chopped sweet onion, 6 oz.
- Minced garlic cloves, 2.
- Sliced yellow bell pepper, 1.
- Sliced orange bell pepper, 1.
- Salt.
- Pitted and sliced avocado, 1.
- Chopped sun-dried tomatoes, 3 oz.
- Onion powder, 1 tsp.
- Sliced mushrooms, 4 oz.
- Red pepper flakes, 1 tsp.
- Avocado oil, 3 tbsps.

Directions:
1. Combine steak pieces with seasonings and balsamic vinegar to coat evenly then reserve.
2. Set the pan on fire to melt the avocado oil over medium-low heat to cook garlic, mushrooms, onion, salt, and pepper for 20 minutes.
3. Meanwhile, combine lettuce leaves with yellow bell pepper, orange, sun dried tomatoes and avocado in a mixing bowl.
4. Rub the steak pieces with pepper flakes, onion powder, and Italian seasoning then set on a broiling pan.
5. Preheat the broiler then cook the steak for 5 minutes
6. Set the steaks on plate with lettuce and avocado salad on the side topped with onion and mushroom mix.

Nutrition :
calories: 435, fat: 23, fiber: 7, carbs: 10, protein: 35

Bisque of Lobster

Prep Time + Cook Time: 1 hour 14 minutes Servings: 5

Ingredients:

- Lobster chunks-24 ounces (pre-cooked)
- Tomato paste-1/2 cup
- Garlic cloves-4 (minced)
- Red onion-1 small (chopped)
- Thyme-1 tsp. (dried)
- Peppercorns-1 tsp.
- Paprika-1 tsp.
- Xanthan gum-1 tsp.
- Carrots-2 (finely chopped)
- Celery stalks-4 (chopped)
- Seafood stock-1 quart
- Olive oil-1 tbsp.
- Heavy cream-1 cup
- Bay leaves-3
- Parsley-A handful (chopped)
- Lemon juice-1 tbsp.
- Salt and black pepper-To taste

Directions:

1. Take a pot. Fill it with the oil.
2. Put it over medium heat.
3. Add onion and stir.
4. Then prepare and cook for 4 minutes.
5. Add garlic and stir again.
6. Cook for another minute.
7. Add celery and carrot.
8. Stir and cook for 1 minute.
9. Combine tomato paste and stock and stir everything.
10. Mix the bay leaves, salt, pepper, peppercorns, paprika, thyme and xanthan gum.
11. Stir and simmer over medium heat for 1 hour.
12. Discard the bay leaves and add cream.
13. Bring it to a simmer.
14. Then, again blend using an immersion blender.
15. Shake and toss the lobster chunks.
16. Fry for a few more minutes.
17. Put in the lemon juice.
18. Stir and distribute them into bowls.
19. Finally sprinkle the parsley on top.

Nutrition :

Calories:- 200; Fat : 12; Fiber : 7; Carbs : 6; Protein : 12

Broccoli with Parmesan Cheese

Prep Time + Cook Time: 27 minutes Servings: 4

Ingredients:

- Broccoli florets: 1 pound
- Minced garlic: ½ tbsp.
- Salt: to taste
- Ground black pepper: to taste
- Olive oil: 5 tbsps.
- Grated parmesan cheese: 1 tbsp.

Directions:

1. Place a medium saucepan half full with water over medium-high heat, stir in salt and bring to boil.
2. Add broccoli florets, cook for 5 minutes and then drain into a

colander, set aside in a bowl until required.

3. Place a skillet pan over medium-high heat, add oil and when hot, add garlic and cook for 2 minutes or until fragrant.

4. Then add broccoli, stir well and cook for 15 minutes.

5. Remove pan from heat, sprinkle cheese on florets and divide evenly between serving plate.

6. Serve straightaway.

Nutrition:
Calories: 195, Fat: 18.2, Fiber: 3, Carbs: 7.8, Protein: 3.8

Butternut Squash and Zucchini Indian Salad

Prep Time + Cook Time: 1 hour and 5 minutes Servings: 6

Ingredients:
- Butternut squash, peeled and grated: 7 ounce
- Zucchini, sliced thin: 2
- Bunch of radishes, finely sliced: 1
- Medium white onion, peeled and chopped: ½
- Mint leaves, chopped: 6

For the salad dressing:
- Mustard: 1 tsp.
- Homemade mayo: 1 tbsp.
- Balsamic vinegar: 1 tbsp.
- Olive oil: 2 tbsps.
- Salt: to taste
- Ground black pepper: to taste

Directions:

1. Whisk together salt, black pepper, vinegar, mayonnaise and mustard in a bowl and stir well and then slowly whisk in oil.

2. Place squash in a salad bowl, add remaining ingredients and toss until mixed.

3. Drizzle with salad dressing, toss until evenly coated and then place in refrigerator until chilled.

4. Serve straightaway.

Nutrition:
Calories: 71, Fat: 4.8, Fiber: 1.8, Carbs: 7.3, Protein: 1.3

Buttery Grilled Onions

Prep Time + Cook Time: 1 hour and 10 minutes Servings: 8

Ingredients:
- White onions: 4
- Salt: to taste
- Ground black pepper: to taste
- Unsalted butter: ½ cup
- Chicken bouillon cubes: 4

Direction:

1. Peel onion, then cut their tops, create a hole in the middle.

2. Stuff the hole evenly with butter and chicken bouillon and then season with salt and black pepper.
3. Wrap the stuffed onion in aluminum foil.
4. Set a kitchen grill, let preheat, then add wrapped onions and grill for 1 hour.
5. When done, uncover onions, then chop into bite-size pieces and serve.

Nutrition:
Calories: 256, Fat: 23.5, Fiber: 2.4, Carbs: 11.1, Protein: 2

Cajun Spaghetti Squash Pasta

Prep Time + Cook Time: 50 minutes Servings: 4

Ingredients:

- Spaghetti squash: 1
- Salt: to taste
- Ground black pepper: to taste
- Cajun seasoning: 1 tsp.
- Cayenne pepper: 1/8 tsp.
- Unsalted butter: 2 tbsps.
- Heavy cream: 2 cups

Directions:

1. Set oven to 350 0F and let preheat.
2. Use a form to prick squash and spread in a single layer on a baking sheet lined with parchment sheet.
3. Place the baking sheet into the oven and bake for 15 minutes.
4. When done, remove baking sheet from the oven and let butternut squash cool for 15 minutes.
5. Then cut butternut squash into half and scoop out its flesh.
6. Place a medium skillet pan over medium heat, add butter and when it melts, add squash and cook for 3 minutes.
7. Season with salt and black pepper, add cayenne pepper and Cajun seasoning, stir well and cook for another minute.
8. Add heavy cream, stir well and cook for 10 minutes.
9. When done, evenly divide squash between serving plates and serve.

Nutrition:
Calories: 289, Fat: 28.5, Fiber: 0, Carbs: 8.7, Protein: 1.9

Cauliflower and Hazelnuts Polenta

Prep Time + Cook Time: 1 hour and 10 minutes Servings: 2

Ingredients:

- Medium cauliflower head, separated into florets and chopped: 1
- Medium white onion, peeled and chopped: 1
- Shiitake mushrooms, chopped: 3 cups
- Hazelnuts: ¼ cup
- Olive oil: 1 tbsp. and 2 tsps.
- Minced garlic: 2 tsps.
- Nutritional yeast: 3 tbsps.

- Water: ½ cup
- Parsley, chopped: 1 tbsp.

Directions:

1. Set oven to 350 0F and let preheat.
2. Then spread nuts on a baking sheet lined with parchment sheet and place into the oven to bake for 10 minutes.
3. When done, remove baking sheet from the oven, let cool completely and chop.
4. Spread cauliflower florets on the baking sheet in a single layer, drizzle with 1 tsp. oil and place it into the oven.
5. Bake cauliflower for 30 minutes at 400 0F and then transfer into a bowl.
6. In the meantime, place onions in a bowl and drizzle with ½ tsp. oil and toss until coated.
7. Place garlic cloves on a piece of aluminum foil, drizzle ½ tsp. oil and wrap it.
8. When cauliflower florets baking time is over, spread onions next to them, add garlic and bake for 20 minutes.
9. Meanwhile, place a skillet pan over medium-high heat, add remaining oil and when hot, add mushrooms and cook for 8 minutes.
10. When cauliflower is done, transfer them into a food processor along with onion, season with salt and black pepper and add yeast.
11. Unwrap garlic, peel the cloves, then add to food processor and pulse for 1 to 2 minutes or until blended.
12. Divide polenta evenly between serving plates, top with cooked mushrooms and nuts, garnish with parsley and serve.

Nutrition:
Calories: 534, Fat: 35.2, Fiber: 13.9, Carbs: 52.6, Protein: 15.3

Cauliflower rice with hot dogs

Prep Time + Cook Time: 25 minutes Serves: 4

Ingredients:
- Steamed cauliflower rice- 2½ cups
- Scallions: sliced- 2
- Minced garlic clove- 1
- Hot dogs: sliced- 2
- Melted ghee- 1 tbsp.
- Avocado oil- 1 tbsp.
- Chopped yellow onion- 1
- Coconut aminos- 2 tbsp.
- Eggs: whisked- 2

Directions

1. Dissolve ghee in a pan on medium heat.
2. Mix in hot dogs, garlic and onions and let it cook for 5 minutes covered.
3. Mix in the avocado oil and cauliflower rice and let it cook for another 5 minutes.
4. Mix in the eggs and fold everything with each other. Let it

cook for another 5 minutes until the eggs are scrambled.

5. Add the scallions and the aminos and mix well.

6. Serve.

Nutrition:

Calories- 200, carbs- 13, protein- 8, fiber-5, fats- 3

Cauliflower, Avocado and Spinach Dip with Sour Cream

Prep Time + Cook Time: 25 minutes Servings: 6

Ingredients:

- Avocado, pitted and peeled: 1
- Spinach leaves: 1 cup
- Cauliflower florets: 3 cups
- Salt: to taste
- Ground black pepper: to taste
- Cream: ¼ cup
- Unsalted butter: 4 tbsps.
- Sour cream: ½ cup

Directions:

1. Place spinach and florets in a heatproof bowl, then place it into the microwave and cook for 15 minutes.

2. In the meantime, place the avocado in a bowl and mash with a fork.

3. Then add it to cooked spinach mixture, season with salt and black pepper and toss until mixed.

4. Add butter, cream and sour cream and blend using an immersion blender until smooth.

5. Serve straightaway.

Nutrition:

Calories: 197, Fat: 18.9, Fiber: 3.6, Carbs: 6.9, Protein: 2.5

Cheesy asparagus

Prep Time + Cook Time: 40 minutes Serves: 6

Ingredients:

- Trimmed asparagus- 2 Ib.
- Minced garlic cloves- 3
- Grated parmesan- 1 cup
- Shredded mozzarella- 1 cup
- Coconut cream- ¾ cup
- Salt
- Black pepper

Directions:

1. Mix asparagus with cream, mozzarella, garlic, salt, and

pepper in a baking tray and sprinkle with parmesan.

2. Bake in the oven for 30 minutes at 400°F.

3. Serve.

Nutrition:

Calories- 200, carbs- 12, protein- 9, fiber- 6, fats- 3

Cheesy creamy garlic mushrooms

Prep Time + Cook Time: 25 minutes Serves: 4

Ingredients:

- Sliced mushrooms- 15 oz.
- Melted ghee- 2 tbsp.
- Coconut cream- ⅓ cup
- Minced garlic cloves- 3
- Grated Parmesan: 2 tbsp.
- Chopped parsley- 2 tbsp.
- Dried oregano- ½ tsp.

Directions:

1. Dissolve ghee on a pan on medium heat and mix in the garlic
2. Let it fry for 2 minutes and add the mushrooms, salt, pepper, and oregano.
3. Cook for 10 minutes.
4. Add in the parmesan and the parsley. Cook for 3 minutes and remove.

Nutrition:

Calories 212, carbs 14, protein 9, fiber 7, fats 4

Cheesy Twice-Baked Stuffed Zucchini

Prep Time + Cook Time: 40 minutes Servings: 4

Ingredients:

- Zucchinis, cut into half and each half in half lengthwise: 2
- White onion, peeled and chopped: ¼ cup
- Shredded cheddar cheese: ½ cup
- Bacon strips, cooked and crumbled: 4
- Sour cream: ¼ cup
- Cream cheese, softened: 2 ounces
- Jalapeno pepper, chopped: 1 tbsp.
- Salt: to taste
- Ground black pepper: to taste
- Unsalted butter: 2 tbsps.

Directions:

1. Set oven to 350 0F and let preheat.
2. In the meantime, use a spoon to scoop zucchini, then place its flesh in a bowl and place its cups in a baking sheet.
3. Add remaining ingredients, stir until combined and fill zucchini cups with this mixture.
4. Place the baking sheet into the oven and bake for 30 minutes.
5. Serve straightaway.

Nutrition:

Calories: 237, Fat: 21.3, Fiber: 1.2, Carbs: 5.1, Protein: 7.6

Cheesy zucchini with parsley

Prep Time + Cook Time: 25 minutes Serves: 4

Ingredients:

- Zucchini: quartered lengthwise- 4
- Parmesan: grated- ½ cup
- Dried thyme- ½ tsp.
- Dried basil- ½ tsp.
- Garlic powder- ¼ tsp.
- Dried oregano- ½ tsp.
- Chopped parsley 2 tbsp.
- Olive oil- 2 tbsp.
- Cooking spray
- Salt
- Black pepper

Directions:

1. Spray the baking sheet with a cooking spray and lay the zucchini on it.
2. Season with thyme, oil, salt, pepper, garlic powder, basil, parsley, parmesan, and oregano.
3. Bake in the oven for 15 minutes at 350°F.

Nutrition:

Calories 200, carbs 11, protein 7, fiber 4, fats 2

Coco Keto Soup

Prep Time + Cook Time: 47 minutes Servings: 3

Ingredients:

- Chicken stock-4 cups
- Lime leaves-3
- Coconut milk-1-1/2 cups
- Shrimp-4 ounces (raw, peeled and de veined)
- Red onion-2 tbsps. (chopped)
- Coconut oil-1 tbsp.
- Mushrooms-2 tbsp. (chopped)
- Lemongrass-1 tsp. (dried)
- Cilantro-1 cup (chopped)
- Ginger-1 inch piece (grated)
- Fish sauce-1 tbsp.
- Cilantro-1 tbsp. (chopped)
- Lime-1 (Juiced)
- Thai chilies-4 (dried and chopped)
- Salt and black pepper-To taste

Directions:

1. Take a pot.
2. Mix chicken stock with coconut milk, lime leaves, lemongrass, Thai chilies, a cup of cilantro, ginger, salt and pepper.
3. Stir and bring it to a simmer over medium heat.
4. Cook it for 20 minutes.
5. Drain and return to pot.
6. Make the soup warm again over the medium heat.
7. Combine the coconut oil, shrimp, fish sauce, mushrooms and onions.
8. Add and cook for 10 minutes more.
9. Put in the lime juice and a tbsp. of cilantro.
10. Whisk and ladle into bowls to serve for lunch!

Nutrition :

Calories:- 450; Fat : 34; Fiber : 4; Carbs : 8; Protein : 12

Coco Meal Soup

Prep Time + Cook Time: 42 minutes Servings: 5

Ingredients:

- Halibut-1 pound (cut into medium chunks)
- Carrots-1 pound (sliced)
- Coconut oil-1 tbsp.
- Ginger-2 tbsps. (minced)
- Chicken stock-12 cups
- Yellow onion-1 (chopped)
- Water-1 cup
- Salt and black pepper-To taste

Directions:

1. Take a pot and heat up with the oil over medium heat.
2. Stir in the onion and stir again.
3. Cook for 6 minutes.
4. Coat ginger, carrots, water and stock.
5. Toss in to bring it to a simmer.
6. Slow down the temperature and cook for 20 minutes.
7. Blend soup using an immersion blender.
8. Then season with salt and pepper.
9. Add all the halibut pieces.
10. Stir gently.
11. Let it simmer as soup for 5 more minutes.
12. Divide into bowls.
13. Serve.

Nutrition :

Calories:- 140; Fat : 6; Fiber : 1; Carbs : 4; Protein : 14

Coconut Cauliflower Rice

Prep Time + Cook Time: 40 minutesServes: 4

Ingredients:

- Toasted coconut shreds, 2 tbsps.
- Black pepper
- Coconut milk, 10 oz.
- Cauliflower head, 1
- Water, ½ cup
- Salt
- Ginger slices, 2

Directions:

1. Take your blender and add in the cauliflower to process
2. Press the cauliflower rice in a clean kitchen towel and reserve
3. Over medium heat, warm the coconut milk in a pot
4. Mix in ginger and water as you stir gently.
5. Allow cooking for 30 minutes
6. Remove the ginger the season and top the coconut shreds.
7. Give it a gentle stir and enjoy

Nutrition:

Calories: 223, Fat: 19.5, Fiber: 3.8, Carbs: 12.4, Protein: 3.4

Creamy Broccoli with Lemon and Almonds

Prep Time + Cook Time: 20 minutes Servings: 4

Ingredients:

- Medium broccoli head, separated into florets: 1
- Salt: to taste
- Ground black pepper: to taste
- Almonds, blanched: ¼ cup
- Lemon zest: 1 tsp.
- Coconut butter, melted: ¼ cup
- Lemon juice: 2 tbsps.

Directions:

1. Place a medium saucepan half full with water over medium-high heat, stir in salt and bring to boil.
2. Then place broccoli florets in a steamer, insert it into the saucepan and cover it.
3. Steam broccoli florets for 8 minutes, then remove them from the saucepan, drain thoroughly and transfer into a bowl.
4. Put water in a saucepan, add the salt, and bring to a boil over medium-high heat.
5. Place a skillet pan over medium heat, add butter and when it melts, add almonds, lemon zest and juice, and stir.
6. Remove pan from the heat, add steamed florets and toss until evenly coated with butter mixture.
7. Divide broccoli florets evenly among the plates and serve.

Nutrition:
Calories: 168, Fat: 12.4, Fiber: 6.3, Carbs: 12.6, Protein: 5.5

Creamy Cheese Sauce

Prep Time + Cook Time: 45 minutes Servings: 8

Ingredients:

- Salt: 1/8 tsp.
- Cayenne pepper: ¼ tsp.
- Sweet paprika: ½ tsp.
- Onion powder: ½ tsp.
- Garlic powder: ½ tsp.
- Unsalted butter: 2 tbsps.
- Grated cheddar cheese: ¼ cup
- Cream cheese, softened: ¼ cup
- Whipping cream: ¼ cup
- Water: 2 tbsps.
- Chopped parsley: 4 tbsps.

Directions:

1. Place a skillet pan over medium heat, add butter and when hot, add butter and when it melts, add cream and stir well.
2. Stir in cream cheese and bring the mixture to simmer.
3. Then remove the pan from heat, stir in cheddar cheese and return pan to heat to cook for 3 to 4 minutes.
4. Add remaining ingredients, stir well and remove the pan from heat.
5. Spoon sauce into a medium bowl and serve.

Nutrition:
Calories: 77, Fat: 7.8, Fiber: 0.1, Carbs: 0.5, Protein: 1.6

Creamy Coconut Cauliflower Mash

Prep Time + Cook Time: 10 minutes
Cooking time: 10 minutes Servings: 2

Ingredients:
- cauliflower head, florets separated-1
- coconut cream-1/6 cup
- coconut milk -1/6 cup
- chives, chopped - ½ tbsp
- Salt and black pepper - to taste

Directions:
1. Fill 2/3 of a cooking pot with water and let it boil over medium-high heat.
2. Add cauliflower florets then cook them for 10 minutes until al dente.
3. Drain the florets and place them in a suitable bowl.
4. Mash them using a potato masher.
5. Stir in cream, pepper, salt, coconut milk, and chives.
6. Mix well and serve.

Nutrition:
Calories: 200, Fat: 2, Fiber: 3, Carbs: 9, Protein: 5

Creamy Endive and Watercress Salad with Chives

Prep Time + Cook Time: 15 minutes Servings: 4

Ingredients:
- Watercress, chopped: 4 ounces
- Medium endives, roots, and ends cut and sliced thin crosswise: 4
- Medium shallot, peeled and diced: 1
- Salt: to taste
- Ground black pepper: to taste
- Fresh chervil, chopped: 1 tbsp.
- Fresh tarragon, chopped: 1 tbsp.
- Fresh chives, chopped: 1 tbsp.
- Almonds, chopped: ⅓ cup
- Lemon juice: 1 tbsp.
- Balsamic vinegar: 1 tbsp.
- Olive oil: 2 tbsps.
- Heavy cream: 6 tbsps.
- Fresh parsley, chopped: 1 tbsp.

Directions:
1. Place shallots in a bowl, add salt, vinegar, lemon juice, and then stir until mixed and set aside for 10 minutes.
2. Then add pepper and olive oil and set aside for 2 minutes.
3. Add remaining ingredients except for cream and vinaigrette and toss to coat.
4. Add cream and prepared shallot vinaigrette to the salad and toss to coat.
5. Top salad with almonds and serve.

Nutrition:
Calories: 204, Fat: 19.6, Fiber: 2.3, Carbs: 5.2, Protein: 3.8

Creamy Sausage Gravy

Prep Time + Cook Time: 12 minutes Servings: 4

Ingredients:

- Sausages, chopped: 4 ounces
- Salt: to taste
- Ground black pepper: to taste
- Unsalted butter: 2 tbsps.
- Guar gum: ½ tsp.
- Heavy cream: 1 cup

Directions:

1. Place a medium skillet pan over medium heat, let heat and when hot, add sausage pieces and cook for 4 minutes.
2. When done, transfer sausage pieces to a plate and set aside until required.
3. Add butter into the pan and when it melts, add remaining ingredients, and stir well.
4. Cook for 3 to 5 minutes or until sauce begins to thicken.
5. Then return sausage pieces into the pan, stir well until coated and remove the pan from heat.
6. Serve straightaway.

Nutrition:

Calories: 251, Fat: 24.9, Fiber: 0, Carbs: 0.8, Protein: 6.2

Crispy Turnip Sticks

Prep Time + Cook Time: 35 minutes Servings: 4

Ingredients:

- Turnips, peeled and cut into sticks: 2 pounds
- Salt: to taste
- Olive oil: ¼ cup

For the seasoning mix:

- Onion powder: 1½ tsps.
- Garlic powder: 1 tsp.
- Red Chili powder: 2 tbsps.
- Dried oregano: ½ tsp.
- Cumin: 1½ tbsps.

Directions:

1. Set oven to 350 0F and let preheat.
2. Mix onion powder, garlic powder, red chili powder, cumin and oregano in a shallow dish until combined.
3. Add parsnip stick, toss until evenly coated and place on a baking sheet lined with parchment sheet.
4. Place the baking sheet into the oven and bake parsnip for 25 minutes until nicely golden brown.
5. When done, let fries cool for 5 minutes and then serve.

Nutrition:

Calories: 230, Fat: 15.1, Fiber: 6.2, Carbs: 23.9, Protein: 4.3

Curried Zucchini Noodles Soup

Prep Time + Cook Time: 25 minutes Serves: 8

Ingredients:

- Minced garlic cloves, 2.
- Sliced red bell pepper, 1.
- Canned coconut milk, 15 oz.
- Curry paste, 1½ tbsps.
- Sliced zucchinis, 2.
- Chopped small yellow onion, 1.
- Fish sauce, 2 tbsps.
- Sliced chicken breasts, 1 lb.
- Chicken stock, 6 cup
- Chopped jalapeno pepper, 1.
- Coconut oil, 1 tbsp.
- Lime wedges.
- Chopped cilantro, ½ cup

Directions:

1. Set the pot on fire with oil to cook onions for 5 minutes over medium heat stirring gently.

2. Stir in curry paste, garlic, and jalapeno to cook for 1 minute

3. Mix in coconut milk and stock to boil for a few minutes.

4. Stir in chicken, red bell pepper, and fish sauce to simmer for 4 minutes

5. Gently stir in cilantro to cook for 1 minute then remove from heat.

6. Set zucchini noodles into soup bowls, add soup on top and serve with lime wedges on the side

Nutrition :

calories: 287, fat: 14, fiber: 2, carbs: 7, protein: 25

Fried Bacon and Swiss Chard

Prep Time + Cook Time: 8 minutes Servings: 2

Ingredients:

- Bacon slices, chopped: 4
- Swiss chard, chopped: 1 bunch
- Minced garlic: ½ tsp.
- Salt: to taste
- Ground black pepper: to taste
- Lemon juice: 3 tbsps.
- Unsalted butter: 2 tbsps.

Directions:

1. Place a skillet pan over medium heat and when hot, add bacon pieces and cook for 3 to 5 minutes or until crispy.

2. Add butter, stir well and continue cooking for 2 minutes or until it melts.

3. Stir in garlic and lemon juice and cook for 1 minute until fragrant.

4. Add chard, cook for 4 minutes and then season with salt and black pepper.

5. When done, remove the pan from heat, divide chard and bacon evenly between serving plates and serve.

Nutrition:

Calories: 317, Fat: 27.6, Fiber: 0.4, Carbs: 1.9, Protein: 14.7

Fried Mushroom and Spinach

Prep Time + Cook Time: 20 minutes Servings: 4

Ingredients:

- spinach leaves - 10 ounces, chopped
- Salt and ground black pepper, to taste
- Mushrooms - 14 ounces, chopped
- garlic cloves - 2, peeled and minced
- fresh parsley - ½ cup, chopped
- onion - 1, peeled and chopped
- olive oil - 4 tbsps.
- balsamic vinegar - 2 tbsps.

Directions:

1. Heat a pan containing oil over medium-high heat, then add garlic and onion and stir gently, and cook for about 4 minutes.
2. Pour some mushrooms into the mixture, stir gently, and cook for about 3 minutes.
3. Then pour spinach, stir gently, and cook for about 3 minutes.
4. Then add vinegar, salt, pepper, stir, and cook for about 1 minute.
5. Add parsley, stir gently, and divide on different plates.
6. Then serve.

Nutrition:

Calories: 175, Fat: 14.7, Fiber: 3.4, Carbs: 9.4, Protein: 5.8

Garlic chili with cabbage and radish

Prep Time + Cook Time: 55 minutes Serves: 6

Ingredients:

- Chopped Napa cabbage- 1 Ib.
- Chopped radish- 1 cup
- Minced garlic cloves- 3
- Veggie stock- 2 tbsp.
- Olive oil- 1 tbsp.
- Chopped green onion stalks- 3
- Coconut aminos- 1 tbsp.
- Chili flakes- 3 tbsp.
- Black pepper and salt

Directions:

1. Mix the cabbage head with pepper and salt in a bowl and let it be well seasoned for 10 minutes.
2. Set aside for 30 minutes well covered.
3. Whisk oil, chili flakes, garlic, and coconut aminos together in a bowl.
4. Pour the chili mixture into a pan over medium high and mix in the stock, radish, and cabbage.
5. Close the lid and let it cook for 15 minutes.

Nutrition:

Calories 200, carbs 15, protein 8, fiber 4, fats 3

Garlicky Brussels Sprouts with Mustard

Prep Time + Cook Time: 50 minutes Servings: 4

Ingredients:

- Brussels sprouts, trimmed, and halved: 1 pound
- Garlic bulb, cloves peeled, and separated: 1
- Salt: to taste
- Ground black pepper: to taste
- Coconut aminos: 1 tbsp.
- Dijon mustard: 1 tbsp.
- Minced garlic: 1 tbsp.
- Unsalted butter: 1 tbsp.
- Caraway seeds: 1 tbsp.

Directions:

1. Set oven to 400 0F and let preheat.
2. In the meantime, take a baking sheet lined with parchment sheet, add Brussel sprouts, season with salt and black pepper, then add remaining ingredients and toss until well coated.
3. Place the baking sheet into the oven and bake for 40 minutes or until cooked through.
4. Serve straightaway.

Nutrition:
Calories: 87, Fat: 3.7, Fiber: 5.1, Carbs: 12.3, Protein: 4.5

Green Beans And Vinaigrette Mix

Prep Time + Cook Time: 22 minutes Servings: 8

Ingredients:

- green beans - 2 pound
- chorizo - 2 ounces, chopped.
- garlic clove - 1, minced
- coconut oil - 2 tbsps.
- beef stock - 2 tbsps.
- macadamia nut oil - 4 tbsps.
- lemon juice - 1 tsp.
- smoked paprika - 2 tsps.
- coconut vinegar - 1/2 cup
- coriander - 1/4 tsp., ground
- Salt and black pepper to the taste.

Directions:

1. Mix chorizo with salt, pepper, vinegar, garlic, lemon juice, paprika and coriander in a blender and pulse well.
2. Add the stock and the macadamia nut oil to the mixture and continue to blend..
3. Add heat to a pan with the coconut oil over medium-high heat source.
4. Then add green beans and chorizo mix
5. Stir gently and cook for another 10 minutes
6. Divide into different plates and serve

Nutrition :
Calories:- 160; Fat : 12; Fiber : 4; Carbs : 6; Protein : 4

Green Beans with Mashed Avocado

Prep Time + Cook Time: 10 minutes Servings: 4

Ingredients:

- Green beans, trimmed: ⅔ pound
- Avocados, pitted and peeled: 2
- Scallions, chopped: 5
- Salt: to taste
- Ground black pepper: to taste
- Olive oil: 3 tbsps.
- Fresh cilantro, chopped: ½ cup

Directions:

1. Place a skillet pan over medium heat, add oil and when hot, add beans and cook for 4 minutes, stirring frequently.
2. Season with salt and black pepper, then remove the pan from heat and transfer beans into a bowl.
3. Place avocados in another bowl, season with salt and black pepper and mash with a fork.
4. Add onion, stir well and then top mashed avocado over beans.
5. Toss beans and avocado and serve straightaway.

Nutrition:

Calories: 325, Fat: 30.2, Fiber: 9.9, Carbs: 15.5, Protein: 3.7

Hot Green Beans: Side Dish

Prep Time + Cook Time: 20 minutes Servings: 4

Ingredients:

- green beans - 12 ounces
- garlic powder - 1/2 tsp.
- paprika - 1/4 tsp.
- parmesan - 2/3 cup, grated
- egg - 1
- Salt and black pepper to the taste.

Directions:

1. Mix parmesan with salt, pepper, garlic powder and paprika in a clean bowl; then stir.
2. Whisk the egg with salt and pepper in a bowl.
3. Mix the green beans in egg and then in parmesan mix.
4. Place the green beans on a lined baking sheet.
5. Then transfer to an oven set a temperature of 400 0F for 10 minutes
6. Serve hot as a side dish.

Nutritions:

Calories:- 114; Fat : 5; Fiber : 7; Carbs : 3; Protein : 9

Hot Special Side Dish

Prep Time + Cook Time: 4 hours 30 minutes Servings: 8

Ingredients:

- almond flour - 2 cups
- coconut flour - 1/4 cup
- whey protein powder - 2 tbsps.
- cheddar cheese - 1¼ cups, shredded
- garlic powder - 1/2 tsp.
- baking powder - 2 tsps.
- eggs - 2
- melted ghee - 1/4 cup
- water - ¾ cup

For the stuffing:

- yellow onion - 1/2 cup, chopped.
- ghee - 2 tbsps.
- red bell pepper - 1, chopped.
- whipping cream - 1/4 cup
- jalapeno pepper - 1, chopped.
- Sausage - 12 ounces, chopped.
- eggs - 2
- chicken stock - ¾ cup
- Salt and black pepper to the taste.

Directions:

1. Mix coconut flour with whey protein, almond flour, garlic powder, baking powder and 1 cup cheddar cheese in a clean bowl and stir the mixture gently.
2. Then pour some water, 2 eggs and 1/4 cup ghee and stir properly.
3. Move this to a greased baking pan, then sprinkle the remaining cheddar cheese.
4. Move to an oven set at a temperature of 325 °F and bake for about30 minutes
5. Leave the bread, and allow it to cool down for about 15 minutes and cube it.
6. Arrange the bread cubes on a lined baking sheet.
7. Then move to the oven set at 200 0F and bake for another 3 hours
8. Remove the bread cubes out of the oven and keep it away for a while.
9. Heat up a pan containing 2 tbsps. ghee over medium- high heat source; then add onion to the mixture and stir.
10. Cook this for 4 minutes
11. Then add jalapeno and red bell pepper; stir and cook for 5 minutes
12. Sprinkle some salt and pepper and stir, then move everything to a bowl.
13. Add heat to the same pan over medium-high source before adding sausage.
14. Then stir and cook for 10 minutes
15. Move to the bowl containing the veggies, and also add stock, bread and stir everything.
16. Whisk 2 eggs with some salt, pepper and whipping cream in a clean bowl.
17. Add this to sausage and bread mix; stir, move to a baking pan that has been greased.
18. Put it in an oven set at 325 0F and bake for 30 minutes
19. Serve hot as a side

Nutrition :

Calories:- 340; Fat : 4; Fiber : 6; Carbs : 3. 4; Protein : 7

Irish Side Dish with Steak

Prep Time + Cook Time: 25 minutes Servings: 6

Ingredients:

- cream - 1/4 cup
- ghee - 4 tbsps.
- spinach leaves - 1 cup
- cauliflower florets - 3 cups
- sour cream - 1/2 cup
- Avocado: 1; pitted and peeled
- Salt and black pepper to the taste.

Directions:

1. Mix spinach with cauliflower florets in heatproof bowl.
2. Then place inside the microwave and cook for 15 minutes
3. Use a fork to mash and crush the avocado and add to spinach mix.
4. Also sprinkle salt, pepper, and add cream, ghee and sour cream.
5. Blend the mixture using an immersion blender.
6. Move to plates
7. Use steak as servings.

Nutrition :

Calories:- 190; Fat : 16; Fiber : 7; Carbs : 3; Protein : 5

Italian Flavored Zucchini and Tomatoes

Prep Time + Cook Time: 15 minutes Servings: 6

Ingredients:

- Medium zucchini, sliced: 4
- Medium onion, peeled and chopped: 1
- Tomatoes, cored and chopped: ½ pound
- Salt: to taste
- Ground black pepper: to taste
- Minced garlic: ½ tsp.
- Italian seasoning: 1 tsp.

Directions:

1. Place a medium skillet pan over medium heat, add oil and when hot, add the onion.
2. Season with salt and black pepper and cook onions for 2 minutes.
3. Add zucchini and mushroom, stir well and cook for 5 minutes.
4. Then add remaining ingredients and continue cooking for 6 minutes.
5. When done, remove the pan from heat, divide vegetables evenly between serving plates and serve.

Nutrition:

Calories: 42, Fat: 0.6, Fiber: 2.6, Carbs: 8.7, Protein: 2.4

236

Keto Chowder Recipe

Prep Time + Cook Time: 4 hours 16 minutes Servings: 3

Ingredients:

- Chicken thighs-1 pound (skinless and boneless)
- Canned tomatoes-10 ounces (chopped)
- Jalapeno pepper-1 (chopped)
- Yellow onion-1 (chopped)
- Cilantro-2 tbsps. (chopped)
- Chicken stock-1 cup
- Cream cheese-8 ounces
- Lime-1 (Juiced)
- Garlic clove-1 (minced)
- Cheddar cheese-for serving (Shredded)
- Lime wedges-for serving
- Salt and black pepper-To taste

Directions:

1. Take a crock-pot.
2. Then mix chicken with tomatoes, stock, cream cheese, salt, pepper, lime juice, jalapeno, onion, garlic and cilantro.
3. Mix and cover to cook on High for 4 hours.
4. Do uncover the pot.
5. Shred the meat into the pot.
6. Divide into bowls.
7. Serve with cheddar cheese on top.
8. Present the lime wedges on the side of the dish.

Nutrition :

Calories:- 300; Fat : 5; Fiber : 6; Carbs : 3; Protein : 26

Keto Eggplant Salad with Toppings

Prep Time + Cook Time: 20 minutes Servings: 4

Ingredients:

- Eggplant - 1, sliced
- Avocado: 1; pitted and chopped.
- mustard - 1 tsp.
- balsamic vinegar - 1 tbsp.
- Zest from 1 lemon
- red onion - 1, sliced
- A drizzle of canola oil
- Some parsley sprigs, chopped for serving
- fresh oregano - 1 tbsp., chopped.
- A drizzle of olive oil
- Salt and black pepper to the taste.

Directions:

1. Drizzle canola oil on some red onion slices and eggplant ones then place them on a pre-heated grill; cook this till they get soft.
2. Move them to a cutting board, let it cool down, cut them into smaller pieces and put them in a bowl.
3. Then add avocado and stir well.
4. Stir a mixture of vinegar with mustard, oregano, olive oil in a

bowl and sprinkle a pinch of salt and pepper as seasoning.

5. Finally, you can add the mixture to the eggplant, avocado and onion mix
6. Toss to ensure it is well coated

7. Then add lemon zest and parsley on top and serve

Nutrition :

Calories:- 120; Fat : 3; Fiber : 2; Carbs : 1; Protein : 8

Keto Mushrooms: Side Dish

Prep Time + Cook Time: 40 minutes Servings: 4

Ingredients:

- baby mushrooms - 16 ounces
- onion - 3 tbsps., dried
- parsley flakes - 3 tbsps.
- garlic powder - 1 tsp.
- ghee - 4 tbsps.
- Salt and black pepper to the taste.

Directions:

1. Mix parsley flakes with onion, salt, pepper and garlic powder in a clean bowl and stir.
2. Then mix mushroom with melted ghee in another bowl and toss to coat.

3. Continue by adding seasoning mix, then toss well to keep it well coated.
4. Arrange neatly on a lined baking sheet, then place in an oven at 300 0F and bake for 30 minutes
5. Serve tasty keto roast as a side dish.

Nutrition :

Calories:- 152; Fat : 12; Fiber : 5; Carbs : 6; Protein : 4

Keto Rice Dish - Side Dish

Prep Time + Cook Time: 40 minutes Servings: 4

Ingredients:

- cauliflower head - 1, florets separated
- ginger slices - 2
- coconut milk - 10 ounces
- water - 1/2 cup
- coconut shreds - 2 tbsps., toasted
- Salt and black pepper to the taste.

Directions:

1. Transfer cauliflower into your food processor and blend.
2. Then move the cauliflower rice to a kitchen towel and press well.
3. Keep it aside for a while.
4. Place a pot containing coconut milk over medium-high heat.

5. Pour some water and ginger; stir gently and bring to a simmer.
6. Add cauliflower; stir gently and cook for another 30 minutes
7. Do away with the ginger, add salt, pepper and coconut shreds.
8. Stir gently, and divide into different plates
9. Serve as a side for a poultry based dish.

Nutrition :
Calories:- 108; Fat : 3; Fiber : 6; Carbs : 5; Protein : 9

Keto Stuffed Peppers

Prep Time + Cook Time: 50 minutes Serves: 4

Ingredients:

- Herbs de Provence, ½ tsp.
- Marinara sauce.
- Black pepper.
- Ghee, 1 tbsp.
- Chopped yellow onions, 3 tbsps.
- Chopped sweet sausage, 1 lb.
- Salt.
- Sliced big banana peppers, 4.
- Olive oil

Directions:
1. Rub the banana peppers with seasonings then drizzle the oil.
2. Set the oven for 20 minutes at 350ºF, allow them to bake
3. In the meantime, set the pan on fire to cook the sausages for 5 minutes over medium heat.
4. Stir in the herbs de Provence, onion, salt, ghee, and pepper to cook for 5 minutes
5. Remove the peppers from the oven.
6. Stuff them with the sausage mix, place them in an oven-proof dish then drizzle marinara sauce over them.
7. Put in the oven again to bake for 10 minutes

Nutrition:
calories: 320, fiber: 4, protein: 10, fat: 8, carbs: 3

Mushroom and Arugula Salad with Prosciutto

Prep Time + Cook Time: 10 minutes Servings: 4

Ingredients:

- Slices of prosciutto: 8
- Sundried tomatoes in oil, drained and chopped: 8
- Cremini mushrooms, chopped: 1 pound
- Bunches of arugula: 4
- Salt: to taste
- Ground black pepper: to taste
- Unsalted butter: 2 tbsps.
- Olive oil: 4 tbsps.
- Apple cider vinegar: 2 tbsps.
- Grated Parmesan cheese: 4 tbsps.

- Chopped parsley leaves: 2 tbsps.

Directions:

1. Place a skillet pan over medium-high heat, add butter and half of oil and when hot, add mushrooms.
2. Season mushroom with salt and black pepper and cook for 3 minutes.
3. Then reduce heat to medium-low level, stir the mushrooms and cook for another 3 minutes.
4. Add vinegar and remaining oil, stir well and cook for 1 minute, set aside.
5. Assemble salad and for this evenly divide arugula evenly between serving plates, then top with prosciutto and mushroom mixture evenly, tomatoes, adjust seasoning, sprinkle with cheese and parsley and serve.

Nutrition:
Calories: 352, Fat: 24.8, Fiber: 2.4, Carbs: 15.5, Protein: 16.3

Mushroom Salad with Parmesan

Prep Time + Cook Time: 20 minutes Servings: 4

Ingredients:

- ghee - 2 tbsps.
- cremini mushrooms - 1 pound, chopped.
- slices prosciutto - 8
- apple cider vinegar - 2 tbsps.
- sun-dried tomatoes in oil: 8; drained and chopped.
- extra virgin olive oil - 4 tbsps.
- bunches arugula - 4
- Some parmesan shavings
- Some parsley leaves, chopped.
- Salt and black pepper to the taste.

Instructions:

1. Add heat to a pan containing ghee and half of the oil over medium high heat source.
2. Then add mushrooms, salt and pepper; stir gently and cook for 3 minutes
3. Reduce the heat; and stir again. Cook for another 3 minutes.
4. Add the remaining oil and vinegar; stir and cook another minute.
5. Place arugula on a serving platter, then add prosciutto on top.
6. Also, add mushroom mix, sun-dried tomatoes, as well as more salt and pepper.
7. Finally, add parmesan shavings and parsley.
8. Now you can serve

Nutrition :
Calories:- 160; Fat : 4; Fiber : 2; Carbs : 2; Protein : 6

Mushroom, Almonds and Hemp Pilaf

Preparation and Cooking Time 35 minutes Servings: 4

Ingredients:

- Mushrooms, chopped: 3
- Hemp seeds: 1 cup
- Almonds, sliced: ¼ cup
- Garlic powder: ½ tsp.
- Salt: to taste
- Ground black pepper: to taste
- Unsalted butter: 2 tbsps.
- Chicken stock: ½ cup
- Dried parsley: ¼ tsp.

Directions:

1. Place a skillet pan over medium heat, add butter and when it melts, add almonds and mushrooms and cook for 4 minutes, stirring frequently.
2. Stir in hempseeds, season with salt and black pepper and add remaining ingredients.
3. Reduce heat to medium-low level, cover the pan and simmer for 20 to 25 minutes or until all the cooking liquid is absorbed.
4. Serve straightaway.

Nutrition:

Calories: 196, Fat: 17.4, Fiber: 1.5, Carbs: 3.3, Protein: 8.2

Okra and Tomatoes with Crispy Bacon

Prep Time + Cook Time: 20 minutes Servings: 6

Ingredients:

- canned stewed tomatoes - 14 ounces; cored and chopped
- Salt and ground black pepper, to taste
- celery stalks: 2; chopped
- onion: 1; peeled and chopped
- okra: 1 pound; trimmed and sliced
- bacon slices: 2; chopped
- small green bell peppers: 1; seeded and chopped

Directions:

1. Heat a pan over medium-high heat, add bacon, stir, brown for a few minutes
2. Move to paper towels and keep it aside for a while.
3. Heat the pan again and ensure heat source is on medium.
4. Pour okra, bell pepper, onion, and celery into the pan, stir, gently and cook for about 2 minutes.
5. Then add tomatoes, salt, and pepper; ensure it is well stirred and cook for 3 minutes.
6. Divide on different plates, and garnish with crispy bacon
7. Then serve.

Nutrition:

Calories: 91, Fat: 3, Fiber: 14, Carbs: 11.7, Protein: 4.7

Oven baked Baby Mushrooms

Prep Time + Cook Time: 40 minutes Serves: 4

Ingredients:

- Garlic powder, 1 tsp.
- Butter, 4 tbsps.
- Baby mushrooms, 16 oz.
- Salt and Black pepper
- Dried parsley, 3 tbsps.
- Dried onion flakes, 3 tbsps.

Directions:

1. Mix onion, parsley flakes, garlic powder, and pepper in a medium bowl
2. On the other hand, combine melted butter with mushrooms to coat
3. Season the mixture then arrange in a well-lined baking sheet.
4. Set the oven for 30 minutes at 300° F.
5. Allow to bake and serve hot.

Nutrition:

Calories: 139, Fat: 11.5, Fiber: 0, Carbs: 3.8, Protein: 3.9

Oven baked zucchini and cream

Prep Time + Cook Time: 30 minutes Serves: 4

Ingredients:

- Zucchini- 1½ Ib.
- Coconut cream- ¼ cup
- Chopped thyme- 1 tsp.
- Chopped shallots- 3
- Olive oil- 2 tbsp.
- Salt
- Black pepper

Directions:

1. Mix zucchini with cream, shallots, thyme, salt, oil, and pepper.
2. Bake in the oven for 20 minutes at 425°F.

Nutrition:

Calories- 199, carbs 9, protein 5, fiber 5, fats 2

Pan-fried bacon with lemony chard

Prep Time + Cook Time: 25 minutes Serves: 2

Ingredients:

- Swiss chard: roughly chopped- 1 bunch
- Chopped bacon slices- 4
- Melted ghee- 2 tbsp.
- Minced garlic cloves- 2
- Lemon juice- 3 tbsp.
- Chicken stock- ½ cup
- Black pepper and salt

Directions:

1. Dissolve the ghee in a pan over medium heat and mix in the bacon to fry for 5 minutes.
2. Mix in the chard, stock, lemon juice, garlic, pepper, and salt and let it cook for 10 minutes.

Nutrition:

Calories 200, carbs 6, protein 4, fiber 3, fats 7

Parmesan sprinkled garlic beans

Prep Time + Cook Time: 20 minutes Serves: 4

Ingredients:

- Trimmed green beans- 1½ Ib.
- Olive oil- 3 tbsp.
- Minced garlic cloves- 4
- Grated parmesan: 2 tbsp.
- Red pepper flakes- ½ tsp.

Directions:

1. Cover beans with water in a pot and simmer over medium-high for 5 minutes.
2. Remove the water and set aside in a bowl.
3. Pour oil in an over medium-high and add pepper flakes, garlic, and beans and cook for 6 minutes.
4. Serve topped with parmesan.

Nutrition:

Calories 200, carbs 11, protein 6, fiber 6, fats 3

Roast green beans with cranberries

Prep Time + Cook Time: 30 minutes Serves: 4

Ingredients:

- Halved green beans- 2 Ib.
- Dried cranberries- ¼ cup
- Chopped almonds -¼ cup
- Olive oil- 3 tbsp.
- Salt
- Black pepper

Directions:

1. Arrange the green beans on a baking sheet and sprinkle oil, salt, and pepper on it.
2. Mix and roast in the oven for 15 minutes at 425°F.
3. Stir in the almonds and cranberries and cook for 5 minutes.
4. Serve.

Nutrition:

Calories 181, carbs 10, protein 6, fiber 5, fats 3

Roasted cheesy mushrooms

Prep Time + Cook Time: 25 minutes Serves: 4

Ingredients:

- Sliced cremini mushrooms- 1½ Ib.
- Grated zest of 1 lemon
- Grated parmesan - ¼ cup
- Dried thyme- 2 tsp.
- Minced garlic cloves- 3
- Lemon juice- ¼ cup
- Olive oil- 3 tbsp.
- Salt
- Black pepper

Directions:

1. Coat the baking dish with oil and mix mushrooms with zest, juice,

Parmesan, thyme, salt, pepper, and garlic
2. Bake in the oven for 15 minutes at 375°F.

Nutrition:
Calories 199, carbs 12, protein 7, fiber 7, fats 2

Roasted Mixed Olives

Preparation and Cooking Time 40 minutes Servings: 6
Ingredients:

- Black olives, pitted: 1 cup
- Kalamata olives, pitted: 1 cup
- Green olives, stuffed with almonds and garlic: 1 cup
- Garlic cloves, peeled: 10
- Olive oil: ¼ cup
- Herbs de Provence: 1 tbsp.
- Lemon zest, grated: 1 tsp.
- Ground black pepper: to taste
- Chopped thyme, for serving: ½ tsp.

Directions:
1. Set oven to 425 °F and let preheat.
2. In the meantime, place all olives on a baking sheet lined with parchment paper, then add garlic and herbs de Provence, drizzle with oil and toss until coated.
3. Place the baking sheet into the oven and bake for 10 minutes.
4. Then add olives and continue baking for 20 minutes, stirring halfway through.
5. When done, divide olives evenly between serving plates, season with black pepper, sprinkle with lemon zest and thyme and toss until evenly coated.
6. Serve immediately.

Nutrition:
Calories: 189, Fat: 18.3, Fiber: 2.5, Carbs: 6.4, Protein: 0.5

Rolls of Sausage Pizzas

Prep Time + Cook Time: 40 minutes Serves: 6
Ingredients:

- Pizza sauce, ¼ cup
- Shredded mozzarella cheese, 2 cup
- Cooked sausage, ½ cup
- Salt.
- Pizza seasoning, 1 tsp.
- Chopped onion, 2 tbsps.
- Black pepper.
- Chopped red and green bell peppers, ¼ cup
- Chopped tomato, 1.

Directions:
1. Line a baking sheet. Grease it slightly. Over the sheet, spread mozzarella cheese and top with sprinkles of pizza seasoning. Set in an oven preheated to 400 0F and bake until done for 20 minutes.
2. Remove the pizza crust from the oven. Spread it with tomatoes,

sausage, bell peppers and onion. Top with tomato sauce drizzling.

3. Take back to the oven and bake for another 10 minutes.

4. Remove the pizza from oven and allow to cool. Slice into 6 equal parts and roll. Enjoy your lunch.

Nutrition :

calories: 117, fiber: 1, carbs: 2, fat: 7, protein: 11

Salad Bowl of Caprese With Tomato

Prep Time + Cook Time: 7 minutes Servings: 3

Ingredients:

- Mozzarella cheese-1/2 pound (sliced)
- Balsamic vinegar-1 tbsp.
- Olive oil-1 tbsp.
- Tomato-1 (sliced)
- Basil leaves-4 (torn)
- Salt and black pepper-To taste

Instructions:

1. Settle the tomato and mozzarella slices alternatively.

2. Display on 2 plates.
3. Season with the salt and pepper.
4. Drizzle the vinegar and olive oil.
5. Sprinkle the basil leaves at the end.
6. And serve.

Nutrition :

Calories:- 150; Fat : 12; Fiber : 5; Carbs : 6; Protein : 9

Sauté Cabbage with Butter

Preparation and Cooking Time 20 minutes. .Servings: 4

Ingredients:

- Green cabbage, shredded: 1½ pound
- Salt: to taste
- Ground black pepper: to taste
- Unsalted butter: 3. 5 ounces
- Sweet paprika: 1/8 tsp.

Directions:

1. Place a medium skillet pan over medium heat, add butter and when it melts, add cabbage.

2. Cook cabbage for 15 minutes, stirring often and then season with salt, black pepper, and paprika.
3. Continue cooking for 1 minute, then divide evenly between plates and serve.

Nutrition:

Calories: 805, Fat: 86.4, Fiber: 4.3, Carbs: 9.9, Protein: 3.1

Saute Edamame with Mint

Preparation and Cooking Time 10 minutes Servings: 4

Ingredients:

- Edamame: ¾ pound
- Salt: to taste
- Ground black pepper: to taste
- Mint leaves, chopped: 1 tbsp.
- Olive oil: 2 tsps.
- Green onions, chopped: 3
- Minced garlic: ½ tsp.

Directions:

1. Place a pan over medium heat, add oil and when hot, add edamame beans.

2. Season with salt and black pepper, then add remaining ingredients and stir until well mixed.
3. Cook edamame for 5 minutes until heated through, then divide evenly between serving plates and serve.

Nutrition:

Calories: 91, Fat: 3, Fiber: 4, Carbs: 11.7, Protein: 4.7

Sauteed Broccoli with Parmesan

Prep Time + Cook Time: 32 minutes Servings: 4

Ingredients:

- broccoli florets - 1 pound
- garlic clove - 1, minced
- parmesan - 1 tbsp., grated
- olive oil - 5 tbsps.
- Salt and black pepper to the taste.

Instructions:

1. Pour some water in a pot, then add a little salt and bring to a boil over medium high heat source.
2. Then add broccoli, cook for 5 minutes before removing the water.

3. Heat up a pan containing the oil over medium high heat source; then add garlic Stir and cook for about 2 more minutes
4. Add broccoli; stir and cook for another 15 minutes
5. Remove the heat; sprinkle parmesan.
6. Divide into clean plates and serve

Nutrition :

Calories:- 193; Fat : 14; Fiber : 3; Carbs : 6; Protein : 5

Sautéed Kohlrabi with Parsley

Preparation and Cooking Time 15 minutes Servings: 4

Ingredients:

- Kohlrabi, trimmed and sliced thin: 2
- Salt: to taste
- Ground black pepper: to taste
- Chopped parsley: 1 tbsp.

- Unsalted butter: 1 tbsp.
- Minced garlic: 1 tsp.

Directions:

1. Place kohlrabi in a medium saucepan, pour in enough water to cover it, then

place the pan over medium heat and bring to boil.

2. Then cook for 5 minutes, drain kohlrabi and transfer into a bowl.

3. Place a medium skillet pan over medium heat, add butter and when it melts, add garlic and cook for 1 minute or until fragrant.

4. Add kohlrabi, season with salt and black pepper and cook for 3 minutes per side or until nicely golden brown on both sides.

5. Add parsley, toss until mixed and remove pan from heat.

6. Divide kohlrabi evenly between serving plates and serve straight away.

Nutrition:
Calories: 55, Fat: 3, Fiber: 3.7, Carbs: 6.8, Protein: 1.9

Sautéed Mixed Vegetable with Pumpkin Seeds

Preparation and Cooking Time 10 minutes Servings: 4

Ingredients:
- Mushrooms, sliced: 14 ounces
- Broccoli florets: 3 ounces
- Red bell pepper, seeded and cut into strips: 3 ounces
- Spinach, torn: 3 ounces
- Garlic, minced: 2 tbsps.
- Salt: to taste
- Ground black pepper: to taste
- Red pepper flakes: 1/8 tsp.
- Olive oil: 6 tbsps.
- Pumpkin seeds: 2 tbsps.

Directions:
1. Place a skillet pan over medium-high heat, add oil and when hot, add garlic and cook for 1 minute or until fragrant.

2. Add mushrooms and cook for 3 minutes.

3. Then add broccoli florets and pepper, stir well, season with salt and black pepper, add pepper flakes and pumpkin seeds and cook for 3 minutes.

4. Add spinach, stir until just mixed, cook for 3 minutes and remove the pan from heat.

5. Serve straightaway.

Nutrition:
Calories: 271, Fat: 23.7, Fiber: 3.5, Carbs: 14.4, Protein: 6.6

Side Cauliflower Salad

Prep Time + Cook Time: 15 minutes Serves: 10

Ingredients:
- Mayonnaise. 1 c
- Salt
- Chopped hard-boiled eggs, 4
- Black pepper
- Chopped celery, 1 cup
- Cauliflower florets, 21 oz.

- Cider vinegar, 2 tbsps.
- Erythritol, 1 tsp.
- Water, 1 tbsp.
- Chopped onion, 1 cup

Directions:
1. Microwave the cauliflower florets with water in a heatproof bowl for 5 minutes
2. Set the salad in a bowl
3. Mix in the onions, celery, and eggs as you stir gently.
4. Combine salt, mayonnaise, pepper, vinegar, and erythritol in another bowl.
5. Add the mixture to the cauliflower, toss and enjoy.

Nutrition:
Calories: 139, Fat: 9.7, Fiber: 1.9, Carbs: 10.8, Protein: 3.8

Spicy Green Beans and Vinaigrette

Prep Time + Cook Time: 22 minutes Serves: 8

Ingredients:
- Minced garlic clove, 1
- Macadamia nut oil, 4 tbsps.
- Lemon juice, 1 tsp.
- Green beans, 2 lbs.
- Smoked paprika, 2 tsps.
- Salt
- Chopped chorizo, 2 oz.
- Black pepper
- Coconut oil, 2 tbsps.
- Coriander, ¼ tsp.
- Beef stock, 2 tbsps.
- Coconut vinegar, ½ cup

Directions:
1. Put lemon juice, chorizo, vinegar, pepper, paprika, garlic, and salt in a blender to pulse until smooth.
2. Mix in macadamia nut oil and stock to blend again
3. Allow the coconut oil to melt over medium heat to sauté the green beans and chorizo mixture.
4. Cook for 10 minutes as you stir gently
5. Enjoy this wonderful meal

Nutrition:
Calories: 159, Fat: 13.1, Fiber: 4.1, Carbs: 8.8, Protein: 3.9

Stuffed Sausage with Bacon Wrappings

Prep Time + Cook Time: 40 minutes Serves: 4

Ingredients:
- Onion powder
- Bacon strips, 8.
- Salt.
- Garlic powder.
- Black pepper.
- Sausages, 8.
- Sweet paprika, ½ tsp.
- Pepper jack cheese slices, 16.

Directions:

1. Ensure you have a medium high source of heat. Set a grill on it. Add sausages to cook until done all sides and set on a plate to cool.
2. Slice a pocket opening in the sausages. Each to be stuffed with 2 slices of pepper jack cheese. Apply a seasoning of onion, pepper, garlic powder, paprika and salt.
3. Each stuffed sausage should be wrapped in a bacon strip and grip using a toothpick. Set them on the baking sheet and transfer to the oven to bake at 400 °F for almost 15 minutes.
4. Serve immediately and enjoy.

Nutrition :

calories: 500, fat: 37, fiber: 12, carbs: 4, protein: 40

Tasty Lunch Pizza

Prep Time + Cook Time: 17 minutes Serves: 4

Ingredients:

- Mascarpone cheese, ¼ cup
- Clive oil, 1 tbsp.
- Shredded pizza cheese mix, 1 cup
- Ghee, 2 tbsps.
- Heavy cream, 1 tbsp.
- Lemon pepper
- Shredded mozzarella cheese, 1 cup
- Steamed broccoli florets, 1/3 cup
- Salt.
- Minced garlic, 1 tsp.
- Black pepper.
- Shaved asiago cheese

Directions:

1. Set the pan on fire to heat the oil to cook pizza mix then spread into a circle over medium heat
2. Spread the mozzarella cheese into a circle also
3. Allow everything to cook for 5 minutes and set on a plate
4. Set the pan on fire to melt the ghee for cooking lemon pepper, mascarpone cheese, cream, salt, pepper, and garlic for 5 minutes over medium heat.
5. Spread half of this mix over cheese crust.
6. Mix in broccoli florets to the pan with the remaining mascarpone mix to cook for 1 minute
7. Top the mixture on the pizza, sprinkle asiago cheese at the end and serve

Nutrition :

calories: 250, fat: 15, fiber: 1, carbs: 3, protein: 10

Turkey and Collard Greens Soup

Prep Time + Cook Time 2 hours and 30 minutes Servings: 10

Ingredients:

- Collard greens, chopped: 5 bunches
- Salt: to taste
- Ground black pepper: to taste
- Red pepper flakes: 1 tbsp.
- Chicken stock: 5 cups
- Turkey leg: 1
- Minced garlic: 2 tbsps.

- Olive oil: ¼ cup

Directions:

1. Place a large pot over medium heat, add oil and when hot, add garlic
2. Cook garlic for 1 minute, then turkey, season with salt and black pepper and then pout in stock.
3. Stir the mixture and simmer the soup for 30 minutes, covering the pot.
4. Add collard greens, stir until just mixed and cook for 45 minutes, covering the pot.
5. Then reduce heat to medium level, taste soup to adjust seasoning and continue cooking for 1 hour, covering the pot.
6. When done, take out greens from the soup using a slotted spoon, then take out the chicken and transfer to a cutting board.
7. Let the turkey cool for 10 minutes, then chop into bite size pieces and add into the soup.
8. Return greens into the soup, season with red pepper flakes and ladle evenly into serving bowls.
9. Serve immediately.

Nutrition:

Calories: 171, Fat: 10.9, Fiber: 0.8, Carbs: 2.2, Protein: 16.1

Warm Delicious Roasted Olives

Prep Time + Cook Time: 30 minutes Servings: 6

Ingredients:

- kalamata olives - 1 cup, pitted
- black olives - 1 cup, pitted
- garlic cloves - 10
- herbs de Provence - 1 tbsp.
- lemon zest - 1 tsp., grated
- green olives - 1 cup, stuffed with almonds and garlic
- olive oil - 1/4 cup
- Black pepper to the taste.
- Some chopped thyme for serving

Instructions:

1. Spread black, kalamata and green olives on a lined baking sheet neatly, and drizzle some oil on them as well as on garlic and herbs de Provence,
2. Then toss to keep it well coated.
3. Transfer into an oven set at a temperature of 425 ºF and bake for 10 minutes
4. Stir the olives and bake for 10 another minutes.
5. Cut the olives on different plates, sprinkle lemon zest, black pepper and thyme on top.
6. Toss to ensure it is coated
7. Serve warm.

Nutrition :

Calories:- 200; Fat : 20; Fiber : 4; Carbs : 3; Protein : 1

Yummy Creamy Spaghetti Pasta: Side Dish

Prep Time + Cook Time: 50 minutes Servings: 4

Ingredients:

- spaghetti squash - 1
- ghee - 2 tbsps.
- heavy cream - 2 cups
- Cajun seasoning - 1 tsp.
- A pinch of cayenne pepper
- Salt and black pepper to the taste.

Instructions:

1. Prick spaghetti with a fork, then arrange neatly on a lined baking sheet.
2. Move to an oven at 350 0F and bake for 15 minutes
3. Remove the spaghetti squash from the oven, keep it aside for a while and let it cool down. Scoop squash noodles
4. Heat up a pan containing ghee over medium heat; before adding spaghetti squash.
5. Then stir gently and cook for a couple of minutes
6. Sprinkle a pinch of salt, pepper, cayenne pepper and Cajun seasoning.
7. Then stir and cook for about a minute
8. Add heavy cream; stir, cook for 10 another 10 minutes.
9. Cut into different plates and serve as a keto side dish.

Nutrition :

Calories:- 200; Fat : 2; Fiber : 1; Carbs : 5; Protein : 8

Yummy Muffins

Prep Time + Cook Time: 55 minutes Serves: 13

Ingredients:

- Egg yolks, 6
- Coconut flour, ¾ cup
- Mushrooms, ½ lb.
- Salt.
- Ground beef, 1 lb.
- Coconut aminos, 2 tbsps.

Directions:

1. Combine egg yolks, coconut aminos and salt in a blender. Process well until the desired consistency is attained.
2. In a separate bowl, stir in salt and beef. Stir in mushroom mixture to combine.
3. Stir in coconut flour.
4. Set the mixture into 13 cupcake cups and transfer into an oven preheated at 350 ºF. bake the cups until done for 45 minutes
5. Allow to cool and enjoy your lunch

Nutritional :

calories: 160, fiber: 3, carbs: 1, fat: 10, protein: 12

Zucchini and Squash Noodles with Peppers

Preparation and Cooking Time 30 minutes Servings: 6

Ingredients:

- Medium zucchinis, cut with a spiralizer: 1 ½
- Medium summer squash, cut with a spiralizer: 1
- Butternut squash, cut with a spiralizer: 4 ounce
- Medium white onion, peeled and chopped: 4 ounces
- Mixed bell peppers, seeded and cut into thin strips: 6 ounces
- Minced garlic: 1 ½ tsp.
- Salt: to taste
- Ground black pepper: to taste
- Bacon fat: 4 tbsps.

Directions:

1. Set oven to 400 0F and let preheat.

2. In the meantime, place zucchini noodles on a baking sheet lined with parchment paper and then add onion and bell peppers.

3. Add garlic, season with salt and black pepper and toss until evenly coated.

4. Add bacon fat, toss until coated and place the baking sheet into an oven.

5. Bake for 20 minutes or until done and serve straightaway.

Nutrition:
Calories: 179, Fat: 8.6, Fiber: 3.6, Carbs: 17.9, Protein: 10

Chapter 9 Ketogenic Dessert Recipes

Almond Lime Cheesecake

Prep Time + Cook Time: 12 minutes Serves: 10

Ingredients:

- Melted butter, 2 tbsps.
- Granulated stevia, 2 tsps.
- Almond meal, 4 oz.
- Unsweetened coconut, ¼ cup

For the filling:

- Boiling water, 2 cup
- Lime juice.
- Sugar–free lime jelly, 2 sachets
- Lime zest
- Cream cheese, 1 lb.

Directions:

1. Set a small pan on fire to melt the butter over medium heat.
2. Set up a mixing bowl to combine almond meal, coconut, stevia, and butter
3. Set the mixture on a baking pan to fit well and refrigerate.
4. Heat a small pan over medium heat to melt the butter.
5. Set up a bowl of hot water and add jelly sachets to dissolve.
6. Stir cream cheese to the jelly.
7. Combine lime zest and lime juice in a blender to process.
8. Spread the mixture over the base and refrigerate the cheesecake.
9. Serve and enjoy.

Nutrition:

Calories: 253 ,Fat: 24.5 ,Fiber: 1.8 ,Carbs: 4.7 ,Protein: 6

Almond Mug Cake

Prep Time + Cook Time: 5 minutes Serves: 1

Ingredients:

- Vanilla extract, ¼ tsp.
- Egg, 1
- Stevia, 1 tsp.
- Coconut flour, 1 tbsp.
- Unsweetened cocoa powder, 1 tsp.
- Almond meal, 4 tbsps.
- Butter, 2 tbsps.
- Baking powder, ½ tsp.

Directions:

1. Set the butter in a mug to microwave until it melts.
2. Stir in the egg, coconut flour, cocoa powder, stevia, vanilla extract, and baking powder.
3. Gently stir in the almond meal to microwave for 2 minutes.
4. Serve the cake topped with berries
5. Enjoy

Nutrition:

Calories: 476 ,Fat: 41.5 ,Fiber: 10.6 ,Carbs: 18.4 , Protein: 13.8

Almond Peanut Butter and Chocolate Brownies

Prep Time + Cook Time: 40 minutes Servings: 4

Ingredients:

- Walnuts, ¼ cup
- Salt
- Baking powder, ½ tsp.
- Peanut butter, 1 tsp.
- Butter, 7 tbsps.
- Almond flour, ¼ cup
- Egg, 1
- Cocoa powder, ⅓ cup
- Erythritol, ⅓ cup
- Vanilla extract, ½ tsp.

Directions:

1. Set a pan on fire over medium heat to heat erythritol and melt 6 tbsps. of butter and then transfer to a bowl.
2. Whisk in cocoa powder, vanilla extract, and seasonings.
3. Gently mix in the egg, walnuts, almond flour, baking powder, and walnuts and set on a skillet.
4. Microwave peanut butter with 1 tbsp. of butter for a few seconds as you stir gently.
5. Sprinkle over brownie mixture in the skillet
6. Set the oven for 30 minutes at 350°F, allow to bake
7. Allow the brownies cool down before slicing.

Nutrition:

Calories: 300 ,Fat: 30.2 ,Fiber: 3.2 ,Carbs: 9.1 ,Protein: 6.4

Almond Peanut Butter Fudge

Prep Time + Cook Time: 2 hours and 12 minutes Serves: 12

Ingredients:

- Vanilla extract, ½ tsp.
- Almond milk, ¼ cup
- Coconut oil, 1 cup
- Salt
- Unsweetened peanut butter, 1 cup
- Stevia, 2 tsps.

For the topping:

- Melted coconut oil, 2 tbsps.
- Cocoa powder, ¼ cup
- Swerve, 2 tbsps.

Directions:

1. Combine 1 cup of coconut oil and peanut butter in a heatproof bowl to microwave until it melts, approximately one minute.
2. Stir in stevia, salt, and almond milk then pour into a lined loaf pan.
3. Refrigerate for 2 hours before slicing.
4. Set a mixing bowl in place to combine cocoa powder, 2 tbsps. of melted coconut oil, and swerve
5. Spread the mixture over the fudge to serve.
6. Enjoy

Nutrition:

Calories: 312 ,Fat: 31.9 ,Fiber: 1.9 ,Carbs: 6.3 ,Protein: 5.8

Baked stuffed apples

Prep Time + Cook Time: 30 minutes
Serve: 4

Ingredients:

- Goat cheese- 12 oz.
- Cinnamon powder- 1 tbsp.
- Apples: medium sized, cored, with tops cut- 4

Directions:

1. Put 3 oz. goat cheese in each apple and sprinkle the cinnamon powder over it.
2. Lay it on a baking dish and bake in the oven for 20 minutes at 375°F.
3. Serve.

Nutrition:

Calories 200, carbs 6, protein 10, fiber 4, fat 3

Cheesy Berry Mousse

Prep Time + Cook Time: 10 minutes Servings: 12

Ingredients:

- Vanilla extract, ½ tsp.
- Strawberries, ½ pint
- Stevia, ¾ tsp.
- Blueberries, ½ pint
- Mascarpone cheese, 8 oz.
- Whipping cream, 1 cup

Directions:

1. Set up a bowl in place to combine mascarpone, stevia and whipping cream using a mixer
2. Align strawberry and blueberry layers in 12 glasses topped with cream.
3. Serve cold
4. Enjoy.

Nutrition:

Calories: 77 ,Fat: 5.6 ,Fiber: 0.7 ,Carbs: 2.8 ,Protein: 4.6

Cheesy Caramel Custard

Prep Time + Cook Time: 40 minutes Serves: 2

Ingredients:

- Eggs, 2
- Water, 1 cup
- Cream cheese, 2 oz.
- Caramel extract, 1½ tsps.
- Swerve, 1½ tbsps.

For the caramel sauce:

- Caramel extract, ¼ tsp.
- Butter, 2 tbsps.
- Swerve, 2 tbsps.

Directions:

1. Combine 1½ tbsps. swerve, cream cheese, eggs, water, and 1 ½ tsps.

caramel extract in a blender to process till done.

2. Transfer the mixture into 2 greased ramekins.
3. Set the oven for 30 minutes at 350°F, allow to bake.
4. Melt the butter in a saucepan over medium heat.
5. Stir in 2 tbsps. swerve and ¼ tsp. caramel extract to cook until melted.
6. Pour the mixture over caramel custard to cool.
7. Serve and enjoy.

Nutrition:
Calories: 372 ,Fat: 31 ,Fiber: 0.1 ,Carbs: 11.3 ,Protein: 8.9

Chocolate Flavored Biscotti

Prep Time + Cook Time: 22 minutes Serves: 8

Ingredients:
- Egg, 1
- Salt
- Chia seeds, 2 tbsps.
- Stevia, 2 tbsps.
- Baking soda, 1 tsp.
- Coconut oil, ¼ cup
- Shredded coconut, ¼ cup
- Almonds, 2 cup
- Cocoa powder, ¼ cup

Directions:
1. Combine almonds and chia seeds in a food processor to blend until done.
2. Mix in coconut oil, coconut, salt, egg, cocoa powder, stevia, and baking soda, blend again.
3. Mold the dough into 8 biscotti pieces and place on a lined baking sheet
4. Set the oven for 12 minutes at 350°F, allow to bake
5. Serve warm or cold.

Nutrition:
Calories: 236 ,Fat: 21.5 ,Fiber: 5.2 ,Carbs: 8.5 ,Protein: 6.9

Cocoa banana buns

Prep Time + Cook Time: 40 minutes Serves: 6

Ingredients:
- Eggs: whisked- 3
- Stevia- 2 tbsp.
- Vanilla extract- 2 tsp.
- Cocoa powder- ½ cup
- Almond butter- 1 cup
- Banana: chopped- 1

Directions:
1. Combine all the ingredients in a bowl and pour the batter into muffin cups.
2. Bake in an oven for 30 minutes at 375°F.
3. Let it cool and serve.

Nutrition:
Calories:141, carbs 14, protein 10, fiber 3, fat 11

Cocoa Brownies

Prep Time + Cook Time: 30 minutes Serves: 12

Ingredients:

- Cream cheese, 4 oz.
- Vanilla extract, 2 tsps.
- Baking powder, ½ tsp.
- 6 eggs
- Cocoa powder, 3 oz.
- Melted coconut oil, 6 oz.
- Swerve, 5 tbsps.

Directions:

1. Set up a blender to process the coconut oil, eggs, cocoa powder, cream cheese, swerve and vanilla extract.
2. Gently stir using a mixer.
3. Set the mixture into a lined baking tray.
4. Set an oven at for 20 minutes at 350°F, allow to bake.
5. Let the brownies cool before slicing for serving.
6. Enjoy.

Nutrition:

Calories: 202 ,Fat: 20.6 ,Fiber: 2.1 ,Carbs: 4.3 ,Protein: 4.8

Cocoa Walnut Spread

Prep Time + Cook Time: 10 minutes Serves: 6

Ingredients:

- Stevia, 4 tbsps.
- Cocoa powder, 4 tbsps.
- Vanilla extract, 1 tsp.
- Coconut oil, 2 oz.
- Halved walnuts, 1 cup

Directions:

1. Set the food processor in place to blend cocoa powder, stevia, oil, vanilla extract, and walnuts evenly.
2. Refrigerate for a few hours and serve.

Nutrition:

Calories: 220 ,Fat: 22.2 ,Fiber: 2.5 ,Carbs: 4.1 ,Protein: 5.7

Coconut Almond Bars

Prep Time + Cook Time: 2 hours 2 minutes Serves: 12

Ingredients:

- Melted coconut oil, 2 tbsps.
- Almond butter, 1¾ cup
- Shredded coconut, ¾ cup
- Chopped dark chocolate, 4 oz.
- Stevia, ¾ cup

Directions:

1. Combine stevia, almond flour, and coconut in a medium mixing bowl

2. Set the pan with 1 cup of almond butter and coconut oil over medium-low heat and whisk well
3. Stir the mixture to the almond flour
4. Set the mixture on the baking tray and press
5. Set up another pan over medium-high heat to whisk together chocolate and the remaining almond butter
6. Pour the mixture on top of almond mix to spread evenly
7. Allow to refrigerate for 2 hours then divide into 12 bars
8. Enjoy this awesome snack

Nutrition:
Calories: 160, Fat: 2, Fiber: 3, Carbs: 8, Protein: 4

Coconut avocado blend with coconut butter

Prep Time + Cook Time: 5 minutes Serves: 4
Ingredients:
- Coconut butter 1 tbsp.
- Chopped avocado- 1 ½ cups
- Coconut water- ½ cup
- Lime zest- 2 tsp.
- Green tea powder- 2 tbsp.
- Stevia- 1 tbsp.

Directions:
1. Blend all the ingredients in a food processor until smooth.
2. Serve topped with peanut butter.

Nutrition:
Calories:187, carbs 10, protein 7, fiber 8, fats 7

Coconut Avocado Pudding

Prep Time + Cook Time: 10 minutes Serves: 8
Ingredients:
- Lime juice, 1 tbsp.
- Chopped avocados, 2
- Canned coconut milk, 14 oz.
- Stevia, 80 drops
- Vanilla extract, 2 tsps.

Directions:
1. Plug and switch on the blender to process coconut milk, avocado, stevia, vanilla extract, and lime juice until done
2. Set the mixture into dessert bowls to refrigerate until ready to use.
3. Enjoy

Nutrition:
Calories: 221 ,Fat: 21.3 ,Fiber: 4.5 ,Carbs: 7.8 ,Protein: 2.1

Chocolate pudding

Prep Time + Cook Time: 1 hour 10 minutes Serves: 4

Ingredients:

- Melted coconut oil -1 oz.
- Shredded coconut- 1 tbsp.
- Melted dark chocolate- 11 oz.
- Coconut cream- ½ cup
- Grated lemon zest- 1 tbsp.

Directions:

1. Mix the oil, cream, zest, chocolate, and the coconut in a bowl.
2. Separate the pudding mix into cups and cool in the fridge for 1 hour.

Nutrition: Calories 173, carbs 2, protein 3, fiber 3, fat 12

Coconut Chocolate Cups

Prep Time + Cook Time: 35 minutes Serves: 20

Ingredients:

- Swerve, 3 tbsps.
- Shredded coconut, ½ cup
- Cocoa butter, 1. 5 oz.
- Coconut butter, ½ cup
- Vanilla extract, ¼ tsp.
- Coconut oil, ½ cup
- Unsweetened chocolate, 1 oz.
- Cocoa powder, ¼ cup
- Swerve, ¼ cup

Directions:

1. Set a pan on fire to melt coconut oil and coconut butter over medium heat
2. Stir in 3 tbsps. of swerve and coconut then remove from heat.
3. Set the mixture into lined muffins pan and refrigerate for 30 minutes.
4. Set a mixing bowl in place to combine chocolate, vanilla extract, ¼ cup swerve.
5. Set the mixture over a bowl with boiling water stirring occasionally.
6. Spread the mixture over coconut cupcakes then chill for 15 minutes before serving.

Nutrition:

Calories: 201 ,Fat: 21.2 ,Fiber: 1.8 ,Carbs: 4.2 ,Protein: 0.9

Coconut Cookie Balls

Prep Time + Cook Time: 10 minutes Serves: 10

Ingredients:

- Stevia, 15 drops
- Coconut milk, 3 tbsps.
- Coconut sugar, 3 tbsps.
- Ground cinnamon powder, 1 tsp.
- Salt
- Almond butter, ½ cup

- Coconut flour, 3 tbsps.
- Vanilla extract, 1 tsp.

For the topping:
- Granulated swerve, 3 tsps.
- Ground cinnamon, 1½ tsps.

Directions:
1. Set up a mixing bowl to stir together coconut milk, coconut sugar, stevia, vanilla extract, 1 tsp. ground cinnamon and seasonings.
2. Mold balls out of the mixture.
3. Set up a mixing bowl to stir together swerve with 1 ½ tsp. cinnamon.
4. Roll the balls in cinnamon mixture then refrigerate until serving time.
5. Serve and enjoy.

Nutrition:
Calories: 35 ,Fat: 2 ,Fiber: 2.1 ,Carbs: 3.9 ,Protein: 0.9

Creamy Blueberry Scones

Prep Time + Cook Time: 20 minutes Serves: 10

Ingredients:
- Eggs, 2
- Heavy cream, ½ cup
- Butter, ½ cup
- Stevia, 5 tbsps.
- Blueberries, 1 cup
- Coconut flour, ½ cup
- Almond flour, ½ cup
- Salt
- Vanilla extract, 2 tsps.
- Baking powder, 2 tsps.

Directions:
1. Combine salt, almond flour, baking powder, coconut flour, and blueberries in a bowl.
2. Set another bowl in place to combine butter, heavy cream, eggs, butter, vanilla extract, and stevia.
3. Stir the two mixtures together to have a firm dough
4. Mold the mixture into 10 triangles and arrange on a lined baking pan.
5. Set the oven for 10 minutes at 350°F, allow to bake.
6. Serve when cooled.

Nutrition:
Calories: 199 ,Fat: 16.1 ,Fiber: 5.2 ,Carbs: 10.6 ,Protein: 4

Creamy Peach Cake

Prep Time + Cook Time: 30 minutes Serves: 12

Ingredients:
- Swerve, 4 tbsps.
- Orange zest, 2 tbsps.
- Cream cheese, 4 oz.
- Coconut yogurt, 4 oz.
- Vanilla extract, 1 tsp.
- Almond meal, 9 oz.
- Salt
- Eggs, 6

- Baking powder, 1 tsp.
- Stevia, 2 oz.

Directions:
1. Set the peaches in the blender to process well.
2. Mix in the eggs, almond meal, vanilla extract, swerve, baking powder, and salt. Blend again.
3. Set the mixture into 2 spring form pans
4. Set the oven for 20 minutes at 350°F, allow to bake

5. Combine cream cheese with orange zest, stevia, and coconut yogurt in a mixing bowl.
6. Set one cake layer on a plate followed by half of the cream cheese mixture, then the other cake layer topped with the remaining cream cheese mixture.
7. Spread it well, slice, and serve.

Nutrition:
Calories: 207 ,Fat: 16.5 ,Fiber: 3.1 ,Carbs: 8.6 ,Protein: 8.7

Creamy Ricotta Mousse

Prep Time + Cook Time: 2 hours and 10 minutes Serves: 10

Ingredients:
- Espresso powder, 1 tsp.
- Whipping cream, 1 cup
- Vanilla extract, 1½ tsp.
- Hot coffee, ½ cup
- Ricotta cheese, 2 cup
- Salt
- Gelatin, 2½ tsps.
- Stevia, 1 tsp.

Directions:
1. Set up a mixing bowl to combine gelatin and coffee.
2. Reserve the coffee mixture aside to cool.

3. Set up a mixing bowl to stir in stevia, espresso, vanilla extract, ricotta and salt using a mixer.
4. Stir in the coffee mixture.
5. Mix in whipping cream to combine evenly.
6. Set the mixture into dessert bowls and refrigerate for 2 hours before serving.
7. Serve and enjoy.

Nutrition:
Calories: 110 ,Fat: 7.6 ,Fiber: 0 ,Carbs: 3.2 ,Protein: 5.9

Lemon Flavored Mousse

Prep Time + Cook Time: 10 minutes Serves: 5

Ingredients:
- Heavy cream, 1 cup
- Salt
- Lemon juice, ½ cup

- Mascarpone cheese, 8 oz.
- Stevia, 1 tsp.

Directions:

1. Set a mixing bowl in place to stir together mascarpone, heavy cream, and lemon juice using a mixer
2. Mix in the seasonings and stevia.

3. Set into dessert glasses to refrigerate until serving time.

Nutrition:
Calories: 168 ,Fat: 15, ,Fiber: 0.1 ,Carbs: 2.6 ,Protein: 5.8

Lemon rhubarb sauce

Prep Time + Cook Time: 20 minutes Serves: 10
Ingredients:

- Stevia- 1/5 cup
- Vanilla extract- 1 tsp.
- Rhubarbs: cut into medium pieces- 4½ cups
- Lemon: juiced
- Lemon zest- 1 tsp.

Directions:

1. Mix all the ingredients in a pan and cook for 10 minutes.
2. Share into bowls and serve.

Nutrition:
Calories 108, carbs 8, protein 2, fiber 2, fat 1

Lemony cherry jelly

Prep Time + Cook Time: 40 minutes Serves: 12
Ingredients:

- Lemon juice- 1 tbsp.
- Cherries: pitted and chopped- 6 cups
- Stevia- ¼ cup

Directions:

1. On a pan, add the stevia and cherries over medium heat and let it simmer.

2. Add the lemon juice and let it cook for 30 minutes.
3. Share into cups and serve.

Nutrition: Calories 50, carbs 12, protein 7, fiber 1, fats 0

Lemony fairy cakes

Prep Time + Cook Time: 40 minutes Serves: 4
Ingredients:

- Eggs- 3
- Almond milk- 1 cup
- Stevia- ¼ cup
- Almond flour- 2½ cups
- Grated lemon zest- 2 tbsp.

- Baking powder- 1 tsp.
- Melted ghee- 2 tbsp.
- Lemon extract- 2 tsp.
- Vanilla extract- 1 tbsp.
- Coconut cream- 3 tbsp.

- Lemon juice- 1 tsp.

Directions:

1. Whisk all the ingredients together in a small bowl.

2. Pour the mixture into a fairy cake pan and bake it in the oven for 30 minutes at 350°F.

3. Serve cold.

Nutrition: Calories 332, carbs 6, protein 8, fiber 5, fat 14

Lemony plum and dates blend

Prep Time + Cook Time: 2 hours Serves: 4

Ingredients:

- Lemon juice- 1 tsp.
- Plums: chopped- 3 cups
- Dates: pitted and chopped- 1 cup
- Water- 2½ cups

Directions:

1. Add all the ingredients to the food processor and blend until smooth.

2. Freeze for 2 hours.

3. Serve in cups.

Nutrition:

Calories 85, carbs 13, protein 1, fiber 1, fat 0

Nutmeg Spiced Coconut Granola

Prep Time + Cook Time: 45 minutes Serves: 4

Ingredients:

- Pumpkin seeds, ½ cup
- Cinnamon, ½ tsp.
- Coconut oil, 2 tsps.
- Ground allspice, 1/8 tsp.
- Sunflower seeds, ½ cup
- Ground nutmeg, 1 tsp.
- Unsweetened coconut, 1c
- Chopped almonds and pecans, 1 cup
- Stevia, 2 tbsps.
- Ground nutmeg, 1/8 tsp.

Directions:

1. Stir in pumpkin seeds, pecans, almonds, sunflower seeds, 1/8 tsp. ground nutmeg, ground allspice, and ½ tsp. cinnamon in a mixing bowl.

2. Set the pan on fire to melt coconut oil and stevia over medium heat stirring gently.

3. Stir together coconut mixture and nuts.

4. Set the mixture on a lined baking sheet.

5. Set the oven for 30 minutes at 300°F, allow to bake the mixture.

6. Allow granola to cool.

7. Cut and serve.

8. Enjoy.

Nutrition:

Calories: 394 ,Fat: 36.2 ,Fiber: 5.9 ,Carbs: 12.4 , Protein: 11.1

Quick bake cookies

Prep Time + Cook Time: 50 minutes Serves: 4

Ingredients:
- Lemon juice- 1 tsp.
- Egg white- 1
- Lemon zest- 1 tsp.
- Coconut flakes- 3 cups
- Almond milk- ⅔ cup
- Vanilla extract- ½ tsp.

Directions:
1. Mix almond milk, lemon zest, juice, vanilla extract, and coconut flakes in a bowl.
2. Mold it into small cookies and lay it on a lined baking sheet.
3. Bake in an oven for 20 minutes at 325°F.
4. Serve on a platter.

Nutrition:
Calories 100, carbs 11, protein 1, fiber 3, fats 4

Slow cook blueberry lemon curd

Prep Time + Cook Time: 15 minutes Serves: 6

Ingredients:
- Lemon juice- ¼ cup
- Grated lemon zest- 2 tsp.
- Egg yolks: whisked- 3
- Stevia- 1/5 cup
- Coconut butter: softened- 4 tbsp.
- Blueberries- 1 cup

Directions:
1. Pour the lemon juice and the blueberries on a small pan over medium heat.
2. Boil slowly then drain the liquid then mash it.
3. Whisk in the zest, yolks, butter, and sugar and pour it into the pan.
4. Let it cook for 5 minutes over medium-low.
5. Serve into cups.

Nutrition:
Calories 140, carbs 6, protein 7, fiber 3, fat 3

Strawberries and cashew blend

Prep Time + Cook Time: 2 hours 10 minutes Serves: 9

Ingredients:
- Strawberries- 2 cups
- Cashew: soaked for 3 hours- 3 cups
- Lime juice- ¼ cup
- Melted coconut oil- ¾ cup
- Almond milk- ½ cup
- Strawberries- 2 cups
- Sliced strawberries for serving

Directions:
1. Pulse lime juice, cashews, almond milk, coconut oil, strawberries and stevia in the food processor until smooth.
2. Pour the cream into a smaller cup and put it in the freezer for 2 hours.
3. Serve with sliced strawberries.

Nutrition:
Calories 140, carbs 8, protein 6, fiber 1, fats 2

Strawberry Coconut Dessert

Prep Time + Cook Time: 10 minutes   Serves: 4

Ingredients:

- Granulated stevia, 2 tsps.
- Strawberries, 1 cup
- Coconut cream, 1¾ cup

Directions:

1. Set up a mixing bowl to combine stevia and coconut cream.
2. Set the mixture in an immersion blender to process until done.
3. Pour the mixture into dessert glasses then chill
4. Serve cold and enjoy.

Nutrition:

Calories: 460 ,Fat: 46.6 ,Fiber: 5 ,Carbs: 13.6 ,Protein: 4.7

Strawberry Tart

Prep Time + Cook Time: 40 minutes Serves: 4

Ingredients:

- Coconut oil- 3½ tbsp.
- Water- ½ cup
- Stevia- ¾ cup
- Coconut flour- ½ cup
- Strawberries: halved- 6 cups
- Baking soda- ⅛ tsp.
- Lemon juice- 1 tbsp.
- Baking powder-⅛ tsp.

Directions:

1. Mix lemon juice, stevia, and strawberries in a bowl and flip to coat.
2. Lay it in an oiled baking tray.
3. Mix baking soda, powder, coconut flour, and water and pour it over the strawberries.
4. Bake in the oven for 30 minutes for 375°F.
5. Cool and serve.

Nutrition:

Calories 205, carbs 9, protein 4, fiber 4, fats 4

Sweet and sour stew

Prep Time + Cook Time: 30 minutes Serves: 4

Ingredients:

- Lime juice- 3 tbsp.
- Water- 1 cup
- Cubed lemon- 4 cups
- Stevia- 6 tbsp.

Directions:

1. Put all the ingredients in a pot and simmer on medium heat for 20 minutes.
2. Pour into bowls.
3. Serve cold.

Nutrition:

Calories 180, carbs 6, protein 2, fiber 2, fat 2

Tasty Chocolate Pudding

Prep Time + Cook Time: 55 minutes Serves: 2

Ingredients:

- Coconut milk, 1 cup
- Water, 2 tbsps.
- Cocoa powder, 2 tbsps.
- Gelatin, 1 tbsp.
- Erythritol,2 tbsps.
- Stevia powder, ½ tsp.

Directions:

1. Set a pan on fire to heat the coconut milk over medium heat.
2. Stir in cocoa powder and stevia.
3. Set a medium bowl in a clean working surface to combine water and gelatin to mix on the pan
4. Whisk in erythritol then divide into ramekins
5. Refrigerate for 45 minutes to serve cold.
6. Enjoy.

Nutrition:

Calories: 300 ,Fat: 29.3 ,Fiber: 4.3 ,Carbs: 9.6 ,Protein: 6.7

Tasty cookie

Prep Time + Cook Time: 35 minutes Serves: 4

Ingredients:

- Eggs- 3
- Swerve- ¼ cup
- Melted ghee- 4 tbsp.
- Mascarpone cheese- ¼ cup
- Melted chocolate- 5 oz.
- Cocoa powder- ¼ cup

Directions:

1. Whisk all the ingredients together well.
2. Pour the mixture into a pan and bake in the oven for 25 minutes at 375°F.
3. Cut into medium sized brownie squares.
4. Serve.

Nutrition:

Calories 120, carbs 3, protein 3, fiber 4, fat 8

Vanilla Cheesecake

Prep Time + Cook Time: 30 minutes Serves: 9

Ingredients:

- 6 eggs
- Vanilla extract, 1 tsp.
- Baking powder, ½ tsp.
- Blueberries, ½ cup
- Melted coconut oil, 5 oz.
- Swerve, 4 tbsps.
- Cream cheese, 4 oz.

Directions:

1. Set up a bowl to mix cream cheese, vanilla extract, coconut oil, eggs, swerve and baking powder.
2. Connect an immersion blender to process the mixture until done
3. Fold in the blueberries.
4. Set the mixture into a baking tray

5. Set the oven for 20 minutes at 320ºF, allow to bake.
6. Allow cooling before slicing to serve.

Nutrition:
Calories: 228 ,Fat: 23.1 ,Fiber: 0.2 ,Carbs: 4.2 ,Protein: 4.7

Vanilla Chocolate Cookies

Prep Time + Cook Time: 1 hour Serves: 12

Ingredients:
- Almond flour, 2 cup
- Monk fruit sweetener, 2 tbsps.
- Swerve, ¼ cup
- Salt
- Butter, ½ cup
- Vanilla extract, 1 tsp.
- Egg, 1
- Unsweetened chocolate chips, ½ cup

Directions:
1. Set the pan on fire to brown the butter over medium heat then set aside for 5 minutes

2. Set a mixing bowl in place to combine the egg with swerve, vanilla extract, and monk fruit extract.
3. Stir in flour, melted butter, half of the chocolate chips, and salt.
4. Spread the mixture on a pan topped with the remaining chocolate chips.
5. Set the oven for 30 minutes at 350ºF, allow to bake
6. Let it cool before slicing then serve.

Nutrition:
Calories: 172 ,Fat: 15.8 ,Fiber: 1.8 ,Carbs: 3.8 ,Protein: 3.4

Vanilla Flavored Ice Cream

Prep Time + Cook Time: 3 hours and 10 minutes Serves: 6

Ingredients:
- Swerve, ½ cup
- Vanilla extract, 1 tbsp.
- Cream of tartar, ¼ tsp.
- Heavy whipping cream, 1¼ cup
- 4 eggs

Directions:
1. Set up a mixing bowl in place to stir together tartar cream, swerve and egg whites using a mixer.

2. Set another mixing bowl in position to whisk together vanilla extract and cream.
3. Gently stir the two mixtures together.
4. Set up another medium bowl to whisk the egg yolks followed by two egg whites mixture then give it a gentle stir.

5. Set the mixture into a container to refrigerate for 3 hours.
6. Serve then enjoy.

Nutrition:
Calories: 238 ,Fat: 23.3 ,Fiber: 0 ,Carbs: 8.8 ,Protein: 4.8

Vanilla pumpkin cookie

Prep Time + Cook Time: 25 minutes Serves: 12

Ingredients:
- Almond flour- 2½ cups
- Pumpkin: mashed- ½ cup
- Vanilla extract- 1 tsp.
- Water- 3 tbsp.
- Coconut butter- 2 tbsp.
- Baking soda- ½ tsp.
- Flaxseed- 1 tbsp.
- salt

Directions:
1. Mix water and flax seed together in a bowl.
2. Mix the salt, baking powder and flour in another bowl.
3. Mix the flaxseed, butter, pumpkin puree, and vanilla extract in a different bowl.
4. Mix in the flour and arrange spoon scoops on a lined sheet.
5. Bake in the oven for 15 minutes at 350°F.
6. Serve when it cools.

Nutrition:
Calories 140, carbs 7, protein 6, fiber 2, fat 2

Vanilla Spiced Macaroons

Prep Time + Cook Time: 20 minutes Serves: 20

Ingredients:
- Shredded coconut, 2 cup
- Egg whites, 4
- Vanilla extract, 1 tsp.
- Stevia, 2 tbsps.

Directions:
- Set up a mixing bowl to beat together the egg whites and stevia using a mixer.
- Stir in vanilla extract and coconut.
- Mold the mixture into small balls then set them into a lined baking sheet.
- Set the oven for 10 minutes at 350°F then, allow to bake.
- Let it cool before serving.
- Enjoy.

Nutrition:
Calories: 32 ,Fat: 2.7 ,Fiber: 0.7 ,Carbs: 1.3 ,Protein: 1

CPSIA information can be obtained
at www.ICGtesting.com
Printed in the USA
BVHW010234040121
596922BV00019B/774